Contents

Practical radiotherapy planning
3rd edition

JANE DOBBS FRCP, FRCR

Consultant in Clinical Oncology, Guy's, King's and St Thomas' Cancer Centre, Guy's and St Thomas' Hospital Trust, London

ANN BARRETT MD, FRCP, FRCR

Professor of Radiation Oncology, Beatson Oncology Centre, Western Infirmary, Glasgow

DAN ASH FRCP, FRCR

Consultant in Clinical Oncology, Yorkshire Regional Centre for Cancer Treatment, Cookridge Hospital, Leeds

ARNOLD

A member of the Hodder Headline Group
LONDON • SYDNEY • AUCKLAND
Distributed in the United States of America
by Oxford University Press Inc., New York

First published in Great Britain in 1985
First published in paperback in 1987
Reprinted 1989
Second edition 1992
Third edition published in Great Britain in 1999 by
Arnold, a member of the Hodder Headline Group,
338 Euston Road, London NW1 3BH

http://www.arnoldpublishers.com

Distributed in the United States of America by
Oxford University Press Inc.,
198 Madison Avenue, New York, NY 10016
Oxford is a registered trademark of Oxford University Press

Whilst the advice and information in this book is believed to be true and accurate at the date of
going to press, neither the authors nor the publisher can accept any legal responsibility or liability
for any errors or omissions that may be made. In particular (but without limiting the generality of
the preceding disclaimer) every effort has been made to check drug and radiation dosages;
however, it is still possible that errors have been missed. Furthermore, dosage schedules are
constantly being revised and new side-effects recognized. For these reasons the reader is strongly
urged to consult the drug companies' printed instructions before administering any of the drugs
recommended in this book.

British Library Cataloguing in Publication Data
A catalogue record for this book is available from the British Library

Library of Congress Cataloging-in-Publication Data
A catalog record for this book is available from the Library of Congress

ISBN 0 340 70631 7

5 6 7 8 9 10

Typeset in 10/11pt Times by
J&L Composition, Filey, N. Yorks

Printed and bound in Malta

What do you think about this book? Or any other Arnold title?
Please send your comments to feedback.arnold@hodder.co.uk

Preface to the third edition

The first edition of this book described radiotherapy planning techniques at the Royal Marsden Hospital in London (where both authors of that edition then worked). In the second edition, the authors, now working in different centres, incorporated their experience of other techniques and added Dr Ash's contribution on brachytherapy.

The book has been rewritten for this third edition in the new era of evidence-based practice to include rationales and techniques for treatment which have proven benefit. We have consulted widely and have added chapters on three dimensional planning and conformal therapy, quality assurance and radio-biological principles of treatment planning, but our aim is still to provide a guide which is based on sound anatomical and pathological principles. As a previous reviewer said, we are concerned with 'the nuts and bolts' of planning and do not attempt to cover the same ground as the large textbooks of cancer management. Suggestions for further reading have been added to each chapter in this new edition.

Although many useful radiotherapy trials have been carried out, areas of uncertainty remain, and we are very conscious of differences in practice elsewhere in the world. We have adopted the recommendations of the International Commission on Radiological Units and Measurements (ICRU) for definitions of volumes, dose specification and reporting. We have attempted to consider techniques of the planning process from basic (level 1) to developmental (level 3) levels in order to give the book wide applicability. Although details of technique vary from centre to centre, we hope that, using our book, any trainee radiation oncologist will be able to produce a safe and adequate plan for most common tumours.

Linear accelerators with energies of 5–6 MV are in wide general use, but there are some situations where higher-energy photons (8–20 MV) may offer advantages. We have chosen to use 5 MV as our standard photon energy, but plans at higher energies have been included where review has shown an improved dose distribution. Field widths are given first in bold type.

Altered fractionation schemes are still largely under investigation and, unless there are definitive randomized trial results, we have mostly used the long-established practice of 2 Gy fractionation. At the same time, we have tried to give practical guidelines for the application of other schedules.

In the UK, past experience and workload have restricted the practice of radiotherapy for benign disease, which we have therefore largely excluded from this book.

We have been greatly helped in the production of this edition by many people whom we would like to thank most sincerely, including the following: our patients who have provided illustrations; our colleagues in our own departments for advice freely given, especially Frances Calman, Sarah Harris, Martin Leslie, Mary O'Connell and Roy Rampling; colleagues in other centres, including Anna Gregor and Jill Ainslie, Head of the Skin Unit at Peter MacCallum Cancer Institute, Melbourne; our physics colleagues, including Maeve Filby, Tony Greener, Martin Robb and especially Stuart McNee for preparation of new isodose distributions and illustrations, and for helpful discussions; Annette Thain, Jane Garrud and Mike Messer for help with references and illustrations; Dr Tom Wheldon for the new chapter on radiobiological principles; Dr George Mikhaeel for reviewing the text and making many helpful suggestions; Tres Stafford for her cheerful patience and hard work in producing the manuscript; and Dr Mac Cochrane for arranging sabbatical leave for Jane Dobbs from the United Medical Dental School and the Special Trustees of Guy's and St Thomas' Hospital.

Jane Dobbs
Ann Barrett
Dan Ash
1998

Basic principles of treatment planning

Introduction

The aim of radiotherapy is to deliver a tumoricidal dose of radiation to a well-defined target volume whilst sparing the surrounding normal tissue, thereby achieving an optimum therapeutic ratio with the minimum level of morbidity. This goal can be achieved using different levels of technical complexity, as described in ICRU Report No. 50, depending on the available planning and therapy equipment and staff expertise. Chapter 1 describes the basic principles of all aspects of the treatment planning process (Fig. 1.1), and Chapter 2 outlines the three-dimensional aspects of treatment planning and delivery.

Single-field treatments are often set up using fixed focus skin distance (FSD), whereas opposing fields may use fixed FSD or an isocentric technique. Simulator guide wires define the 50 per cent isodose. For a single field, divergence of the beam ensures adequate cover of the tumour at depth. When opposing fields are used to encompass the target volume within the 95 per cent isodose, inward bowing of the isodoses (see Fig. 18.4) occurs and field sizes at the skin will therefore be larger than the target volume (by approximately 1 cm) when seen on the simulator check films.

Pre-planning

For many tumour sites, multidisciplinary clinical meetings are held with radiologists, pathologists, surgeons, physicians, radiation oncologists, nurses and radiographers to discuss the clinical and imaging data and histopathology details in order to devise a management plan for the individual patient. This enables accurate staging of the tumour (using TNM, FIGO, etc., as shown in Fig. 1.2) and a decision as to whether the planned treatment is curative or palliative. The role and scheduling of surgery and/or chemotherapy in relation to a course of radiotherapy are defined at the start, and may influence the site and size of the target volume as well as the radiation dose. For example, patients with high-risk bulky stage IIA Hodgkin's disease are treated with primary chemotherapy. Subsequently, radiotherapy is given to sites of initial involvement. Radiation doses may be lowered to take account of the potential toxicity of combined chemotherapy/radiotherapy (e.g. lung morbidity from bleomycin, cardiac morbidity from adriamycin), and precise shielding of the lungs and heart is of great importance.

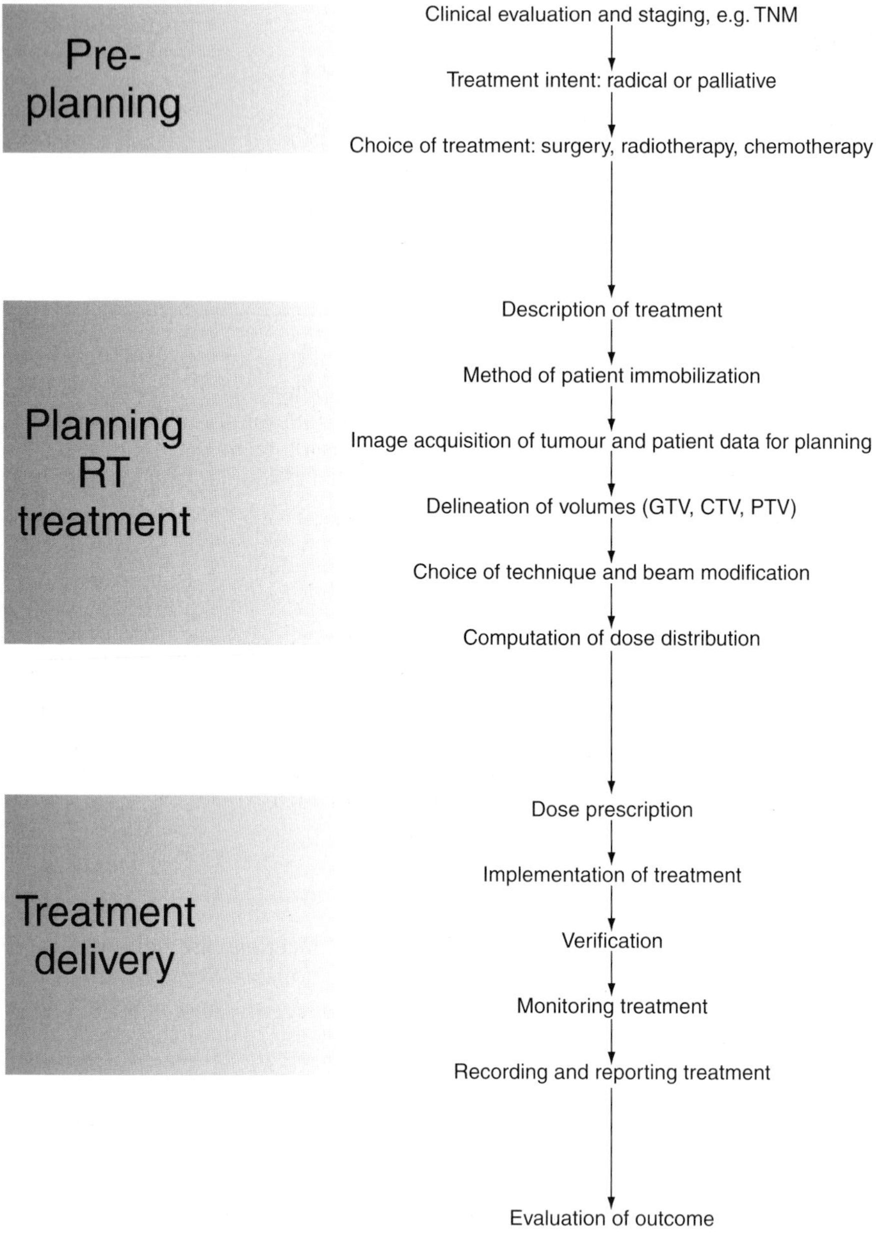

Pre-planning

Planning RT treatment

Treatment delivery

Clinical evaluation and staging, e.g. TNM

Treatment intent: radical or palliative

Choice of treatment: surgery, radiotherapy, chemotherapy

Description of treatment

Method of patient immobilization

Image acquisition of tumour and patient data for planning

Delineation of volumes (GTV, CTV, PTV)

Choice of technique and beam modification

Computation of dose distribution

Dose prescription

Implementation of treatment

Verification

Monitoring treatment

Recording and reporting treatment

Evaluation of outcome

Fig. 1.1   Radiotherapy planning processes.

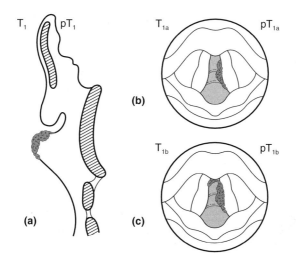

Fig. 1.2 Staging of the larynx. (a) Glottis tumours T_1 – tumour limited to vocal cord(s) with normal mobility. (b) T_{1a} – limited to one vocal cord. (c) T_{1b} – involves both vocal cords with invasion of the anterior commissure. (Adapted, with permission, from *TNM Atlas. Illustrated Guide to TNM Classification of Malignant Tumours*, Fourth Edition, 1997. Heidelberg: Springer-Verlag.)

Once a decision to treat with radiotherapy has been made, a preliminary plan of action is devised for the choice of target volume, method of patient immobilization, treatment technique, treatment machine and energy and dose prescription. Each of these steps requires detailed specialist knowledge and close collaboration with other members of the team, e.g. radiologists, mould-room technicians, physicists, radiographers and dosimetrists, to ensure accurate execution of a complex set of procedures.

Planning

PATIENT POSITION

The position of the patient for treatment must be technically ideal and yet comfortable. It is important that the patient be treated in one position only, as changes result in alterations in internal and external anatomy and risk of over- or underdosage. The choice of position for treatment may be constrained by equipment limitations, e.g. the arm position may be restricted by the limited aperture size of the CT scanner, and the distance between the patient and the head of the therapy machine may affect positioning. CT planning of breast radiotherapy demands that the patient lies supine, flat on the couch with her arms directly above her head to enter the CT aperture, whereas the simulator planning position often uses an inclined wedge or board with the patient's arms abducted holding arm poles for better fixation.

The position of the patient, all positioning aids and anatomical measurements should be documented accurately in writing with a diagram and polaroid photograph to ensure reproducibility through all stages of the planning process and subsequent treatment. The degree of immobilization required varies according to the technique being used. Complex fixation is essential for high-dose small-volume techniques (e.g. in the case of the CNS), where a high degree of precision is needed. On the other hand, a large-volume technique such as total body irradiation (TBI) can accommodate a margin of movement into the mode of treatment delivery. Immobilization can be achieved with perspex shells or casts for tumours of the head and neck or limbs, or with vacuum-moulded bags of polystyrene beads for the trunk and limbs (Fig. 1.3). Field markings can be made on the shell or vacuum bag, thereby avoiding marking the patient's skin. Verification studies have shown that other devices also ensure good reproducibility, e.g. inclined chest board with foot rest and arm poles fixing the arms in abduction for breast treatments, foam blocks of varying shapes used as head rests, chest wedges, or knee or ankle restraints for pelvic treatments. Lasers are used in the mid-line to align the patient in the longitudinal axis of the beam with opposing lateral lasers for horizontal alignment during both localization and treatment. Where the patient has kyphosis, scoliosis, frozen shoulder or limitation of joint movement (as with fixed deformity of the hips), extra limb pads or immobilization devices may be necessary. Metallic prostheses, abdominal stomata and the batteries of pacemakers must be located and excluded from the radiation volume where possible.

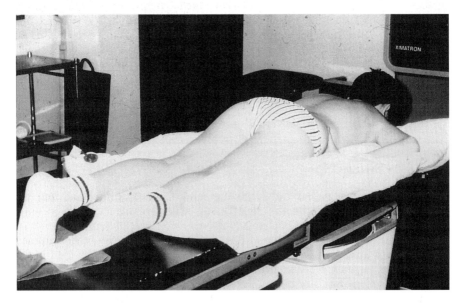

Fig. 1.3 Vacuum-moulded bag of polystyrene beads for trunk immobilization.

It is important that the technician who is preparing the shell is given details of the tumour site to be treated, e.g. the position of the patient (prone, supine, flexion or extension of neck, arm position, etc.). An impression of the relevant area (made using quick-setting dental alginate or plaster of Paris) is filled with plaster, and this form is used to make a perspex shell by vacuum moulding (Fig. 1.4). The shell fits over the patient and fastens to a device on the couch with perspex straps and pegs. Verification studies have shown that a perspex shell provides accurate localization of target volumes in the brain to within 2 mm. Relocatable stereotactic frames (e.g. Gill Thomas) are secured to the head by insertion of a dental impression of the upper teeth into the mouth and an occipital impression on the head frame, and are used for stereotactic radiotherapy with a reproducibility of 1 mm or less.

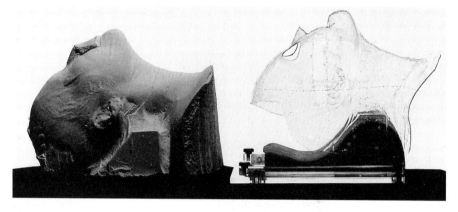

Fig. 1.4   Construction of perspex shell from plaster cast.

METHODS OF TUMOUR LOCALIZATION

Localization of the target volume within the patient in relation to external reference points should be done under exactly the same conditions as subsequent treatments. For example, the patient positioning should be identical, respiration and bladder filling should be constant, and couch tops should be flat without the use of a curved CT or MRI couch or a flexible 'tennis-racket' insert for therapy, any of which would change body contour or organ position. Acquisition of tumour data involves the use of optimum imaging modalities defined in tumour site protocols developed in collaboration with diagnostic imaging experts. Tumour information may be available from ultrasound, CT, MRI, PET or SPECT, as well as from clinical observation and palpation and surgical findings. The choice of imaging modality and collation of data with subsequent localization requires interpretation of the data by a radiologist and/or registration of images with those used for target localization and dosimetry. Current methods of target localization include the use of a simulator, CT scanning and simulator-CT and CT-simulator facilities.

USE OF A SIMULATOR

A simulator is an isocentrically mounted diagnostic X-ray machine which can reproduce treatment conditions and has the facility for screening by means of an image intensifier linked to a closed-circuit television. It has a couch which is capable of all the movements of a treatment unit, a gantry which can be rotated through 360°, and two pairs of cross-wires mounted in the beam which can be set to any field size following the 50 per cent isodose line of the beam. Any X-ray beam of diagnostic quality gives well-defined images, whilst screening shows organ movements and allows rapid adjustment of fields.

Treatment machines may be operated at a fixed *d*istance between the *s*ource and the *s*kin (SSD) or the *f*ocal spot and the *s*kin (FSD). Alternatively, the machine may rotate around the patient on an axis centred on a fixed point (the isocentre) which is 100 cm from the focal spot (FAD) and is usually placed at the centre of the target volume. The depth of the isocentre below the skin is called the 'pin depth', and the focus to skin distance is called the 'pin setting' (Fig. 1.5). Alternatively, the isocentre can be located by reference to the couch top using the couch height scale to measure the distance from the isocentre to the couch. For some patients this distance may be less variable than the pin depth measurement.

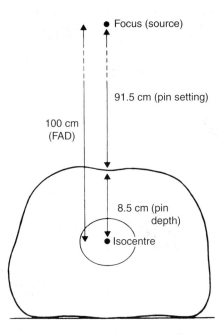

Fig. 1.5 Diagram to show pin depth and pin setting for an isocentric technique.

To determine the target volume, any palpable masses are marked with wire and contrast medium may be placed in the bladder, rectum, vagina or oesophagus. A skin tattoo is placed over an immobile bony landmark, such as the pubic symphysis or xiphisternum, to act as a reference point. Additional tattoos may also be needed to align irregularly shaped fields such as the 'mantle' (see Chapter 22). For chest, abdominal or pelvic treatments, lateral rotation can be minimized by marking two lateral points on the skin at fixed distances up from the couch on each side. Laser positioning lights should be available in the simulator to align the patient using these reference tattoos (Fig. 1.6). If treatment will use a beam coming posteriorly through the couch, a 'tennis-racket' insert or other window in the couch may be considered to avoid attenuation of the beam. This can lead to inaccuracy of patient positioning, and a rigid carbon-fibre insert may be used instead.

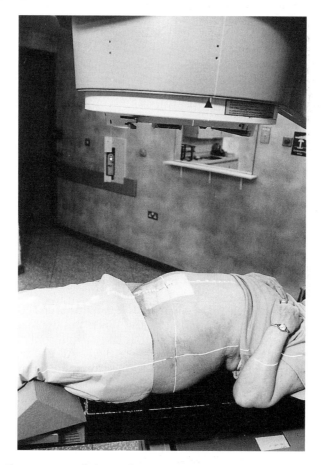

Fig. 1.6 Laser lights in the sagittal and coronal plane to align a patient using reference skin tattoos.

When more than two beams will be used for treatment, a transverse outline of the body contour through the centre of the simulated volume is taken, using an automated contouring device, plaster of Paris or wire. Mid-line and lateral skin reference points are marked on this contour. By convention, outlines are orientated looking up from the feet to the head. The lateral separation between two fixed points, measured with callipers, is marked on to a base line on a sheet of paper, and a perpendicular line is drawn at the mid-point. The outline is then transferred, aligning the mid-line and lateral points. The right and left sides are also recorded (Fig. 1.7). The length of the perpendicular line (XY) should correspond to the interplanar distance (IPD) or separation measured on the patient.

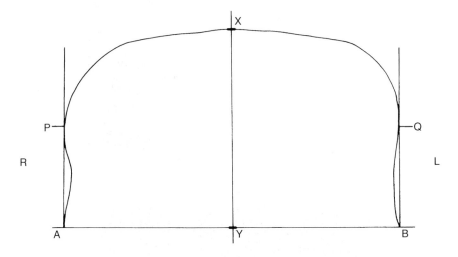

Fig. 1.7 Transverse outline of patient contour. AB = lateral separation measured from patient using callipers; P,Q = lateral tattoos; XY = mid-line.

Where the skin surfaces are parallel, the IPD is determined with a sliding rod as shown in Fig. 1.8, and for areas of irregular contour, such as the neck, callipers are used (Fig. 1.9).

Open films may be taken on the simulator (often for head and neck treatments) and the target volume defined subsequently. When this approach is used for single or AP-PA opposing fields, an AP film is taken as a record of the treatment localization. For treatment with three or more fields, AP and lateral films are taken with rulers, magnification rings or a simulator graticule ruler to indicate the magnification factor. For the lateral film a mid-line ruler is used. The width of the target volume is drawn on to the AP simulator film and transferred to the transverse outline using the mid-line for alignment and magnification markers (Fig. 1.10a). Using the lateral film (Fig. 1.10b), the AP dimension of the target volume and the distance of its anterior border from the skin surface are determined in the treatment plane and transferred to the outline using a sagittal mid-line magnification indicator. The position of adjacent structures such as the lens, spinal cord, lungs, kidneys and rectum should also be marked on the outline

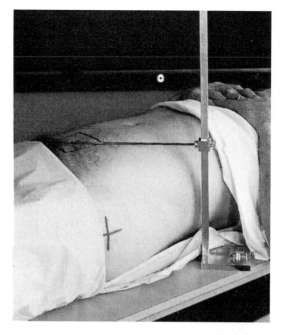

Fig. 1.8   Measurement of interplanar distance (IPD) using a sliding rod.

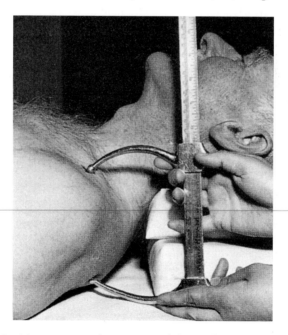

Fig. 1.9   Measurement of separation of skin surfaces using callipers.

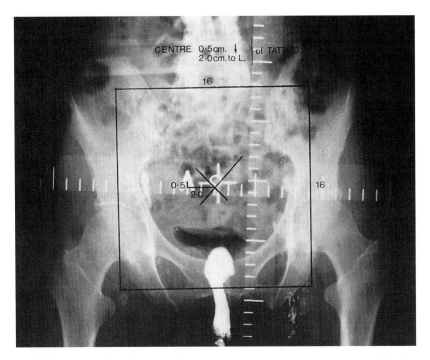

Fig. 1.10a   Localization of the target volume shown by AP simulator film.

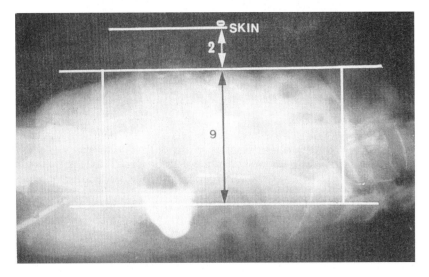

Fig. 1.10b   Localization of the target volume shown by lateral simulator film.

(Fig. 1.10c). When multiple fields are used, a dose distribution is then produced using a computerized planning system.

Alternatively, the target volume at depth may be defined directly using the simulator guide wire and a plan constructed as described above.

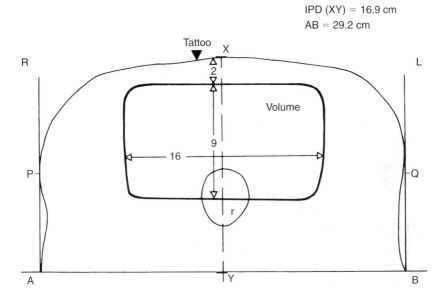

Fig. 1.10c Localization of the target volume marked on transverse outline using information from (a) and (b), r = rectum.

CT LOCALIZATION

Clinical studies show that from 30 to 80 per cent of patients undergoing radiotherapy may benefit from CT planning, because the additional information increases the accuracy of definition of the target volume compared with conventional simulation. Use of CT has been estimated to improve overall 5-year survival rates by around 3.5 per cent, and has the greatest impact in small-volume treatments in the brain, thorax, pelvis and abdomen. CT images also provide density data for dose calculations by conversion of CT matrix numbers into relative electron densities using calibration curves. Compton scattering is the dominant tissue interaction process for megavoltage beams, and is directly proportional to electron density. Hence CT provides detailed density information for dose calculations of tissue inhomogeneity, such as the lung, as well as unique anatomical and tumour data.

CT scans taken for radiotherapy treatment planning are usually different from those taken for diagnostic use. The scanner should have the largest possible aperture to aid therapy positioning, and must have internal or external positioning lights in the mid-line and lateral planes in the scanner room, as in the simulator and therapy rooms. Accurate couch registration to better than 1 mm is important, as the length of the target volume is taken from longitudinal CT couch measurements. The CT couch must be flat topped, and the patient is positioned using supporting aids, immobilization devices and laser lights identical to those for subsequent radiotherapy treatment. A tattoo is made on the skin over the nearest immobile bony landmark to the centre of the target volume, e.g. the pubic symphysis. It is marked with radio-opaque material such as a catheter or barium paste for visualization on the CT image and topogram. Additional lateral tattoos are used to prevent lateral rotation of the patient, and are aligned using horizontal lasers.

Oral contrast medium may be used to outline small bowel, oesophagus or stomach, and rectal instillation or a vaginal tampon are used for other hollow viscera. Structures such as the introitus, anal margin, stomata and any tumour masses or surgical scars are outlined with radio-opaque barium or catheters. It should be remembered that oral contrast media can affect dose calculations if these are based on CT density data. For bladder treatments, patients should empty their bladder before CT scanning and treatment. If the rectum contains excess gas distorting the prostate, a repeat CT on another day should be performed for planning prostate treatments.

With the patient breathing normally as for treatment, a scout view (topogram) is obtained over the tumour-bearing region (Fig. 1.11) and CT scans are taken at 5- to 10-mm intervals. Divergence of the CT beam occurs only in the transverse plane, and is therefore not comparable with a simulator or treatment beam where there is divergence in all directions. Scout views should not therefore be used for planning, but only to record the levels of CT scans obtained. The size of the circle of reconstruction is chosen to obtain maximum resolution, but must include the patient's full body contour.

Ideally, the CT scanner and treatment planning computer are networked to allow for direct transfer of CT images. Outlining of body contour, tumour, target volume and normal organs takes place at the planning computer, marking each CT slice using a tracker ball or mouse with interactive software program. The final target volume must encompass the tumour with appropriate margins at all levels. For two-dimensional planning, a dose distribution is calculated on the CT image corresponding to the centre of the proposed target volume (Figs 1.12 and 1.13). Off-axis beam data can be used to determine the dose distribution at other levels within the target volume, in order to record the homogeneity of the dose throughout the entire volume. Three-dimensional treatment planning involves three-dimensional localization of target volume and normal structures on contiguous thin CT slices with three-dimensional dose computation and the possibility of conformal therapy as discussed in Chapter 2.

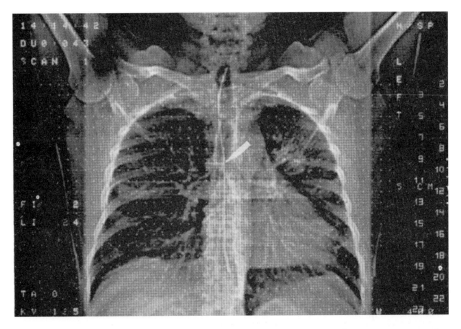

Fig. 1.11 CT topogram of chest to show levels of CT images. Skin tattoo (arrowed) defined by crossed radio-opaque catheters.

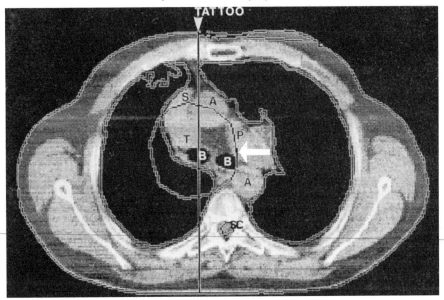

Fig. 1.12 CT image just below carina through the centre of the target volume (arrowed) showing body contour, tumour (T), spinal cord (SC), aorta (A), bronchi (B), superior vena cava (S) and pulmonary trunk (P).

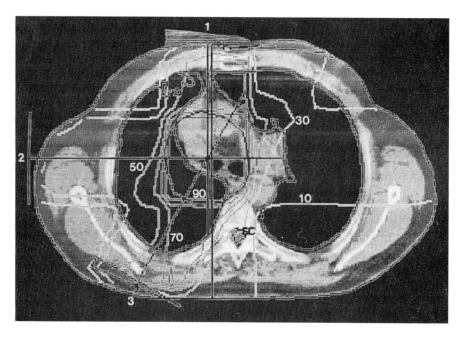

Fig. 1.13 Dose distribution from three fields produced by integrated CT treatment planning system.

SIMULATOR-CT

A CT mode attached to the simulator gantry can be used to produce images with a relatively limited resolution during the simulation process. This provides both external contouring and some internal normal anatomical data, such as lung and chest wall thickness, for simple inhomogeneity corrections. Images do not produce detailed tumour information or accurate CT numbers. They are time-consuming to obtain, and are therefore usually limited to the central, superior and inferior axes of the target volume. However, the cost is low compared with that of the CT scanner, and there is less restriction on aperture size, making the facility particularly appropriate for breast techniques and mantle and TBI irradiation. The advantage of simulator-CT for breast techniques is that it gives greater freedom of choice of patient positioning, and a 3-slice target localization which improves breast dose homogeneity.

CT-SIMULATOR

State-of-the-art CT scanners can be combined with software to generate images from a beam's-eye perspective which are equivalent to conventional simulator images. These can be used to replace the simulation process, but have to be related to an internal isocentre for anchoring data to external landmarks. The practical issues of how to perform simulation from the CT data have yet to be resolved. However, the ability to derive CT scans, and to provide target volume definition, margin generation, dose calculation and simulation all on one work station is a major advance. The CT-simulator provides maximum tumour information as well as full three-dimensional capabilities (unlike the simulator-CT facility).

IMAGE REGISTRATION

For some tumour sites, MRI, PET, ultrasound and SPECT may provide the optimum tumour information. At present, CT remains the gold standard for acquisition of anatomical data, and correlation of CT numbers with electron densities (which is impossible with MRI) makes it ideal for radiotherapy treatment planning. It has therefore become imperative to find methods of combining optimum tumour imaging data with CT data for treatment planning. This correlation is complicated by differences in patient positioning, geometrical distortions of magnetic resonance images, varying anatomical boundaries and differences in spatial resolution, and is discussed further in Chapter 2.

DEFINITION OF TARGET VOLUME

ICRU Report 50 recommends international definitions of tumour, target and normal organ volumes for comparison of clinical results. The gross tumour volume (GTV) is defined as the demonstrable macroscopic extent of tumour that is either palpable, visible or detectable by conventional radiography, ultrasound, radioisotope scans, CT or MRI. Staging systems such as the TNM classification attempt to describe the site, size and extent of this GTV prior to policy decisions for local treatment, i.e. radical or palliative, and surgery or radiotherapy.

For radiation treatments, the aim is to give a tumoricidal dose to the macroscopic disease and/or the estimated extent of the microscopic spread. Subclinical disease is determined by knowledge of the tumour histology and its natural history, including local invasive capacity and potential to spread to adjacent tissues and lymph nodes. To encompass this potential microscopic spread, a margin must be allowed around the GTV to produce the clinical target volume (CTV). However, precise data for quantifying this margin are lacking, and its definition is based on knowledge from surgical and post-mortem specimens and patterns of tumour recurrence, as well as from clinical experience and clinical trials. It is perhaps the most difficult and subjective step in the entire planning process. Other factors, such as the age of the patient and considerations of normal tissue tolerance, may influence the maximum volume considered to be appropriate for treatment.

In practice, there are some situations in which the CTV may move due to physiological or technical factors. For instance, respiration or swallowing may lead to movement of a bronchial or laryngeal tumour, and bladder or rectal fill-ing may lead to movement of a prostate tumour. Clinical studies have reported organ motion varying from 15 mm for bladder wall, to 8 mm for the prostate, 3 mm for the breast and 0.1 mm for the brain as 2 standard deviations from the mean. An internal margin (IM) has to be added to the CTV to compensate for expected movements and variations in the shape, position and size of the CTV, thereby defining the internal target volume (ITV). During a fractionated course of radiotherapy, day-to-day variation in patient position and in alignment of the beams with external marks will occur. To account for these inaccuracies, a set-up margin (SM) for each technique can be defined using verification studies or a programme of quality assurance. For example, set-up variations of 10 mm for the pelvis, 13 mm for the breast and 2–4 mm for the head and neck are reported as 2 standard deviations from the mean. Combining the internal margin for phys-iological changes and the set-up margin for technical variations with the CTV leads to the planning target volume (PTV) (Fig. 1.14). The PTV is a geometri-cal concept used for treatment planning, and is defined to select appropriate beam sizes and beam arrangements so as to ensure that the prescribed dose is actually delivered to the CTV.

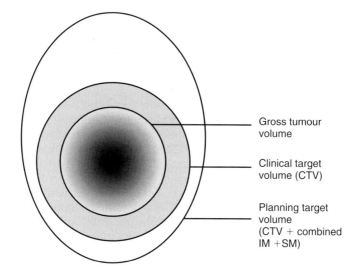

Gross tumour volume

Clinical target volume (CTV)

Planning target volume (CTV + combined IM + SM)

Fig. 1.14   Target volume definitions according to ICRU Report No. 50. IM = internal margin; SM = set-up margin. (Reproduced with permission from International Commission on Radiation Units 1993: *ICRU Report 50. Prescribing, recording and reporting photon beam therapy*. Bethesda, MD: International Commission on Radiation Units.)

It is not usually realistic to add up all of the uncertainties linearly. If random uncertainties (class A) are probability distributed, and systematic uncertainties (class B) are estimated by approximate standard deviations, then their combined effect can be estimated. The total standard deviation is then the root of the sum of the squares of all class A and B uncertainties. This final margin means that the PTV is located within the enveloping isodose with a confidence interval of 70 per cent (or 90 per cent with 2 standard deviations). In practice, there is a tendency to use standard cumulative margins added to the CTV to define the PTV. However, for a lung tumour the margin may be 6 mm in the transverse direction and 15 mm in the cranio-caudal direction due to the effect of respiration. It is recommended that each institution should evaluate local variations and uncertainties and define a reasonable level of probability for the different components.

NORMAL ORGAN VOLUMES

Whenever radiotherapy is given, both tumour and normal tissues will be irradiated. There is wide variation in the intrinsic radiosensitivity of different normal tissues and susceptibility to changes in fraction size. The amount of dose delivered to all adjacent normal organs must be quantified and recorded, either as maximum organ doses (two-dimensional) or as dose–volume histograms (three-dimensional). The site and volume of normal organs must therefore be defined using the same localization procedures and in the same way as the PTV, and indeed the two may overlap. A margin must be defined to take into account physiological movement of the organ and variations in patient position both inter- and intra-fractionally during a course of radiotherapy. The concept of a planning organ at risk volume (PRV) is used to be analogous to the PTV, and the size of the combined margins around the organ is stated in different directions. Increased shielding of parts of normal organs is now feasible with the use of conformal blocks and multileaf collimators, with calculation of dose–volume histograms for description of normal tissue doses.

CHOICE OF TREATMENT MACHINE AND TECHNIQUE

Once the PTV and normal organs have been defined in either two or three dimensions, the optimum dose distribution for treating the tumour is sought. Liaison with a dosimetrist is vital to obtain the best selection of parameters. For example, a treatment machine must be chosen according to percentage depth dose characteristics and build-up depth, which will vary with energy and beam size (Table 1.1). Other factors to be considered are the effect of penumbra on beam definition, the availability of independent or multileaf collimators, and the facilities for beam modification and portal imaging.

Discussions with the dosimetrist should include an exploration of the cell density pattern within the PTV, requirements for homogeneity of dose distribution (e.g. ± 5 per cent), avoidance of areas for maximum or minimum dose spots, tolerance doses of adjacent normal organs in relation to part or total organ volumes, and a preliminary plan of likely beam arrangements.

Table 1.1   Data from treatment machines in common use, showing variation of D_{max} and percentage depth dose with energy

Machine	Energy (MV)	FSD (cm)	10 × 10 cm field*	
			D_{max} depth (cm)	%DD at 10 cm
^{60}Cobalt	1.25	100	0.5	58.7
Linear accelerator	5	100	1.25	65
Linear accelerator	10	100	2.3	73
Linear accelerator	16	100	2.8	76.8

*Maximum field size at 100 cm is 40 × 40 cm.

DOSE SPECIFICATION

The biological effect of a given dose is difficult to predict because of variations in cell density at the centre and periphery of the target volume, heterogeneity of tumour cell populations, and inadequate knowledge of cellular radiosensitivity. Nevertheless, one must attempt to specify a dose which is representative of the absorbed dose in the target volume as a whole, in order to assess the effectiveness of treatment and to allow intercomparison between radiotherapy centres.

In this book, the ICRU dose specification point at the centre of the target volume has been chosen because it is easy to determine, it is representative of the dose distribution and it does not lie in a peripheral steep dose gradient. This point frequently lies on the central axis of the beam where the dose is more accurately defined (Table 1.2).

Table 1.2   Dose specification points for simple beam arrangements

Single beam	Centre of target volume
Two opposed coaxial equally weighted beams	Mid-plane point
Two opposed coaxial unequally weighted beams	Centre of target volume
Two or more intersecting beams	Intersection of central axes
Rotation therapy (270–360°) Rotation therapy with smaller arcs	Centre of rotation (1) Centre of rotation (2) Centre of target volume
Electrons	Maximum target absorbed dose with 90 per cent isodose enclosing target volume

It is essential that this dose specification point is accompanied by a statement of the homogeneity of the irradiation (Fig. 1.15) as defined by maximum and minimum target doses. Ideally, variation should be limited to ± 5 per cent, although this will vary with the exact clinical situation, and usually a maximum of up to 7 per cent is acceptable. The maximum target dose is the highest dose in the target volume which is clinically significant (greater than $15\,mm^3$ unless in a critical tissue where special considerations apply). The minimum target dose is an important parameter because it correlates with the probability of tumour control. The level of minimum dose (95 per cent, 90 per cent, etc.), the volume of the tissue irradiated to this dose, and its position relative to the macroscopic tumour should be assessed.

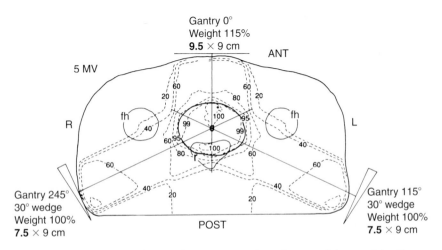

Fig. 1.15 Isodose distribution for treatment of carcinoma of the prostate. Dose specification point – intersection of central axes (ICRU) = 100 per cent; maximum tumour dose = 100 per cent; minimum tumour dose = 95 per cent; average tumour dose = 99 per cent; fh = femoral head; r = rectum.

Many centres still use the minimum isodose around the target volume as a target specification dose. However, this approach has several disadvantages. First, the homogeneity of the distribution may not be stated, and the maximum dose may be 10 to 15 per cent higher than the minimum dose. Second, the minimum isodose frequently lies in a region of steep dose gradient at the periphery of the volume. It also lies at the edge of the beam, where calculation of dose is less accurate than on the central axis of the beam. Finally, the minimum isodose lies on the edge of the target volume which, as previously discussed, is the most difficult parameter to define in the planning process. Use of the ICRU dose specification points (Table 1.2) will minimize these problems and should be adopted for reporting doses to allow comparison between treatment centres.

CHOICE OF BEAM ARRANGEMENT

Single beam

Superficial skin tumours are treated using a single beam (see Chapter 16), and the dose is prescribed as an applied dose, i.e. 100 per cent at the D_{max} which is at the skin surface for superficial therapy. Most superficial machines have energy ranges of 50–150 kV with appropriate filtration which defines percentage depth doses. An appropriate energy is selected from tables or charts for different beam sizes for a given FSD in order to encompass the target volume, both on the skin and at depth, with a 90 per cent isodose. When a single megavoltage beam is used, the dose is prescribed to the ICRU point at the centre of the target volume, rather than being given as an applied dose. For example, when using a Cobalt 60 beam to treat a vertebral metastasis, if an applied dose is used giving 100 per cent at 0.5 cm D_{max}, the front of the vertebral body situated at a depth of around 6 cm will receive only about 70 per cent of the dose. If the dose is prescribed to the centre of the vertebra, the spinal cord dose must be calculated to check that it is within tolerance. Whichever method is used, the dose received by tumour and homogeneity across the target volume must be carefully considered and the dose variation recorded. It is assumed that beam sizes are defined as the width of the 50 per cent isodose at the isocentric distance (the definition recommended by the ICRU).

Opposing beams

Opposing beams may be used for speed and ease of set-up for palliative treatments (e.g. for lung) or for target volumes of small separation (e.g. for larynx) or tangential volumes (e.g. for breast). Beam modification with the use of wedges alters the dose distribution to compensate for missing tissue and produce a more homogeneous result.

For coaxial opposing beams, doses are prescribed at the mid-plane point on the central axis of the beam. Isodose distributions show that the 95 per cent isodose does not conform closely to the target volume (see Fig. 18.4), the distribution of dose is not homogenous, and much normal tissue, including spinal cord, is irradiated to the same dose as the tumour. These factors make this simple technique suitable mainly for lower-dose palliative treatments. An isodose distribution is only prepared if there is concern about the homogeneity of the dose within the target volume, or about the dose to critical normal tissues; otherwise a simple calculation is made of the mid-point dose. The applied (or given) dose for each field is determined from depth dose charts which are available for each beam size and normalized (or fixed) to 100 per cent, at the depth of maximum build-up (D_{max}) for a 10 × 10 cm field at the standard FSD. These data only apply to square fields. If rectangular or irregular fields are used, the contribution from scattered irradiation is different, and tables are consulted to obtain equivalent square fields.

Example

For coaxial opposing fields 12 × 6 cm at a fixed FSD = 100 cm, the equivalent square = 8 cm.

For patient separation (IPD) of 16 cm, the mid-plane lies at 8 cm.

For an 8 × 8 cm field (from 8-MV depth dose charts) the percentage depth dose at 8 cm = 76.5 per cent.

For two opposing fields, the mid-plane dose (MPD)

$$= 76.5 \text{ per cent} \times 2$$

$$= 153 \text{ per cent.}$$

To obtain a 2-Gy mid-plane dose each day, the applied dose to each field

$$= 2 \times \frac{100}{153}$$

$$= 1.3 \text{ Gy.}$$

This example is for a fixed FSD treatment, but many centres treat opposing fields isocentrically. Isocentric treatment means that the centre of the target volume (here the mid-separation of the patient) is positioned so that it is at the centre of rotation of the treatment machine. This means that the FSD is non-standard (in the above example 100 − 8 = 92 cm). Alternative output charts are available for isocentric techniques at different FSD normalized to 100 per cent at the isocentre, or a table of tissue maximum ratios is required. The advantage of an isocentric technique is that the second beam is set up simply by rotating the gantry through 180° using the same isocentre, which reduces the setting up time.

Complex beam arrangements

For many tumours seated at depth, a radical tumour dose can only be achieved with a combination of several beams if overdose to the skin and other superficial tissues is to be avoided. Computerized dose planning systems are used to construct an isodose distribution with beams of appropriate energy, size, weighting, gantry angle and wedge to give a homogeneous result over the target volume. This may involve the use of mixed beams (combining photons and electrons for part of each treatment), beam modification using bolus, wedges, compensators, shielding blocks or multileaf collimators, and optimization of skin dose (e.g. skin sparing using higher megavoltage energies or maximized dose to the skin using tissue equivalent bolus).

BEAM MODIFICATION

Wedges

As will be seen from the following chapters, combinations of two or three beams are most commonly used. The effect of a beam of radiation may be modified by the introduction of a wedge which alters the dose distribution, because of greater absorption of radiation through the thick end of the wedge (Figs 1.16a and b). Variable wedges are an integral part of most modern linear accelerators as an alternative to wedges of fixed angles of 15, 30, 45 and 60°, which have to be inserted manually into the treatment unit. Variable wedges can be either a single motorized wedge, or virtual wedges when the collimator is driven across the field for a chosen period of time.

Wedges are used to produce a satisfactory distribution where beams intersect, so that a high dose area can be avoided. They may also be used to compensate for obliquity of body contour or a sloping target volume. When physical wedges are in place, they attenuate the beam. To achieve the same dose at the patient, the number of monitor units set will have to be increased compared with those for an open field.

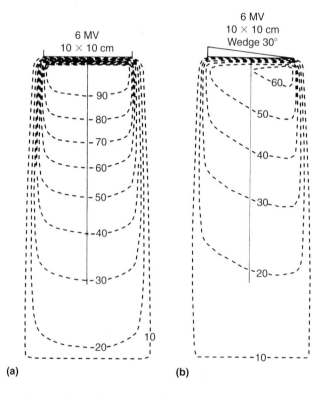

Fig. 1.16 (a) Open field (b) Modification of isodose curve by insertion of 30° wedge into the beam (including wedge attenuation factor).

Compensators

A compensator may be placed in the beam to correct dose inhomogeneity due to varying depth of target volume or obliquity of contour. It must be inserted in the beam at a sufficient distance from the skin to ensure that contamination by secondary electrons is avoided. Any material may be used as a compensator, so long as it provides similar X-ray attenuation to the amount of 'missing' tissue. Aluminium alloy is commonly chosen because the resultant compensator is small and light to handle (Figs 1.17a and b). Alternatively, compensators can be made from sheets of lead using an automated milling machine programmed by a computer planning system.

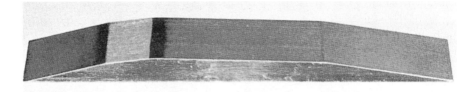

Fig. 1.17a   Compensator to correct for sloping body contour.

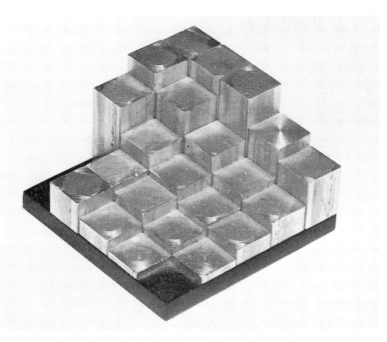

Fig. 1.17b   Individually designed stepped compensator.

Sometimes a better dose distribution can be obtained by 'weighting' one of the treatment beams, so that more radiation is given, for example, by an anterior field than by lateral fields. The effect of weighting is shown in Figs 1.18a and b.

If the field enters the skin surface obliquely, a dose gradient will be produced, since part of the beam will pass through air with less absorption than that part

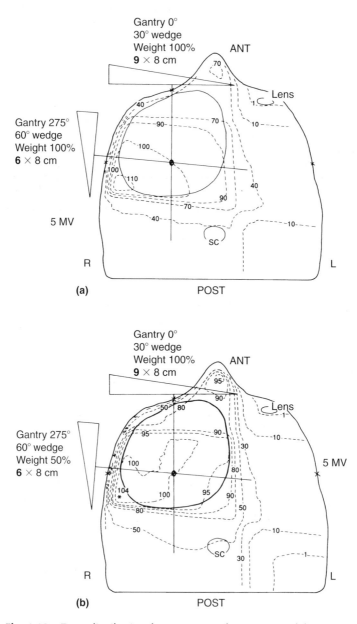

Fig. 1.18 Dose distribution for treatment of carcinoma of the antrum using (a) equally weighted fields and (b) with anterior : lateral weighting of 2:1; sc = spinal cord. Weighting defined at ICRU point.

which passes entirely through tissue. This can be corrected by using a wedge or compensator.

Beam shaping

Low-melting-point alloy blocks may be used to shape fields and reduce the amount of normal tissue irradiated. They are placed on to a tray attached to the machine head, and they usually have a thickness of four to five half value layers (HVLs). From first principles, four HVLs would result in 6 per cent transmission and five HVLs in 3 per cent transmission. A technique using alloy blocks designed to allow for beam divergence is described in Chapter 22 (under *'Mantle' technique*). However, linac beams are 'hardened' by filtration, and the HVL increases slightly with each successive HVL, for example 5–6 per cent instead of 3 per cent (5HVLs) and 8 per cent instead of 6 per cent (4HVLs). These transmission values are measured with a small beam and a wide block. In clinical treatments, however, the block usually shields only a small part of the beam, and scattered radiation may substantially increase the dose under the shielding block (e.g. to 15 to 20 per cent).

Multileaf collimators (MLCs) provide detailed and dynamic beam shaping and, when available, may be used instead of alloy blocks. MLC positions for appropriate shielding are defined in the planning system in the beam's-eye view. These positions can be transferred directly to the linac by network or disc. Alternatively, the positions of the leaves could be digitized from a hard copy of the beam's-eye view.

INHOMOGENEITY CORRECTIONS

Attenuation of an X-ray beam is affected by tissue density, being less in lung tissue, which is of low density, than in bone. This variation affects both the shape of the dose distribution and the value of the isodoses. Lung tissue should therefore be localized when planning treatment for tumours of the thorax (e.g. lung, oesophagus or breast). The relative electron density of lung tissue compared with water is in the range 0.2–0.3. These values are used to correct for inhomogeneity. If two-dimensional planning is used, correction is only valid at the planned central slice of the target volume. For example, for breast treatment, a simulator film (central lung distance) or simulator-CT (central or 3 CT slices) may be used to measure lung depth in the tangential beam. For more accurate heterogeneity corrections, three-dimensional planning is needed with localization of lung tissue throughout the three-dimensional volume using CT planning. Using CT scanning, a pixel by pixel correction can be made to take account of all tissue densities within the body contour by conversion of CT numbers into relative electron densities using calibration curves. However, CT numbers are also affected by contrast agents (e.g. those introduced into the bowel or rectum during planning), metal prostheses and immobilization devices and, as these variables may alter between planning and daily treatments, the use of total tissue inhomogeneity corrections may be unwise. During pelvic CT scans, the rectum and bowel may contain variable and large amounts of gas (low density) and contrast media (high density – during planning only) and, because of this variability,

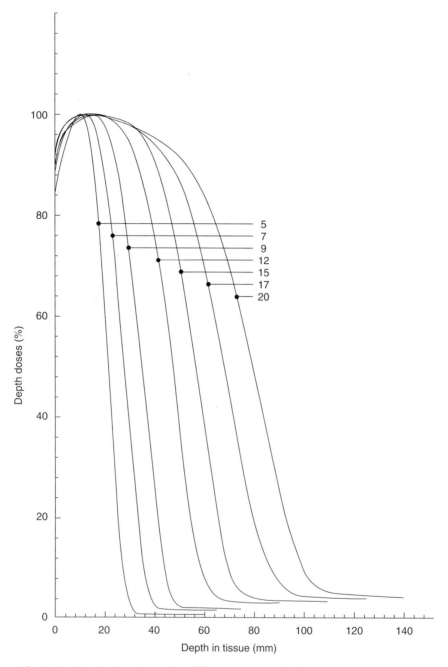

Fig. 1.19 Depth dose charts for different energies of electron beams (MeV) for a 10 × 10 applicator.

inhomogeneity corrections are not normally used in the pelvis. If conditions are stable, the density correction for pelvic bones is in the region of ±3 per cent.

ELECTRON THERAPY

Electron therapy may be used to treat superficial tumours overlying cartilage and bone (at sites such as the nose, ear, scalp and back of the hand). This approach may be preferable to superficial or orthovoltage therapy where there is increased bone absorption because of the photoelectric effect. Single-field electron treatments are useful for treating the tumour bed as a boost dose after tangential breast radiotherapy, because of the electron-beam characteristic of sparing underlying tissue, in this instance the lung (Figs 1.19 and 1.20). There is a sharp fall in dose beyond the 90 per cent isodose (4–12 MeV) and the electron energy is chosen so that the target volume is encompassed by the 90–95 per cent isodose at the deep margin.

Electrons are particularly useful at higher energies (15–25 MeV) for treatment of head and neck tumours, e.g. cervical lymph nodes overlying the spinal cord, small-volume thyroid carcinomas and parotid tumours.

The effective treatment depth in centimetres is about one-third of the beam energy in MeV, and the total range is about half (Fig. 1.19), but this is dependent on field size (especially at <4 cm). There is a tail to the curve due to Bremsstrahlung from the scattering foil, collimating system and patient's tissue. Different tissue densities, such as those of bone and air (as found in ribs overlying lung, and facial bones containing air-filled sinuses), cause non-homogeneous dose distributions. Doses beyond air cavities may be higher than expected even after density corrections, and this may limit the usefulness of electrons for treating in these clinical situations. Electron-beam edges do not diverge geometrically due to lateral scatter, which is greater at low energies, with the characteristic shape shown in Fig. 1.20. Wider margins must be added to the target volume for adequate treatment of tumours at depth. Where there is tumour infiltration of the skin, the skin-sparing characteristic of electron beams below 16 MeV should be removed by adding bolus material, which can also be used to provide tissue-equivalent material for an irregular contour such as the nose or ear.

Field sizes of <4 cm should be avoided because of inadequate depth of penetration and loss of beam flatness.

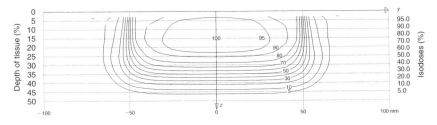

Fig. 1.20 Isodose chart for a 9-MeV electron beam using a 10 × 10 cm applicator at 100 cm SSD.

BEAM JUNCTIONS

When treatment is given to target volumes that lie adjacent to one another, consideration must be given to the non-uniformity of dose in the potential overlap regions caused by divergence of the adjacent beam edges. If the beams are abutting on the skin surface, they will overlap with excess dose at depth. If there is a gap between the beams at the skin, there will be a cold area in the superficial tissues. Clinical examples of this problem include treatment of:

- adjacent vertebrae with single posterior fields which may be separated in time, where there is a risk of overlap of dose at the underlying spinal cord;
- primary head and neck tumour and regional lymph nodes, where photon and electron beams may need to be matched;
- primary breast cancer and adjacent axillary and supraclavicular nodes, where a single isocentric technique centring at the junction has been proposed;
- primary CNS tumours, such as medulloblastoma, where beams are matched at the anterior spinal cord and junctions between fields are shifted during the course of treatment; and
- adjacent mantle and inverted Y coaxial opposed fields which are matched at depth to cover the target volume.

Various techniques have been developed to minimize dose heterogeneity at beam junctions in these different clinical situations. Half-beam blocking using shielding or independent collimator jaws can be used to eliminate divergence up to the match line, but is then dependent on immobilization of the patient's position and reliability of skin marks to reproduce the match perfectly. Couch rotation can be used to remove beam divergence, as described in Chapter 20, when matching breast and lymph node irradiation. However, it is still common to match beams by using a gap on the skin surface between beams, so that the beam edges converge at a planned depth (d) (Fig. 1.21a). The dose in the triangular gap (x) below the skin surface will be lower than that at the point P where the beams converge, because it lies outside the geometric margins of both beams. Doses at y are higher because they include contributions from both beams. The positioning of point P anatomically will vary according to the aim of treatment. If treatment is for medulloblastoma, a homogeneous dose is required to potential tumour cells within the spinal cord, which is therefore placed at point P (Fig. 1.21b), and point P is moved in a cranio-caudal direction at regular intervals to prevent any risk of overdose at junctions. Where treatment is aimed at metastases in adjacent vertebral bodies, it is important to avoid overdosage at the spinal cord, which is therefore placed in the superficial cold triangle x with point P anterior to it. The gap on the skin is the sum of the beam divergence for each beam. It is calculated as the distance from the edge of the beam as defined by the 50 per cent isodose to the point of convergence P measured perpendicular to the central axis and marked s for spread (beam divergence) for each beam. Graphs have been prepared which express beam divergence as a function of the depth below the skin for different field sizes and FSD. Once the gap has been calculated, it may be necessary to increase it slightly to allow for possible movement of patient or skin

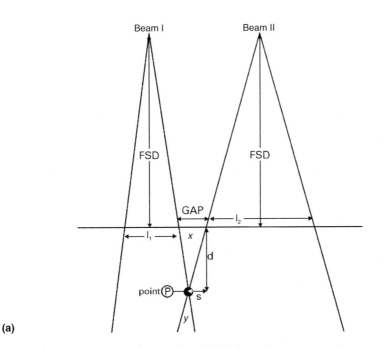

(a)

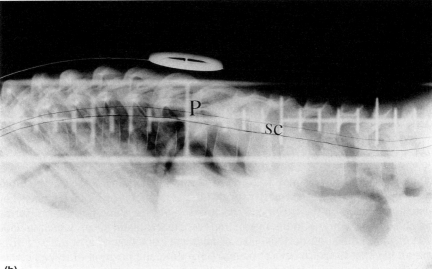

(b)

Fig. 1.21 (a) Technique for matching two beams I and II (length l_1 and l_2) at a point P at depth d by allowing a gap on the skin surface (x, y, s – see text). (b) Lateral simulator film of the spine showing spinal cord (sc) and point P for treatment of medulloblastoma.

tattoos, to ensure that there is no overdosage. Whenever possible, a patient should be treated in the same position (supine or prone) for matching adjacent fields. To accurately match metastatic disease in the spine, previous simulator and beam films and treatment records should be used to reconstruct previous treatment fields, and deliver subsequent treatment in the same position, with the use of an undercouch facility if appropriate.

DOSIMETRY

Beam data from the therapy machines are available as percentage depth dose charts for varying energies and field sizes at fixed FSD for most units. These can be used to calculate doses for treatment using single fields, and to learn the construction of isodose distributions using 'hand' planning. However, most dose computation uses computerized treatment planning systems which have been programmed with beam data from therapy machines and have a careful quality control programme. Following production of a satisfactory isodose distribution to a given target volume using two- or three-dimensional algorithms, the calculations are checked by a physicist and the detailed instructions for delivery are prepared by radiographers on the therapy unit.

DOSE PRESCRIPTION

The dose prescription includes the following factors: total dose to the target volume; number of fractions; dose per fraction; overall time for treatment; number of fractions per week; dose specification points. In this book, all radical radiation doses quoted will be according to the standard fractionation schedule of 2-Gy daily fractions with total doses of 50–70 Gy, as these have been demonstrated by experience to produce good tumour control with tolerable acute reactions and low rates of late complication. The principles of dose–time fractionation are discussed in detail in Chapter 4.

IMPLEMENTATION OF TREATMENT

The beam arrangement may be verified on the simulator, the final instructions then prepared for treatment delivery and the dose prescription signed. The patient is placed on the treatment couch in exactly the same position as during localization, according to the instructions on the treatment sheet, which include use of immobilization devices, size of head pad, position of arm poles, full or empty bladder, measurement of patient separation and position of reference tattoos. Laser lights are used to align the patient in the sagittal and coronal planes to prevent rotation, and photographs are used as a helpful record. The beam parameters are set (beam size, gantry angle, wedges, shielding blocks or collimator settings) and the FSD instructions are checked. The dose prescription is checked and the monitor unit calculations are double-checked before treatment is delivered, ideally under the observation of the responsible clinician on the first day.

VERIFICATION

Verification of the geometrical set-up is obtained on the first day of treatment using beam check films or electronic portal imaging (on- or off-line) as a film record to be compared with the simulator (Figs 1.22a and b) or CT localization films. This comparison can be made by eye or using a computer software program to match either bony landmarks or field margins and measure any deviations. Verification protocols will define the level of action for any deviation, and radiographers and radiation oncologists should review films together.

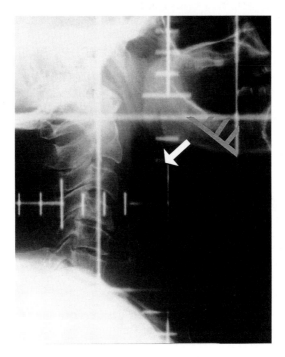

Fig. 1.22a   Simulator film – treatment of epiglottic tumour (see arrow).

The dose to the patient during treatment can be measured using lithium fluoride thermoluminescent dosemeters (TLD) or semiconductor diodes, and comparison made with doses calculated from the isodose distribution. TLD is used for most *in-vivo* dosimetry, because lithium fluoride is supplied in small versatile packages and is cheap and reasonably tissue equivalent, although it is time-consuming to calibrate and read out, and requires care to produce accurate results. Diodes require connection cables, may be temperature and direction dependent, and can produce unreliable results, but they have a high sensitivity and provide instant read-out.

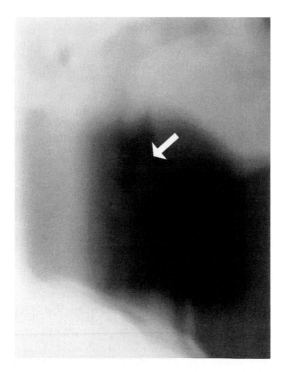

Fig. 1.22b   Beam portal film showing comparison for verification of geometrical set-up.

MONITORING TREATMENT

Patients are reviewed weekly during their treatment in the clinic by a team of radiographers and radiation oncologists. Treatment charts are checked for cumulative data given, verification–simulator film comparisons can be made, TLD results checked and signed, and early normal tissue reactions monitored according to World Health Organization/European Organization for Research and Treatment of Cancer (WHO/EORTC) scales. Instructions can be given to cut out perspex shells to improve skin sparing, blood test results can be checked (e.g. after chemotherapy), and medication can be prescribed for side-effects such as nausea, diarrhoea, oesophagitis, skin reactions and any other acute side-effects. Opportunities are provided for patients and their families to ask any questions and to indicate any need for psychological or social support, and checks are made that they have received all of the information they require about their diagnosis, treatment and likely side-effects.

RECORDING AND REPORTING RADIATION TREATMENTS

When reporting a radiotherapy treatment either locally or for publication, the use of ICRU definitions of volume and dose is recommended. Volumes are described according to ICRU definitions of GTV, CTV and PTV, with adequate descriptions of the margins and imaging modalities used in their construction. The dose at or near the centre of the PTV, as well as the maximum and minimum doses to the PTV, is reported together with fraction size and overall time, and any gaps in treatment. For each organ at risk, the maximum dose and the volume of the organ receiving that dose should be reported whenever possible. The mean dose and its standard deviation and dose–volume histograms are reported when available, as are techniques for any inhomogeneity corrections.

Further reading

Hermanek, P., Hutter, R.V.P., Sobin, L.H., Wagner, G. and Wittekind, C.H. (eds) 1997: *International Union Against Cancer TNM atlas. Illustrated guide to the TNM classification of malignant tumours*, 4th edn. Berlin: Springer-Verlag.

Husband, J.E.S. and Reznek, R.H. (eds) 1998: *Imaging in oncology.* Oxford: ISIS Medical Media Ltd.

International Commission on Radiation Units and Measurements 1993: *ICRU Report No. 50. Prescribing, recording and reporting photon beam therapy*. Bethesda, MD: International Commission on Radiation Units and Measurements (ICRU report 62: Supplement to ICRU Report No. 50; in press).

Pavy, J.J., Denekamp, J., Letschert, J. *et al.* 1995: EORTC Late Effects Working Group. Late effects toxicity scoring: the SOMA scale. *Radiotherapy and Oncology* **35**, 11–15.

CHAPTER 2

Three-dimensional planning and conformal therapy

Introduction

More complex planning and delivery of radiotherapy (level 3, ICRU Report No. 50) is appropriate for some sites to maximize tumour dose and minimize the dose to adjacent normal tissues or organs at risk. This conformal therapy requires the highest achievable degree of immobilization, and three-dimensional imaging using all appropriate techniques. Co-registration of such images is desirable to define the tumour, target volume and normal tissues. Shaped fields are chosen using a beam's-eye view; dose distributions are calculated using three-dimensional algorithms and compared using the information obtained from dose–volume histograms. Treatment is delivered using beams shaped with alloy blocks, and multileaf collimator or stereotactic techniques. Special care must be given to verification of the position of the fields and dose distributions.

The use of conformal therapy is usually restricted to radical treatments. It may be particularly useful in the following situations:

- where the macroscopic tumour remains *in situ* (e.g. pre-operative treatment for carcinoma of the rectum);
- where increasing the total tumour dose is expected to be advantageous (e.g. in prostate, head and neck tumours, or lung cancer);
- where the treatment volume may otherwise include sensitive normal tissues (e.g. brain and lung);
- for paediatric tumours and other special sites such as the breast where limiting the volume of normal tissue irradiated (e.g. growing muscle, heart, etc.) is especially important;
- to treat irregular volumes (especially with concave margins) not easily achieved with conventional planning (e.g. tumours near the spinal cord, and of cervix, or prostate).

While some of these uses, such as reduction of dose to sensitive structures, are likely to be advantageous, others, such as the benefits of dose escalation are less clear and must be tested in rigorous clinical studies.

Accuracy of immobilization

The patient's position for treatment must be comfortable, reproducible and suitable for acquisition of images for planning and treatment delivery. Immobilization devices are used as described in Chapter 1. External movement is minimized using heat-moulded perspex or other shells, vacuum bags or alpha cradles and positioning devices such as foot rests and leg restraints. For stereotactic brain treatments, a relocatable frame or special jaw bites may be used. For single-fraction stereotactic brain treatments, MRI-compatible stereotactic frames held to the skull by means of carbon-fibre pins represent the best achievable immobilization. The use of relocatable masks of rigid material such as plaster bandages or the relocatable Gill Thomas frame provide 1–2 mm of accuracy (Fig. 2.1). Relocatable whole-body fixation systems with a stereotactic table top using vacuum bags restrict movement to 3–4 mm.

The degree of day-to-day variation in patient position differs from one part of the body to another. Movements of the brain within a perspex shell may be as

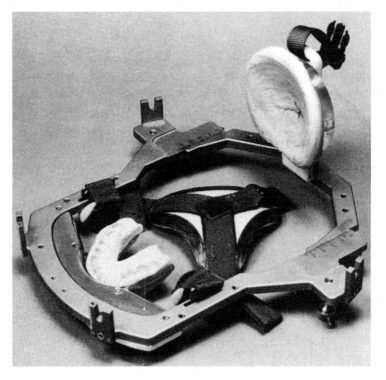

Fig. 2.1 Gill Thomas stereotactic frame used for treatment of brain tumours.
Reprinted from Radiotherapy and Oncology, 21, Graham, J.D. *et al.*, A non-invasive,
relocatable stereotactic frame for fractionated radiotherapy and multiple imaging,
60–2, Copyright 1991, with permission from Elsevier Science.

little as 1–4 mm, whereas pelvic movements may be up to 10–30 mm. These variations must be taken into account when choosing the planning target volume (PTV).

Organ movement

Internal movements must also be considered, the most important of which are changes with respiration and bowel and bladder filling. Voluntary bladder emptying is the most practical way of minimizing day-to-day variations in the pelvis, although it is not very precise. Some recent conformal studies have included daily rectal stenting to minimize the effect of volume changes to the rectum. Inter- and intra-fraction variations must be taken into account, and these may be more than 2 cm. Geometrical errors in set-up are a combination of random or systematic errors, and may be normally distributed or inisotropic. Organ movements may also be non-uniform. For example, in the thorax, movement of the diaphragm may be approximately 1 cm at the dome, while excursions at the posterior part of the diaphragm may be as great as 3 cm. Ways of matching target volumes to these variations are being sought. Treatment may be gated and given in short bursts at one phase of the respiratory cycle only. An alternative technique of active breathing control temporarily immobilizes breathing, and radiotherapy is given only while the breath is being held. Spiral CT tomotherapy is being developed to match planning images with treatment delivery. Similar techniques may also be used for treatment of the liver or kidney, where excursions of up to 3 cm may occur.

Imaging

CT scans are necessary for conformal therapy planning. CT is essential for dose calculation using electron density, but in some situations MRI may give better tissue differentiation. Scans must be obtained with the patient lying in the treatment position with appropriate immobilization on a flat couch. Contiguous thin slices at 3–5 mm for the head and 3–10 mm for the body are obtained. Care must be taken to include complete external body contour and whole organ contours for dose–volume histograms. Important information additional to that obtained from conventional CT scanning may be obtained from ultrasound, MRI, positron emission tomography (PET) or single positron emission computed tomography (SPECT) scanning. Image registration methods must be used to transform the position of a point in the images to the corresponding physical point in the patient, and to find correspondence (or match) between two image sets from different modalities (Plate 2.1). Extrinsic landmarks may be matched using reference points which may be located using fiducial markers and systems, such as stereotactic frames, dental moulds, plastic helmets or ear plugs, for the brain. Markers may be glued to the skin, but the accuracy of this technique is limited by skin movement. Retrospective image registration methods include extracting corresponding structures or features from each data set and trying to minimize the distance between them, and voxel-based methods which maximize the correspondence between pixel grey values in different data sets. Patient data can also be matched to a stereotactic atlas. This may lead to large errors which can be remedied by allowing the atlas to deform locally by a process known as elastic matching.

Acquired images can be transferred to the treatment planning system by means of a digital imaging communication in medicine (DICOM) system which, using a common file format, enables communication between machines, or a picture archiving and communication system (PACS), which can be used for image viewing, transmission, archiving and retrieval. Image-to-patient accuracy is approximately 1 mm (half a slice thickness) for stereotactic frames, 2.5 mm for relocatable frames and 5 mm for skin markers. For image-to-image matching, manual landmarks give 5 mm accuracy, point-based landmarks give 3–4 mm and voxel similarity gives 2–3 mm. The better the immobilization that can be achieved, the tighter the margins that can be used to determine the planning target volume.

Definition of target volumes

Using all of the imaging data available, and taking into account all of the relevant clinical factors, gross tumour volume (GTV) and clinical target volume (CTV) are determined and marked on each scan slice. Images are then viewed in three dimensions and appropriate margins chosen for the PTV (Plate 2.2). Automatic delineation of this margin can be performed by the computer, but since movement of organs may be much greater in one direction than in another, the margins may not be equal in all directions. An automatic contouring facility is available for outlining the body contour and individual structures using density data. Complete organ delineation is essential for the production of dose–volume histograms (Plates 2.3a and b) (see below).

Choice of dose distribution

When the PTV has been defined, a beam's-eye view of it is used to choose beam directions and sizes and to shape fields with appropriate shielding (Plate 2.4). Conventional and much three-dimensional planning uses a 'forward' approach where the best plan is arrived at by repeated trial and error. Another approach is to use 'inverse' planning with computer-assisted optimization. Objectives and constraints are first defined, and then the optimal beam arrangement and weighting are determined by the computer. Possible objectives might, for example, be to treat the PTV homogeneously with an accuracy of 5 per cent to a dose of 60 Gy, at the same time taking into account the constraints of restricting the dose to the kidney to 20 Gy and 50 per cent of its volume, and not exceeding 40 Gy to 4 cm of spinal cord. These dose–volume constraints are chosen using the best available clinical data, but more research is needed in many areas to define them accurately. Beam directions may be coplanar or non-coplanar for optimal dose distribution as decided using the beam's-eye view (Plates 2.5a and b).

Dose distributions are then calculated using a three-dimensional algorithm. This should account for the heterogenous nature of the patient in 3D by accurately determining scatter dose at each calculation point, as well as the primary dose. The pencil beam based method is most common and Monte Carlo calculations which accurately predict dose at tissue interfaces are the way forward.

Multileaf collimation

Appropriate shielding or beam shaping may be achieved with custom-made alloy blocks or by using a multileaf collimator (MLC). The latter has movable leaves or shields which can block part of the radiation field (Fig. 2.2). Typical MLCs have 20–80 leaves arranged in opposing pairs which can be positioned under computer control to create an irregular field that conforms to the tumour shape. As well as eliminating the hazards of production and the use of alloy blocks, this system allows rapid adjustment of field shaping to match the beam's-eye view of the PTV (Plate 2.4). MLCs can be used in arc rotation therapy or to achieve beam intensity modulation by creating a dynamic compensator for a number of fixed gantry exposures or for a continuously arcing fan of beams. The MLC can replace the upper or lower jaws of a linear accelerator, or it can act as tertiary collimation. Beam shaping or tissue compensator can be achieved with the leaves in static mode, with their position determined by computer calculation. MLC may be used to define the beam intensity independently in different regions of each incident beam, to produce the desired uniform distribution of dose or to produce a deliberate non-uniform dose distribution in the target volume (Plate 2.6). This is known as beam intensity modulation or intensity-modulated radiation therapy (IMRT), and is an extension of older techniques for achieving dose homogeneity using compensators, wedges and bolus. The position of the leaves of the MLC can be varied in time with a fixed or moving gantry. A sequence of static MLC fields can be used with the beam switched off between changes in position – this is known as the stop and shoot technique. Each field can then be verified by portal imaging (see below). Alternatively, there may be automatic sequencing of beam segments without stopping treatment. For such dynamic multileaf collimation (DMLC) it is difficult to verify the accuracy of the beam, and very careful quality assurance must be developed. Other methods of DMLC include tomotherapy, where there is intensity-modulated rotational delivery with a fan beam, and devices such as the Peacock Mimic system.

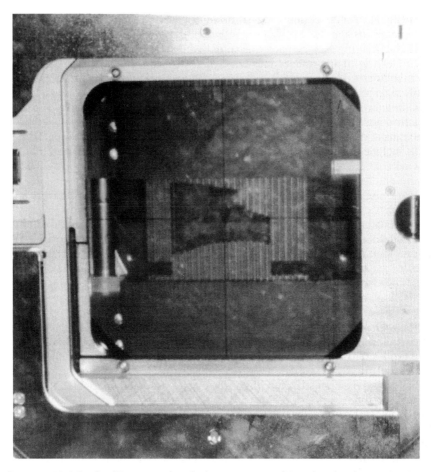

Fig. 2.2 Multileaf collimator in head of treatment machine showing beam shaping.

TREATMENT VERIFICATION

The quality assurance programme for MLC is vital, and must include *in-vivo* dosimetry to check dose delivered, and portal imaging to check the geometric accuracy of the beam. Standard film may be used for verification, but has poor contrast compared with electronic portal imaging. A metal plate–phosphor screen combination can be used. This converts photon beam density into a light image which can be viewed by video camera using an angled mirror or fibre-optic arrangement, or can be scanned with a laser beam off-line to obtain an image. Such images are compared with simulator films and digitally reconstructed radiographs (DRR) which are obtained from the planning system by projection of CT data along the direction of the beam (Plates 2.7a and b). Although these are often of limited resolution because of the large CT slice thickness used, they are valuable for detecting field shifts, and can be refined using smaller slice thicknesses or spiral CT.

Portal imaging may be used to ensure that patient positioning is constant with each fraction of treatment, and that it matches the original plan. Comparison with simulator films or DRR may be made by eye otherwise image evaluation tools may be used for comparison of the position of field boundaries and internal structures. Two methods are possible – either bony landmarks may be matched and field-edge displacements noted, or field edges may be matched and the translation of internal structures measured. Techniques for dealing with this data include manual or automated matching techniques. Field edges are not always easy to define, and a convention may be adopted, such as using the maximum gradient method.

Errors may be systematic and random. Systematic errors may result from incorrect data transfer from planning to dose delivery, or inaccurate placing of devices such as compensators, shields, etc. Such systematic errors can be corrected.

Random errors in set-up may be operator dependent or may result from day-to-day changes in patient anatomy which are impossible to correct. Accuracy of set-up may be improved with implanted opaque markers such as gold seeds whose position can be determined in three dimensions using two film projections at planning, and whose position can be checked during treatment. Translational errors can thereby be reduced to 1 mm and rotational errors to 1°.

As well as assessment of geometric matching of the field, a check of dose distribution must be made. *In-vivo* dosimetry using TLD or semiconductor silicon diodes may be employed. Transit dosimetry is a technique which computes the distribution of dose actually delivered to the patient from a transmission portal image for comparison with the dose distribution computed at the planning stage. The three-dimensional distribution of the electron density of the planned treatment is given by the DRR. This can be registered with the portal image. The portal image can then provide a measure of photon intensity or fluence, indicating the dose to each point.

Complicated physics calculations must take into account field sizes, attenuating materials, skin detector distance, patient thickness, photon beam energy, ratio of scatter to primary irradiation and many other factors before a three-dimensional map of the primary fluence in the patient can be computed by back-projection and thus a determination of the three-dimensional dose distribution can be obtained. Full discussion of this topic is beyond the scope of this book (but see *Further reading* at the end of this chapter). Other developments include the use of radiation-sensitive gels containing either thiosulphate ions or tissue-equivalent polymer gel (bang gel dosimetry), which can be read by magnetic resonance after irradiation in a phantom. The dose at a specific point in the phantom can then be compared with the dose computed at that point from transit dosimetry.

Equally important are the mechanical checks of MLC that are required to ensure safe delivery of treatments. These must include examination of the stability of leaf speed, the effect of acceleration and deceleration of leaves, the accuracy of leaf position, the effect of the shape of leaf ends, and transmission through and between leaves.

PRESCRIBING AND REPORTING

ICRU conventions should be followed as described in Chapter 1. Treatment prescription should define the geometric PTV and the dose to be given. Any report of the treatment should include the relevant value of the isodose selected to define the treated volume normalized to the dose at the ICRU reference point, as well as the size of the PTV and CTV. The size of the integrated margin as well as the sum-up method and probability level used should be reported. The dose at the ICRU reference point and maximum and minimum doses must be stated as must other dose values considered to be relevant (e.g. the mean dose and its standard deviation, dose–volume histograms or biologically weighted doses). A quantitative evaluation of the planning includes a review of the maximum and minimum doses in the target volume and their distribution, and the study of dose–volume histograms (DVHs). DVHs are based on the concept that there is a volume effect for normal tissue damage, and therefore increasing the volume that is receiving the same dose will lead to increased damage. DVHs display in two dimensions what percentage of the volume is raised to a defined dose. Comparison of DVHs may help the clinician to decide which of several different treatment plans with similar dose distributions in the target volume is best in terms of normal tissue exposure (Plates 2.8a, b, c and d). Since such decisions are difficult and may be made subjectively, attempts have been made to produce models which estimate tumour control probability (TCP) and normal tissue complication probability (NTCP), and some planning systems incorporate these models for interpretation of DVH (see Chapter 4). However, as yet there is no general agreement about the reliability of these models and, like automatic organ contouring, they must be used with care until the clinical database is improved.

Further reading

Webb, S. 1993: *The physics of 3D radiotherapy: conformal radiotherapy, radiosurgery and treatment planning*. Bristol: Institute of Physics.
Webb, S. 1997: *The physics of conformal radiotherapy: advances in technology*. Bristol: Institute of Physics.

CHAPTER 3

Quality assurance in radiotherapy

Introduction

A comprehensive quality assurance (QA) programme is needed to ensure that the best possible care is delivered to the patient by defining and documenting all procedures involved in radiotherapy treatments.

A quality assurance policy must be formulated by a radiotherapy manager with overall responsibility for implementation, although large parts of this responsibility may be delegated to other appropriately trained and qualified members of the radiotherapy team.

In recent years, reports of requirements for quality assurance have been published by a number of national and international bodies, including the WHO, the European Organization for Research and Treatment of Cancer (EORTC), the European Society for Therapeutic Radiation Oncology (ESTRO), the American Association of Physicists in Medicine (AAPM) and the British Standards Institute (BSI) (see *Further reading* at the end of this chapter). Quality assurance defines the procedures to be followed in order to test technical aspects of the functioning of a system or subsystem, and quality control (QC) in radiotherapy, which forms part of an overall quality system, is designed to eliminate any inaccuracy or deficiency which would lead to suboptimal treatment. Quality control should ensure accuracy and precision. It is a regulatory process in which actual performance is compared with defined standards or reference values, and it should specify what actions are needed to keep or regain conformity with these standards. It is recommended that each institution should use a recognized externally assessed Quality System that defines procedures to cover all aspects of radiotherapy delivery, and that describes work instructions to carry out those procedures.

There must be periodic complete reviews of the system with documentation of all activities according to a defined protocol. There must be inspection and testing of all equipment. Reference values must be specified, with tolerances and action to be taken if these are exceeded. Provision must be made for staff training. External audit is followed by certification by an appropriate agency, such as the British Standards Institute or the European Society Quality Assurance Network (ESQUAN).

Practical implementation

These issues may be considered under the following headings:

1. machine checks;
2. dosimetry protocols;
3. planning checks;
4. patient documentation.

MACHINE CHECKS

Special procedures must be used to determine the functioning of each treatment machine or item of equipment at the time of installation and acceptance. Data obtained by detailed studies during the phase of commissioning usually provide the reference values against which subsequent checks are assessed. Inter-comparisons between different institutions or with national or international standards are very useful for detecting systematic errors. Quality control should then ensure that the unit performs according to its specification and is safe for both patients and staff. It should guarantee the accuracy of dose delivered, pre-vent major errors, minimize down time of the machine and promote preventative machine maintenance.

There should be a specific QC protocol for each unit which outlines the tests to be performed, the test methods to be used to ensure consistency in the per-formance of each unit, the parameters to be tested, the frequency of measure-ment, staff responsibilities, reference values, tolerances, action to be taken in case of deviation, and rules for documentation.

The frequency of such testing is determined by the severity of the risk in the event of a malfunction, the probability of error affecting the safety of perfor-mance, the expected life and long-term stability of the unit, and the experience of staff. Special testing must be carried out when any change is made to the unit.

Tests should be simple and quick, and should be made in maintenance and therapy mode. Daily, weekly and extended testing of the following is needed:

• dosimetry;
• beam alignment;
• safety checks.

Daily checks are not usually absolute measures, but they test a number of para-meters together. If the system is found to be malfunctioning, independent tests must be carried out to identify the error.

Weekly tests should use absolute measures, but constitute more of a check on the consistency of machine operation than the extended monthly testing, in which each parameter is checked independently. Details of such QC protocols are given in the documents listed at the end of this chapter.

Briefly, regular checks should include the following:

- tests of optical and mechanical systems such as beam alignment, laser systems and couch and collimator movement;
- dose-monitor calibration;
- beam symmetry;
- accessories, e.g. wedges, compensators;
- interlocks and other safety devices;
- computer systems.

TL defines a tolerance level such that when a parameter falls within the range TL, the equipment may be considered suitable for high-quality radiotherapy.

Action levels are defined where correction is needed before treatment can proceed. Values between the tolerance and action levels should be checked and, if consistent, adjustments should be made.

Similar checks must be carried out for all imaging equipment and treatment-planning systems.

The results of daily checks are recorded in a log-book kept in the control room of the treatment unit, in which radiographers can also record any problems with machine functioning. This ensures continuity and facilitates the early recognition of trends in errors. All other checks, actions and maintenance work are recorded in a separate log-book. Good co-operation is needed between all staff groups. A physicist co-ordinates all QC activity, checks that tests are up to standard, and reports any major deviations to the clinician.

DOSIMETRY PROTOCOLS

These include dose-monitor calibration checks, checks of beam quality and symmetry, and evaluation of beam flatness. *In-vivo* dosimetry systems such as thermoluminescent dose meters and silicon diodes must also be regularly checked and calibrated.

PLANNING CHECKS

The treatment prescription must include identification of the patient and a description of the treatment technique, immobilization devices, target volume, doses to specified target volumes or organs at risk, and the fractionation schedule. A copy of any isodose distributions prepared must also be kept. When the plan has been produced, the calculations should be checked by a second physicist. Any transcription of the treatment parameters and plans must again be independently checked, as must the calculation of monitor units. For isocentric treatments, the FSD of each field should be checked frequently in order to detect changes in patient contour.

A patient record card is used to document each treatment, and weekly review of patients and treatment charts should verify cumulative dose calculations and assess treatment responses and clinical problems. Computerized verification systems help to compare set-up parameters with prescribed values. Visual records of simulator films, planning CT scans, photographs and port films should also be kept.

PATIENT DOCUMENTATION

Radiation treatment records are usually maintained separately from other hospital records in order to ensure ready access. They should identify the patient and give information on history and clinical findings, histological diagnosis, staging of the tumour and proposed treatment plan. This should conform to written treatment policies for specific tumour sites, and data should be recorded to enable subsequent evaluation of the outcome of treatment. Written consent for treatment may be required. At the end of treatment, a summary detailing actual treatment parameters should be written and appropriate continuing care of the patient assured.

A departmental procedure for investigation of deviations or errors must be in place for every part of the system.

Staffing

A quality programme as described above is essential for the safe delivery of treatment. It can only be achieved if each member of the team understands clearly the boundaries of responsibility, and if excellent co-ordination of all QC activity can be obtained by a highly qualified physicist acting with the person responsible for overall management of the radiotherapy department. Careful training of all staff members must therefore be an integral part of any effective QA system.

Further reading

Aletti, P. and Bey, P. (eds) 1995: *Recommendations for a quality assurance programme in external radiotherapy*. ESTRO Series on Physics for Clinical Radiotherapists. Booklet 2. Leuven: Garant.

BSI 9000 European Standard EN ISO 9000, published 1994.

Leer, J.W.H., McKenzie, A.L., Scalliet, P., Thwaites, D.I. 1998: *Practical Guidelines for the Implementation of a Quality System in Radiotherapy*. ESTRO. Leuven: Garant.

CHAPTER 4

Radiobiological principles

TOM WHELDON

Radiation and cell kill

Ionizing radiation causes wide-ranging molecular damage throughout cells. In practice, the most important damage is that responsible for double-strand breaks (or more complex lesions) in genomic DNA. It is believed that most clinically significant effects of radiotherapy are due to irreparable DNA lesions which result in *sterilization* – the loss of proliferative cells' ability for sustained cell division. In tumours, loss of proliferative ability by all the cells of the tumour is the necessary condition for tumour cure. Partial sterilization of the tumour cell population results in tumour stasis or regression, perhaps giving a clinical remission, followed by regrowth of the tumour from those cells which have retained their proliferative ability. In self-renewing normal tissues, sterilization of proliferative cells leaves the tissues unable to provide replacements for cells which are ordinarily being lost at a constant rate from the tissue, and initiates a 'run-down' of the mature cells of the tissue. Proliferative sterilization is often referred to as 'cell kill', with those cells that retain long-term proliferative ability being described as 'survivors'.

Cell survival curves

Cell-culture techniques have been very important in allowing the proliferative sterilization of cells to be investigated quantitatively. For an irradiated cell population, the proportion of cells that still retain the ability to proliferate (relative to an unirradiated control population) is called the surviving fraction, and a plot of log surviving fraction against single radiation dose gives a *survival curve* for the cells concerned. Typically, survival curves are continuously bending, with a slope that steepens as the dose increases. Mathematically, a continuously bending curve is most simply described by a *linear quadratic* (LQ) equation of the form

$$SF = Exp(-\alpha d - \beta d^2) \tag{4.1}$$

where SF is the surviving fraction, d is the given single dose and α and β are parameters characteristic of the cells concerned. The ratio α/β gives the relative importance of the linear dose term and the quadratic dose term for those cells, and controls the shape of the survival curve (Fig. 4.1). When α/β is large,

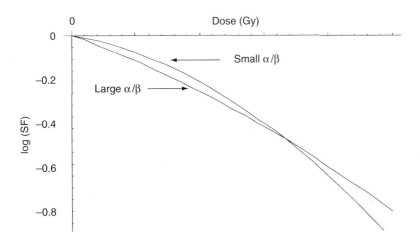

Fig. 4.1 Two contrasting survival curves for irradiated cells, with log of the surviving fraction (SF) plotted against single radiation dose. The more steeply curving survival curve has the lower α/β ratio when fitted to the linear quadratic equation.

the linear term predominates, so a plot of log(SF) against d is (relatively) straight, while if α/β is small, the quadratic term is more important, giving a plot with greater curvature. For cells whose survival curves have a low α/β ratio, doubling the dose leads to more than doubling of the effect on log(SF). Such cells will be particularly sensitive to changes in fraction size when radiation is given as a fractionated schedule.

Acute and late effects on tissues

The dose–response relationship for normal tissue injury depends on the survival curves of the tissue stem cells. The timing of expression of injury depends on the rate of turnover of mature cells in the tissue. Epithelia and haemopoietic tissues have rapid turnover, and so experience *acute effects* (with a time-scale of days or weeks). *Late effects* (with a time-scale of months or years) occur in tissues and organs with slow turnover (e.g. endothelial tissues, neuroglial tissues, and parenchymal tissues of lung, liver and kidney). The risk of major late effects is usually dose-limiting in radiotherapy. Stem cells of late-responding tissues have been found to have much more curved survival curves (low α/β ratio) than cells of acute-responding tissues (higher α/β ratio, less curved survival curve). Radio-biologically, this difference may be related to slow cell turnover in late-responding tissues, allowing many stem cells to remain in resting states where they are highly proficient in the repair of damage caused by small doses. Consequently, late-responding tissues are particularly sensitive to changes in fraction size, larger fractions being more damaging to these tissues, but small fractions being well tolerated.

Acute- and late-responding tissues are also affected differently by changes in the overall treatment time. Because surviving stem cells of acute-responding tissues initiate repopulation during a course of radiotherapy, the time over which the radiation is distributed makes a difference to the final level of damage. Late-responding tissues do not experience repopulation during a course of radiotherapy, and are relatively unaffected by the overall treatment time. These differences are summarized in Table 4.1.

Table 4.1 Summary of differences between acute- and late-responding tissues

Tissue type	Survival curve α/β value	Fraction size sensitivity	Treatment time sensitivity
Acute-responder	High	++	+
Late-responder	Low	++++	0

The linear-quadratic model for tissues

Differences between acute-responding and late-responding tissues and typical tumours are important when we consider the biological consequences of replacing one treatment schedule with a different one. From experience, radiotherapists developed 'rules of thumb' for altering a treatment schedule, e.g. a substantial dose reduction might be necessary if fraction size were increased, increased treatment time allowed skin sparing, etc. Some of these empirical rules were quantified by algebraic formulae, the most popular expression being the nominal standard dose (NSD), which predicted what total dose could be safely given if either fraction size or treatment time were changed. These early formulae have now been superseded by equations based on the linear-quadratic model, which include a recognition that tissues react differently to changes in schedule structure. The application of the LQ model to tissues is based on the idea that the severity of tissue damage is inversely proportional to stem cell survival, and that stem cell survival can be calculated by mathematical development of the LQ survival curve equation to allow it to be applied to fractionated treatments. In particular, two different schedules will have equal biological effects on a tissue (i.e. they will be 'isoeffective' for the tissue) if each schedule produces the same level of stem cell survival in the tissue. We shall not attempt to derive the mathematics of the LQ model in detail, but will state some results which are useful in practice. Consider two treatment schedules, namely total dose D_1 given as fractions sized d_1 and total dose D_2 given as fractions sized d_2. We shall assume for now that both schedules are given in the same overall time period. For a tissue whose cells have a survival curve described by the LQ parameters α and β, it can be shown that the schedules are isoeffective, for that tissue, when

$$D_1(\alpha/\beta + d_1) = D_2(\alpha/\beta + d_2). \tag{4.2}$$

Notice that the survival curve parameters appear as a ratio, the α/β ratio which controls survival curve general shape, in this expression, which means that only this single number need be known for a tissue in order to apply the equation. In fact, α/β estimates have been made and tabulated for many tissues. Late-responding tissues are usually found to have low values of α/β (about 3 Gy), while acute-responding tissues have higher values (about 10 Gy). (This means that the cells of late-responding tissues have more steeply curving survival curves.) Tumours are more variable, but the majority are like acute-responding tissues, with α/β values of 10 Gy or more. In practice, equation (4.2) is often used to compare an unfamiliar schedule with a standard schedule which would have the same effect. Most usefully, the unfamiliar schedule can be assessed by asking what total dose, given as 2-Gy fractions, would have the same effect (on that tissue) as the unfamiliar schedule. This is helpful for determining whether the unfamiliar schedule is 'hot' or 'cold'. For example, consider a schedule which consists of 10 twice-weekly fractions of 4 Gy to a total dose of 40 Gy in 5 weeks. In equation (4.2), let d_1 be 4 Gy and D_1 be 40 Gy. If we now set $d_2 = 2$ Gy, and calculate D_2 (for a particular choice of tissue α/β), we shall get the total dose given as 2-Gy fractions which would have the same effect on that tissue as the schedule D_1, d_1. Notice, however, that the calculation depends on the assumed value of α/β. For this example, we shall repeat the calculation for acute-responding and late-responding tissues. For acute-responding tissues ($\alpha/\beta = 10$ Gy) we find that $D_2 = 47$ Gy, while for late-responding tissues ($\alpha/\beta = 3$ Gy) we find that $D_2 = 56$ Gy. Therefore, the new schedule is expected to be 'hotter' in terms of its effects on late-responding than on acute-responding tissues, but it is no 'hotter' than a conventional radical regimen (e.g. 60 Gy in 2-Gy fractions). It should be noted that the simple LQ model does not allow for differences in total time between the schedules, which are therefore presumed to be given in the same overall time (5 weeks in this case), despite their different fractionation patterns. This restriction is not so important for late-responding tissues (for which the total time is a minor variable), but the results for acute-responding tissues (for which the time factor can be significant) need to be interpreted cautiously with this limitation of the model borne in mind. In recent years, the LQ model has been developed extensively and applied to more complex schedules, including brachytherapy. The standard schedule with which an unfamiliar schedule is to be compared is not necessarily one using 2-Gy fractions. A rather abstract standard schedule, more appealing to mathematicians than to clinicians, is a hypothetical regimen in which a very large number of small fractions are given (mathematically, an infinite number of zero-sized fractions are given, but to a finite total dose). The equivalent total dose calculated on such a schedule is called the *biological effective dose* (BED). It is usually quite a large dose (e.g. 100 Gy for a typical radical regimen) because it represents the limit of tissue sparing by fractionation, i.e. the total dose that could be given if the individual fraction size were vanishingly small. Linear-quadratic calculations performed using BED are mathematically equivalent to those performed with the standard regimen taken to be one using 2-Gy fractions, although the latter has the advantage of clinical familiarity. An important feature of the LQ model in its various forms is the recognition that the cells of different tissues differ in their survival curve shape and therefore respond differently to changes in fraction size. Since a target volume may contain several tissue types as well as the tumour, a change of fractionation regimen will affect these components differently. There is therefore no such thing as a regimen which is 'generally equivalent' to some other regimen – the regimens can only be matched (by choice of total dose) for equivalent effects on each specific tissue. This is now an important consideration in clinical radiobiology, and it is one of the reasons why the LQ model has replaced the NSD and similar isoeffect formulae that were developed before this principle became known.

Volume effects

Together with total dose and fractionation schedule, target volume is a major variable in radiotherapy. For a given fractionation regimen, higher doses can usually be given when volumes at the same site are small rather than large.

Normal tissues are required to perform orchestrated functions which can be impaired in various ways by irradiation. Most normal tissues also cannot regenerate from a single surviving cell. However, tissue recovery may be assisted by immigration of unirradiated neighbouring cells, particularly if the treatment volume is small. Volume is also an important determinant of normal tissue response to a given dose, first because larger volumes provide less opportunity for tissues to draw upon their 'functional reserve' and second because larger irradiated volumes make it more likely that a critical volume element will exceed some upper dose limit. These factors differ according to tissue structure, and they vary from one tissue to another. In general, the normal tissue complication probability (NTCP) increases with dose (for a given fractionation regimen) and with the irradiated volume. It is important to know, at least approximately, how changes in irradiated volume at a particular site will affect the tolerance dose which can safely be given. (The 'tolerance dose' may arbitrarily be taken to be that dose which gives no more than a 5 per cent incidence of significant side-effects, based on clinical experience.) A body of data has been amassed, based on experience, which provides some simple 'rules of thumb' concerning the trade-off between treatment volume and tolerance dose, but these need to be used very cautiously. The Lyman model provides an empirical equation to represent the dose–volume trade-off. This was intended to be a guide to calculating the tolerance dose for a partially irradiated organ relative to the tolerance dose if the whole organ were to be irradiated. Lyman's equation states that

$$TD(V) = TD(1)/V^n \tag{4.3}$$

where $TD(V)$ is the tolerance dose for a partial volume V (expressed as a fraction of the volume of the whole organ), $TD(1)$ is the tolerance dose for full volume (whole organ) and n is a parameter quantifying the dose–volume trade-off, which differs from one organ to another.

Clinical data on dose–volume trade-offs for various organs have been compiled and fitted to the Lyman equation (Table 4.2). Organs appear to differ

Table 4.2   Estimated dose–volume trade-offs for representative normal organs

Organ	Approximate tolerance dose for whole organ irradiation (for conventional treatment regimen using 2-Gy fractions)	Percentage increase in tolerance dose when volume is halved (TD(0.5)/TD(1))
Lung	17–20 Gy	83
Kidney	15–23 Gy	63
Bladder	65 Gy	41
Heart	40 Gy	28
Brain	45 Gy	19
Rectum	60 Gy	9

dramatically in the increase of tolerance dose associated with a halving of the volume, with lung tissue having a high 'exchange rate' for dose–volume trade-off, suggesting that reduced volume conformal radiotherapy may be especially advantageous in irradiation of the thorax.

In some cases, radiation injury may result from an excessively high dose to a small tissue element within the treatment volume. It may then be appropriate to compute figures of merit such as the dose to the 'hottest' 1 per cent or 5 per cent of the volume (or to some biologically significant element) which can be derived from dose–volume histogram (DVH) data, and to seek to correlate these figures with the occurrence of injury.

Radiation dose and tumour cure probability

In radical radiotherapy, the objective is complete sterilization of any tumour cells present, which must be achieved without incurring an unacceptably high risk of serious injury to normal tissues.

Radiation kills cells randomly, which means that each tumour cell has the same probability of surviving irradiation, that probability depending on the given dose. Suppose that SF_2 is the probability of any cell surviving a single dose of 2 Gy, the most commonly used fraction size. For example, SF_2 might be 0.5 for a typical carcinoma. After the first 2-Gy fraction, 50 per cent of the cells survive; after the second dose, 50 per cent of those survivors still survive (i.e. 25 per cent of the original population); after the third dose, 50 per cent of *those* survivors still survive (i.e. 12.5 per cent of the original population), and so on. Generally, after F fractions, the final survival probability will be $(SF_2)^F$. Therefore, for a conventional treatment regimen consisting of 30 treatments of 2 Gy, the final survival probability (in this example) would be 0.5^{30} or 9×10^{-10}.

These relationships have some interesting clinical implications. First, there is no dose which gives zero probability of cell survival – even after a large dose there will be some probability, possibly very small, of survival of each cell. However, a visible tumour will contain a large number of cells, so even if each cell individually has a small chance of surviving, there may be a good chance that at least one cell will survive and could regenerate the tumour. We therefore need to know the relationship between the given dose and the probability that a whole cell population will be sterilized with not a single cell surviving – the basic requirement for tumour cure. This can be computed using the theory of Poisson statistics. We can then calculate the number of treatments necessary to achieve some value of cure probability, such as 90 per cent (remember that 100 per cent cure probability cannot be achieved by any finite dose).

We can repeat the calculation for tumours of different sizes (different cell population numbers) for our example of $SF_2 = 0.5$, and also for other values of SF_2 representing more sensitive or less sensitive tumour types. Figure 4.2 shows these relationships. Although we have used a rather simple model for these calculations, we can observe some features which also turn up in more complex and realistic models.

First, note that the relationship between tumour cell number and number of treatments is logarithmic, i.e. a large change in cell number corresponds to a rather modest change in the number of treatments and hence the total dose required. For example, the number of treatments required for 10^4 cells is just half

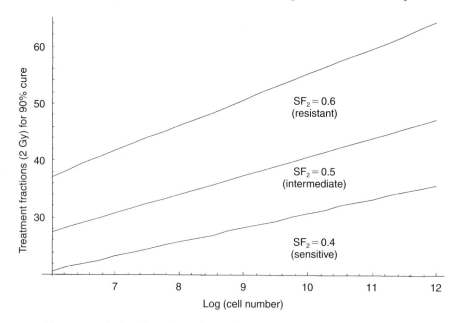

Fig. 4.2 Calculated number of 2-Gy fractions to achieve 90 per cent cure probability, as a function of tumour cell population number, for differing values of cellular intrinsic radiosensitivity (expressed as the surviving fraction following a single 2-Gy treatment, SF_2). Moderate variation in SF_2, as seen between cells of different tumour types, leads to large differences in the number of 2-Gy treatment fractions required for 90 per cent cure probability. In some cases, the predicted number of fractions required is much larger than could be given safely.

the number required for 10^8 cells. It is because of this logarithmic relationship that quite high total doses have to be given to regions containing only microscopic spread (in fact often about half the dose given to the bulk tumour). Within regions of microscopic spread it is likely that the tumour cell density will gradually decrease, on average, with increasing distance from the visible edge. This suggests that the radiotherapy dose should similarly decrease with distance, roughly in proportion to log cell density. Although the cell density distribution will not be known in detail, it is possible that a tapering dose distribution, implemented in practice as a multi-step shrinking field, could be advantageous in some cases.

A second feature of the model is that a small change in SF_2 has quite a large effect on the required total dose (compare the three curves shown in Fig. 4.2). Small variations in the intrinsic radiosensitivity of tumour cells could result in a tumour being easily curable, or completely incurable, by a radiotherapy regimen.

Another feature of the dose–cure relationship is the steepness of the increase in tumour cure probability with total dose, illustrated in Fig. 4.3. In this figure, the solid curves show the dose–cure relationships for a series of tumours with

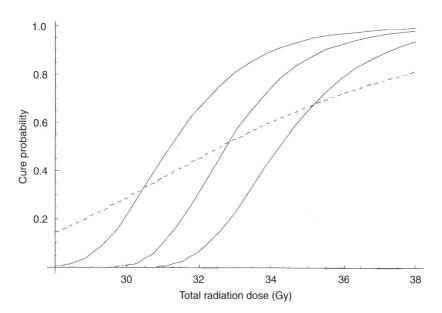

Fig. 4.3 The solid lines in this figure show the expected relationship between total radiation dose and cure probability for individual tumours with differing radiosensitivity and cell number. The curves are sigmoid in shape, located at different positions on the dose axis, and each is quite steep. The broken line shows the much shallower dose response usually seen when proportion cured is plotted against dose for groups of tumours, as in clinical trial studies. The shallower response is thought to result from the heterogeneity of the tumours in each dose group.

slightly different parameters, and they can be seen to be increasing steeply with total dose in all cases. This implies that relatively small differences in total dose could make a significant difference to cure probability for each tumour. However, these steep relationships are not seen in the dose–cure relationships for treatment of groups of tumours with differing parameters, such as occur in clinical studies with patient groups. The broken line in Fig. 4.3 shows the much shallower gradient which is typically observed in such studies. The shallow gradient of the curve for tumour groups is the resultant of a series of steep curves for individual tumours with differing radiosensitivities. This has some significance when we consider the importance of moderate changes in total dose when treating individual patients. The importance of a dose increment in treating an individual tumour depends on how close the treatment regimen has come to achieving cure. For a large or resistant tumour, with cure probability close to zero, a modest dose increment will make little difference. Conversely, for a small or highly sensitive tumour, with cure probability close to unity, a small dose increment again makes little difference. However, if the treatment regimen achieves a cure probability close to 50 per cent, it is in this situation that the dose–response curve is as steep as that calculated from the Poisson model. This means that for any individual patient there is some probability, usually unknown, that a large change in tumour control probability will result from a small change in delivered dose. Even where the average dose–response curve for patient groups is known to be shallow, a minority of patients may benefit substantially from small changes in the given dose. It is these patients for whom the choice of treatment plan may be especially critical.

Tumour radiobiology

It is believed that the main factors controlling tumour response to fractionated radiotherapy are the so-called 'Five R's' of radiobiology (Table 4.3). Currently, the most important of these factors are thought to be the intrinsic radiosensitivity of cells and the kinetics of repopulation of surviving cells.

Intrinsic radiosensitivity varies between different tumour cell lines in culture, with cell lines derived from clinically radioresistant tumour types having a statistical tendency towards higher SF_2 values. It has been reported that SF_2 values for individual tumours in carcinoma of the cervix are predictive of the clinical response to radiotherapy in these patients. However, SF_2 measurements on tumours are technically difficult and time-consuming, and are not easy to implement for predictive radiosensitivity testing. Experimental research is in progress on alternative tests which may prove more suitable.

Although tumours are very diverse, the radiobiological properties of most tumours are similar to those of acute-responding tissues, i.e. a high α/β ratio, moderate sensitivity to changes in fraction size, and some dependence on total treatment time. The role of treatment time has been controversial, but it is now widely believed that many tumours repopulate rapidly during the latter part of a course of radiotherapy, and that any factor which prolongs time in treatment

Table 4.3 Radiobiological factors controlling response to fractionated radiotherapy (the 'Five R's') and their clinical relevance

Radiobiological factor	Mechanism of effect on response	Clinical relevance
Radiosensitivity	Intrinsic radiosensitivity differs between cells of tumours and normal tissue types, and strongly determines final surviving fraction	Can account for variable response of tumours. Curative dose is proportional to the log of cell number (so subclinical disease needs smaller dose)
Repair	Cells differ in their capacity to repair DNA damage, particularly after small doses of radiation. Repair is usually more effective in non-proliferating cells. The repair process takes at least 6 h to complete	Repair is maximal in late-responding tissues given small fractions. Hyperfractionation may be advantageous. Treatments need to be well separated in order to avoid compromising repair
Repopulation	Surviving cells in many tumours and in acute-responding (but not in late-responding) normal tissues proliferate more rapidly once treatment is in progress	Shortened treatment times (accelerated therapy) may be advantageous for some tumours. Acute (but not late) effects will be increased. Gaps should be avoided
Reoxygenation	Hypoxic cells, which occur especially in tumours, are relatively resistant to radiation. Hypoxic surviving cells reoxygenate, becoming radiosensitive, as treatment proceeds	Very short treatment times could lead to resistance due to persistence of hypoxic cells
Redistribution	Cells in certain phases of the proliferative cycle (e.g. late S) are relatively resistant and survive preferentially. With time between fractions, cells redistribute themselves over all phases of the cycle	Closely spaced treatment fractions could lead to resistance due to persistence of cells in less sensitive phases

could lead to significantly reduced tumour cure probability. Attempts are currently being made to identify which tumours are most capable of rapid repopulation by measuring kinetic parameters in individual patients, but is not yet clear whether these parameters have sufficient predictive power.

Avoidance of gaps during treatment

The occurrence of rapid repopulation in irradiated tumours, sometimes with doubling times as short as 3–4 days, has important implications for interruptions of treatment. Unscheduled gaps occur not infrequently in radiotherapy schedules because of machine breakdown or patient intercurrent illness or non-attendance. (We shall exclude from consideration patients whose treatment is deliberately stopped because of unusually severe acute reactions.) Gaps are important because they may lead to prolongation of the total treatment time, allowing opportunities for rapid repopulation by surviving tumour cells towards the end of the schedule. Although prolongation will often spare acute normal tissue reactions, the risk of late effects is not reduced. It has been estimated for squamous carcinomas of the head and neck that reductions in cure probability of 1 to 2 per cent may result from each day of prolongation. If gaps occur, the best management strategy is 'post-gap acceleration', i.e. the use of twice daily treatments (separated by more than 6 h) or weekend treatments to enable 'catching up' so that treatment is nevertheless completed within the originally intended period. This does not require any changes to fraction size or total dose. However, this approach is not always feasible in practice. Now that the deleterious effect of prolongation is recognized, avoidance of gaps is an important consideration for all radiotherapy departments.

Treatment scheduling

Radiotherapists currently use a variety of treatment schedules, but nearly all of these consist of a series of daily doses (e.g. 2 Gy) over a time-scale of several weeks. The total dose is usually limited by anticipated risk of injury to late-responding tissues, although there are situations where acute responses (e.g. mucosal reactions) are the main concern. Treatment schedules with this structure probably take advantage of differences between the survival curves of cells in late-responding tissues (low α/β ratio and fraction size sensitivity) and the survival curves of those in typical tumours. This means that late-responding tissues are spared to a greater extent than most tumours by the use of small fractions, giving a favourable therapeutic ratio. Late responses are not strongly influenced by overall treatment time, and it would be desirable to make the latter as short as possible in order to minimize the opportunities for tumour repopulation, but this is constrained by the need to allow time for reoxygenation of hypoxic tumour cells during therapy, as well as the adverse effects of reduced treatment time on acute-responding tissues (which also have reduced opportunities for repopulation).

Recently, new treatment schedules have been designed based on the principle that the therapeutic ratio could be further improved by reducing the fraction size below 2 Gy and treating two or three times daily in order to give a shortened time-scale. This approach is called *accelerated hyperfractionation*, and there are now several schedules based on the concept, e.g. the continuous hyperfractionated accelerated radiotherapy (CHART) schedule (3 × 1.5 daily to 54 Gy in 12 days).

The rationale depends on the expected α/β ratio difference between tumours and late-responding tissues, and on the need to keep the schedule short in order to offset rapid repopulation in the tumour, with reoxygenation considered to be of lesser importance. In such schemes it is important for treatment fractions to be sufficiently spaced throughout the day to allow cellular repair to occur in late-responding tissues. A minimum time interval of 6 h is recommended, but it is not certain whether this is sufficient. Acute reactions may be increased and need to be monitored.

However, tumours are known to be extremely heterogeneous with regard to cell survival parameters and growth kinetics, as well as other properties. It is unlikely that any one schedule is ideal for treatment of all tumours, even those of a single pathological type, and it would be highly desirable to select treatment schedules for individual patients on the basis of the radiobiological and kinetic parameters for each tumour. Predictive tests are not yet sufficiently reliable to be used in this way, but individualized scheduling based on biological assay is a likely development for the future.

Treatment plans, schedules and 'double trouble'

The design of physical treatment plans usually proceeds without regard to treatment schedule. However, there may be an interplay between dose distributions and treatment schedules, which gives an altered biological effect sometimes described as 'double trouble'. Consider a treatment plan in which the spread of dose within the target volume is 10 per cent, so if the intended treatment is 30 fractions of 2 Gy to give 60 Gy in total, the spread of dose will be from 57 Gy to 63 Gy. However, the low-point and high-point doses will not have been delivered as 2-Gy fractions (the dose variation of 10 per cent affects each dose fraction, so the fraction size will range from 1.9 Gy to 2.1 Gy). A treatment schedule of 30 × 2.1 Gy to 63 Gy is what is 'seen' by cells located close to the high-dose point in this example, and this 63-Gy dose is more damaging, especially to late-responding tissues with a low α/β ratio, than 63 Gy given as 2-Gy fractions (which is what is implied when only the physical total dose is cited). Therefore, the spread of radiobiological damage within a target volume has two components, namely that due to variation in the total dose, and that due to variation in the fraction size by which that total dose is given. The 'double-trouble' effect is most marked for late-responding tissues, for large treatment volumes with considerable dose variation, and for intended treatment schedules where the prescribed fraction size is sometimes large (radiotherapy of breast cancer may be such a situation). Although not yet routine, radiobiological considerations need to be included in the analysis of the dose–response relationship in patients who are experiencing side-effects.

Radiobiological treatment planning

A natural development of the 'double-trouble' concept has been the construction of 'radiobiological treatment plans' with the physical dose mathematically replaced by some radiobiological equivalent which includes the effect of variation in fraction size. For example, the physical dose at each point in the dose matrix could be replaced by the dose calculated by the LQ model to have the same effect on late-responding tissues when given as 2-Gy fractions. Isodose curves can be constructed using the 'radiobiological dose' and compared with more conventional isodose plots using the physical dose. Algorithms have been developed which can be incorporated in commercial treatment planning systems and used to compute 'radiobiological treatment plans'. In clinical examples, these have been used to design plans which would be expected to minimize biological damage to particular structures. Another approach is to employ DVHs rather than complete plans. It is possible to compute LQ-transformed DVHs (which incorporate the biological effects of changing fraction size within the volume) and, from this, to calculate the dose that is biologically equivalent to the 'hottest' and 'coldest' 1 per cent of the volume. Theoretically, radiobiological isodose curves and transformed DVHs should be more representative of the biological damage accumulating in particular tissues as a result of fractionated radiotherapy, and with appropriate experience they may provide better guidelines for treatment planning.

Future directions

It is likely that mainstream developments in clinical radiotherapy over the next few years will include increased use of conformal therapy techniques and the further exploration of novel fractionation schemes such as CHART. Radiobiological treatment planning will become more common, and predictive assays may begin to be introduced. A major weakness of clinical radiobiology at present is the empirical nature of the volume-effect models which predict organ tolerance dose when the target volume is reduced. Realistic biological models are required for each major organ system, and they should be able to make use of data on functional impairment of organs as well as quantitative data such as the proportion of patients who experience a particular side-effect. The acquisition of functional impairment data following radiotherapy (e.g. by lung function tests) is likely to become increasingly important, and will help to improve both volume effects and fractionation models. Theoretically, the conformal radiation dose should be tailored to the distribution of tumour cell density within a target volume, but at present very little is known about cell density distributions, even in typical patients with a particular tumour type. More refined analysis of normal tissue adjacent to excised tumour, perhaps involving the use of molecular techniques that are able to detect small numbers of tumour cells, should be able to provide some estimates. Radiobiological treatment planning techniques will probably need to be run in parallel with physical planning for quite a few years. It is important that adequate patient data be collected during this time, which will most probably require increased use of CT or other imaging techniques to ensure that both physical and radiobiological dose distributions can be accurately mapped to the anatomy of individual patients. Predictive testing techniques, although still at a preclinical stage of development, should eventually allow the identification of the most appropriate treatment strategy for each patient.

Further reading

Bentzen, S.M. 1993: Quantitative clinical radiobiology. *Acta Oncologica* **32**, 259–75.

Burman, C., Kutcher, G.J., Emami, B. and Goitein, M. 1991: Fitting of normal tissue-tolerance data to an analytic function. *International Journal of Radiation Oncology, Biology and Physics* **21**, 123–35.

Steel, G.G. (ed.) 1997: *Basic clinical radiobiology*. London: Edward Arnold.

Withers, H.R. 1992: Biological basis of radiation therapy. In Perez, C.A. and Brady, L.W. (eds), *Principles and practice of radiation oncology*. Philadelphia, PA: Lippincott, 64–96.

CHAPTER 5

Principles of brachytherapy

For brachytherapy treatments, radioactive material is inserted directly into a tumour and concentrates the dose there. The inverse square law states that the dose is inversely proportional to the square of the distance from the source. The dose therefore falls off very rapidly, and the surrounding normal tissues receive substantially lower doses than the tumour. If 65 Gy are delivered at 0.5 cm from the source, then the dose at 2 cm is only 4.06 Gy.

As well as its physical advantages, there are also biological advantages. Low-dose-rate brachytherapy is a type of extreme hyperfractionation, and is therefore relatively sparing to normal tissues. This often allows implants to be used for salvage therapy after failure of previous external beam radiation. Although the dose rate used for brachytherapy may be low, the fact that the radiation is delivered continuously means that the overall treatment time is short. This not only has important practical advantages, but it also reduces the opportunity for tumour repopulation during treatment.

For both physical and biological reasons, brachytherapy should be considered whenever possible for accessible localized tumours that are of relatively small volume. The treatment is contraindicated where tumour infiltrates bone, where the margins of the target volume are not clearly identifiable, and where there is active infection in the tissues to be implanted.

Brachytherapy can be used either as a single modality to deliver a radical dose, or in combination with external beam radiation where the treatment is used to deliver a boost. It can also be used in combination with surgery where an implant can be performed peroperatively to deliver a high dose of radiation to the tumour bed after surgical excision. The treatment is applicable to a wide range of tumour types and sites, many of which are discussed in later chapters.

Brachytherapy was first developed with radium tubes and needles, but these have been abandoned in most centres because of radiation protection problems. For intracavitary treatment, radium has been largely replaced by caesium, which can be used in manual or remote afterloading systems. For interstitial implants, iridium 192 is now the isotope of choice because it can be readily cut to any length and is sufficiently flexible to follow curved planes. It can also be prepared in different strengths so that it can be used for low-dose-rate interstitial implants and for high-dose-rate intraluminal treatments. The relatively short half-life of 74 days means that the stock of wire has to be regularly renewed, but only 2 cm of lead are required for adequate protection, compared with 10 cm for radium (see Table 5.1).

Table 5.1 Isotopes for brachytherapy

Isotope	Half-life	Energy range (MV)
Radium 226	1620 years	0.19–2.43
Caesium 137	30 years	0.66
Iridium 192	74 days	0.30–0.61
Iodine 125	60 days	0.027–0.035
Gold 198	2.7 days	0.41–1.09

The ability to produce high-activity iridium wire which can be afterloaded into narrow catheters has now made it possible to deliver brachytherapy intraluminally for treatment of carcinomas of the bronchus and oesophagus.

For those tumour sites where there may be difficulty in removing implanted sources, or where very low dose rates may be an advantage, an implant can be performed with permanently implanted sources, using iodine 125 seeds or gold grains.

As all implantation techniques involve the use of active sources, care needs to be taken with regard to radiation protection for the patient, the operator and other staff. Manual afterloading techniques have been developed for intracavitary caesium insertions and for iridium-wire implants using the Paris system. These already reduce exposure to very low levels, and even further reductions can be achieved by the use of remote afterloading machines which can be adapted to most of the techniques described.

Before undertaking any interstitial implant, it is important to identify clearly the target volume and to have pre-planned the number and distribution of radioactive sources to be used. The distribution of sources is aimed at achieving as homogeneous a dose as possible, since high doses around each source could cause necrosis and low doses between the sources could result in recurrence. It is recommended that an established set of rules for implantation is followed, and both the Manchester and Paris rules of implantation will ensure that the target volume is relatively homogeneously irradiated. The Paris system was specifically developed for use with iridium-wire afterloading techniques, and is recommended because it provides a means of calculating doses individually for each implant as performed. It also allows an appreciation of the relationship between the dose in the centre of the implant and that at the periphery.

The distribution rules for iridium-192 implants are as follows.

1. Active sources should be parallel and straight.
2. The lines should be equidistant.
3. The line or plane on which the mid-point of the sources lies (central plane) should be at right angles to the axis of the sources.
4. The linear activity of the lines should be uniform along the length of each line, and identical for all lines.

5. The separation of sources may be varied from one implant to another. A minimum of 8 mm separation is acceptable for the smallest volumes, rising to 20 mm for the largest.
6. For volume implants, the distribution of sources in cross-section (central plane) should be either in equilateral triangles or in squares.
7. Because it is not usual to cross the ends of the sources, the average length of active wire must be longer than the target volume by 25 to 30 per cent, depending on the number and separation of sources used.

Dose calculation in the Paris system is based on the distribution of sources in the central plane – that is, the plane which is at right angles to the axis of the mid-point of the sources (Fig. 5.1).

The basal dose rate represents the dose in the centre of the implanted volume, and is defined as the dose rate at a point in the middle of a pair or group of sources where the dose rate is lowest. In the case of a large implant, there may be several pairs or groups of sources arranged in triangles or squares. For these, a mean basal dose rate is taken for the implant as a whole (Fig. 5.2). The basal dose rate at a point is the summation of dose rate contributions from each source obtained from graphs of dose rate variations with distance from the source.

Once the basal dose rate in the centre of the implant has been defined, the reference dose rate is taken as 85 per cent of the basal dose rate. This serves to calculate the duration of the implant, and the 85 per cent isodose defines the treated volume. A value of 85 per cent has been chosen to provide an isodose

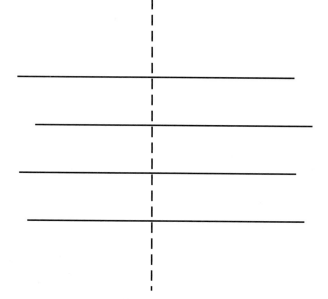

Fig. 5.1   Central plane of an implant at right angles to the axis of the mid-point of the sources.

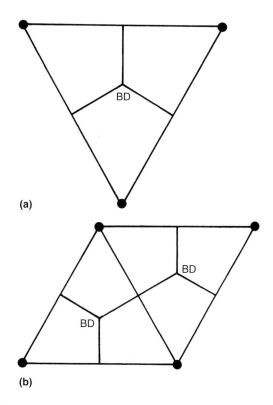

(a)

(b)

Fig. 5.2 Basal dose rate point for two different volume implants arranged in (a) one and (b) two equilateral triangles.

contour that reasonably covers the target volume with an acceptable variation between the dose at the centre and that at the periphery of the target volume. The time for which the implant must be left in place is derived by dividing the prescribed dose by the reference dose rate. Calculations must take into account the actual activity of the iridium wire used for implantation, and correction must be made for radioactive decay during the period of implantation (Table 5.2).

The Manchester and Paris systems of dosimetry were developed in the days before computers were readily available for dose calculation. Now that computerized dosimetry programs are available, there is an increasing tendency to calculate the prescribed dose from computer-derived isodoses, rather than to adhere to the established systems which have the advantage of being tried and tested over many years. This situation is potentially dangerous because the choice of isodose for prescription is at a place where there is a steep gradient of dose. There may therefore be a wide variation between the dose at the periphery and that at the centre of the target volume, and a large proportion of the implanted volume may receive a considerably higher dose than that prescribed at the periphery. For safe treatment, the central dose should be no more than 20 per cent higher than the peripheral dose.

Table 5.2 Calculation for breast implant

Two-plane implant to deliver 25 Gy

Superficial plane = 5-cm wires × 2

Deep plane = 7-cm wires × 3

Separation between sources = 18 mm

Activity of wire (midway through treatment)
= air kerma rate 0.5 μGy/h/mm at 1 m (0.1193 mG/mm)

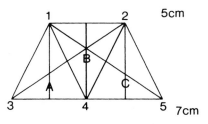

Wire	A		B		C	
	Distance (mm)	Dose rate (Gy/h)	Distance (mm)	Dose rate (Gy/h)	Distance (mm)	Dose rate (Gy/h)
1	10.4	0.1245	10.4	0.1245	20.8	0.0465
2	20.8	0.0465	10.4	0.1245	10.4	0.1245
3	10.4	0.1340	20.8	0.0555	27.5	0.0365
4	10.4	0.1340	10.4	0.1340	10.4	0.1340
5	27.5	0.0365	20.8	0.0555	10.4	0.1340
Total		0.4755		0.4940		0.4755

$$\text{Mean basal dose rate} = \frac{0.4755 + 0.4940 + 0.4755 \text{ Gy/h}}{3}$$

$$= 0.4817 \text{ Gy/h}$$

Reference dose rate (85%)
$$= 0.4817 \times 0.85$$
$$= 0.4095 \text{ Gy/h}$$

Treatment time
$$= \frac{25.00}{0.4095}$$

$$= 61.05 \text{ h}$$

$$= 2 \text{ days } 13 \text{ h}$$

The ICRU Report No. 58 on dose and volume specification in interstitial brachytherapy recommends that, when reporting an interstitial implant, the following information should be provided.

1. *Description of volumes*:
   - gross tumour volume;
   - clinical target volume;
   - treated volume.
2. *Description of sources and techniques*:
   - description of time pattern;
   - total reference air kerma (TRAK) (the sum of the products of the reference air kerma rate and the irradiation time for each source).
3. *Description of doses*:
   - prescribed dose;
   - mean central dose in the central plane (equivalent to basal dose in the Paris system);
   - peripheral dose (equivalent to the reference dose in the Paris system).
4. *Description of high and low dose volumes*.

When performing the implant, it is important to know the relationship between the volume treated and the length and separation of the sources used. This knowledge will help to ensure that the target volume is adequately covered. The following relationships apply to implants performed according to the Paris system.

The length of the treated volume is approximately 70 per cent of the length of the active sources (Fig. 5.3).

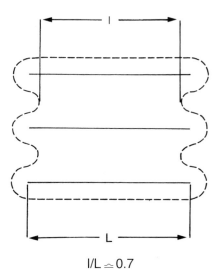

$$l/L \simeq 0.7$$

Fig. 5.3 Relationship between treated volume (l) and length of active sources (L).

The thickness of the treated volume in a single-plane implant is approximately 50 per cent of the separation between the sources (Fig. 5.4).

The treatment margin around a volume implant performed in triangles is 30 to 40 per cent of the distance between the sides of the triangle.

In all of these examples, the ratio of treated volume to source length or separation increases as more sources are used.

The usual aim is to deliver 10–12.5 Gy per day, so that 65 Gy are delivered within 5 to 6 days. This dose rate is a little higher than that recommended in the classic Manchester system. Sometimes, for technical or clinical reasons, the dose rate falls outside these limits. The exact importance of dose rate changes within the range encountered in interstitial therapy is not entirely clear. It may have relatively little effect on tumour control, but this is not the case for normal tissue complications, and it is now recommended that the optimum range of dose rate for interstitial therapy is 0.40–0.60 Gy/hour. This means that implants have

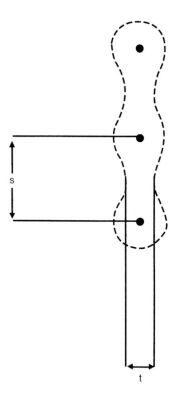

$$t/s \simeq 0.5$$

Fig. 5.4   Relationship between source separation (s) and thickness (t) of treatment volume (not drawn to scale).

to be carefully pre-planned in terms of the lengths and separations of the sources to be used, so that an appropriate activity of iridium-192 wire is ordered to achieve a reference dose rate of 0.40–0.60 Gy/hour.

For intracavitary radiation, most experience has been gained with irradiation at a low dose rate (0.4–2 Gy/hour). A dose rate correction of approximately minus 15 per cent has been necessary when changing to afterloading systems at medium dose rate (2–12 Gy/hour). For high dose rates (>12 Gy/hour), intracavitary radiation must be fractionated in order to avoid normal tissue morbidity.

Further reading

International Commission on Radiological Units and Measurements 1997: *Dose and volume specification in interstitial brachytherapy. ICRU Report No. 58.* Bethesda, MD: International Commission on Radiological Units and Measurements.

Pierquin, B., Wilson, J.F. and Chassagne, D. 1987: *Modern brachytherapy.* New York: Masson.

CHAPTER 6

Head and neck – general considerations for treatment

Introduction

The development of new techniques for surgical reconstruction in the head and neck has markedly reduced the cosmetic and functional deficit previously produced by surgery, and more patients are being treated with a combination of primary surgery and postoperative radiation, rather than primary radiation with surgery for salvage. This approach requires close collaboration, and patients should be reviewed in a multidisciplinary joint clinic before deciding on management.

The decision to give postoperative radiation will depend on the prognostic factors for tumour recurrence, which include initial stage, pattern of spread, adequacy of excision margins, presence of perineural invasion, differentiation and lymph node involvement. The volume irradiated postoperatively may not always be the same as that which might have been used before full surgical staging, particularly in relation to the need for elective lymph-node radiation.

For those patients who have had a neck dissection, the indications for post-operative radiation are as follows:

- incomplete excision;
- involved nodes at more than one level (Fig. 6.1);
- evidence of extra-capsular spread.

Many patients now receive chemotherapy in association with radiation. This may affect tolerance of radiation by increasing the severity of the normal tissue reactions, and may necessitate an unplanned gap in the radiation schedule. It can also modify the tolerance of the spinal cord and other critical normal tissues.

Dose and fractionation

As elsewhere in this book, the standard doses quoted for the different head and neck cancer sites use daily 2-Gy fractions. For those cases where the volume of irradiation is small, it is safe and reasonable to treat with larger fraction sizes over a shorter period, e.g. 50 Gy in 16 fractions over 23 days or 55 Gy in 20 frac-

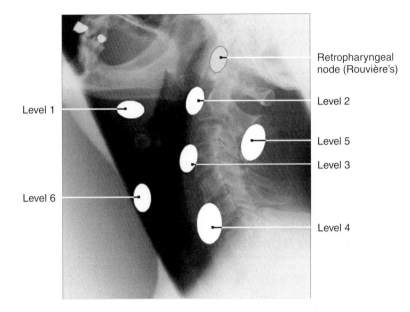

Fig. 6.1   Lateral X-rays illustrating levels of cervical lymph nodes.

tions over 28 days. However, it is important to have some experience of these schedules, and to pay attention to the details of the technique and dose specification used.

Although daily fractionation has been standard for many years, there is increasing evidence that hyperfractionation with or without acceleration improves the local control rate in head and neck cancer, and may result in a reduction in late normal tissue morbidity.

Apart from the fact that large fraction sizes should not be used for large volumes, the pattern of fractionation should not require any modification of the target volume where non-standard fractionation is used.

Localization

The assessment of all patients with tumours of the head and neck region must include a full ear, nose and throat (ENT) examination, not only to delineate the local extent of the primary tumour but also to exclude other lesions. A chest x-ray should be performed to exclude lung disease. All patients are treated in perspex shells to prevent movement during treatment, to ensure accurate reproducibility in the treatment set-up, and to avoid making ink marks on the patient's skin. Requests for individual shells must include details of the treatment site, patient positioning, the degree of flexion or extension of the neck, and the need for mouth-bite, which is used to displace the lower jaw out of the irradiated area in order to spare the mucosa.

Any palpable tumour or lymphadenopathy is marked with radio-opaque material for localization of the target volume, which is performed with the patient wearing the perspex shell. CT scanning may be used and multiple transverse outlines taken for dose planning, or alternatively AP and lateral films may be taken on a simulator and the target volume transferred to a transverse outline taken through the centre of the volume.

In practice, many treatments in the head and neck are given using opposing fields, and it is common to define field sizes on the skin. Since the area outlined by the simulated field is always larger than the high-dose volume for any given field size, care must be taken to encompass the target volume at depth adequately.

The illustrations in the next few chapters show examples of field margins. These are often close to the spinal cord, but their position should be verified with on-treatment check films.

Implementation of plan

Patients are treated with either a linear accelerator or a cobalt unit according to availability. A cobalt unit may be preferable for patients with superficial lesions, in order to reduce skin sparing and avoid high exit radiation doses. The field arrangements described in the following chapters are aligned using an isocentric technique. When such a technique is used, the pin depth is measured from the plan and the appropriate machine FSD (pin setting) adjusted to the entry point on the cast. The patient is aligned using a laser light back-pointer to the exit point. The gantry angle, head twist (collimator angle), couch angle and wedges are then used according to the instructions on the plan. For some anterior fields, back-pointing is not possible because the exit ring would lie on the head pad. Here the cross-wires of the field are aligned with a transverse outline marked on the shell at the level of the entry ring at the centre of the field.

For most head and neck treatments, the full skin-sparing effect of a megavoltage treatment beam is desirable. However, where the tumour is very close to or involves the skin, or where there is an operation scar, the full dose is required at the skin. In some cases the perspex shell may provide sufficient build-up of dose, but additional wax may be needed. Where skin sparing is desired, the shell should be cut out as soon as the check films are approved during the first week of treatment.

For many patients, treatment is given to both the primary tumour and regional lymphadenopathy. Ideally, both target volumes would be treated in continuity, but this may not be possible because of variability of body contour in the head and neck region, obstruction of beams by the shoulders, or the close proximity of the spinal cord to the target volume, which limits the radiation dose. Several special techniques are used in an attempt to overcome these limitations and to provide a homogeneous dose distribution in three dimensions.

Matching of fields in head and neck cancer treatment

Although much of head and neck cancer treatment can be accomplished with two parallel opposed fields, there is a frequent need to match on other fields, and this must be done while avoiding potentially dangerous hot spots and cold spots at field junctions.

The main areas where problems arise are as follows:

- matching orthogonal fields, i.e. lateral parallel opposed fields and anterior fields;
- matching photon and electron fields;
- determining the position of the field junction;
- the use and positioning of lead blocks to protect the spinal cord.

A number of methods of field matching can be considered, and each has its advantages and disadvantages with regard to the above problems. These methods include:

- a 5- to10-mm gap between fields;
- matching divergence of beams from adjacent fields;
- use of a half-beam block to eliminate beam divergence at the junction;
- use of a moving junction;
- simple matching of beams at the 50 per cent margin defined by the light beam.

MATCHING ORTHOGONAL FIELDS

This has commonly been achieved by leaving a 5- to 10-mm gap between fields (Fig. 6.2). However, with this arrangement there is a risk that there will be an

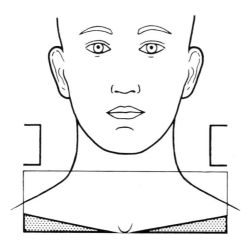

Fig. 6.2 Lateral parallel opposed fields and anterior neck field with a 5–10 mm gap between fields.

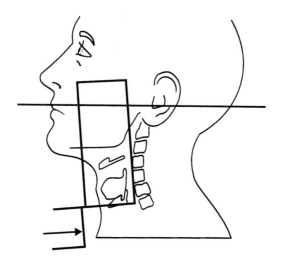

Fig. 6.3   Lateral parallel opposed fields matched to anterior field with no gap. The gantry angle of the superior border of the anterior field is aligned with the inferior border of the parallel opposed lateral fields, taking into account the collimator rotation.

underdose between fields, which may be a cause of recurrence if there is tumour at the junction.

It is preferable to match the divergence of the beams from the lateral parallel opposed fields with that from the anterior field (Fig. 6.3). The matching is done on the treatment simulator so that the 50 per cent light beam from each field is matched directly. The gantry angle of the superior border of the anterior field is chosen to align with the inferior border of the parallel opposed lateral fields, taking into account the collimator rotation. This does not eliminate slight divergence of the lateral field into the anterior field. If the lateral field includes the spinal cord in the first phase of treatment, there is a slight risk of overdose at the level of the spinal cord. It is not usual to use a moving junction for this, but a small lead block can be placed at the lower posterior margin of the lateral field in order to protect the spinal cord, provided that this can be done safely without shielding disease (Fig. 6.4).

MATCHING PHOTON AND ELECTRON FIELDS

Matching is necessary when the posterior neck nodes overlying the spinal cord must be treated. In the first phase of treatment, both anterior and posterior neck are treated with opposed lateral photon fields. In the second phase, the field is split so that the part anterior to the spinal cord continues to be treated by photons, while the posterior part is treated by electrons. The electron energy is chosen so that it is sufficient to include the nodes at risk while avoiding a significant exit dose to the spinal cord.

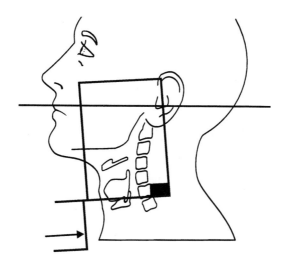

Fig. 6.4 Small block inserted at the infero-posterior margin of the lateral field to protect the cord from possible divergence from the matched anterior field.

The shape of the electron beam isodoses (see Fig. 1.20) means that, if the beams are matched from light to light without a gap, there will be an overdose of up to 20 per cent where the electron beam isodoses bulge into those of the photon field. However, the overdosed volume is small, occurs in non-critical connective tissue, only applies for 20 to 25 per cent of the overall treatment, and does not cause any significant clinical effect. Photon and electron fields are therefore matched to the light beam edges without a gap.

POSITION OF JUNCTION AND SPINAL CORD SHIELDING

If the neck is to be treated with an anterior field, the upper level of the field cannot be above the level of the hyoid unless the neck is hyperextended. This is because the nodes that lie posteriorly in the cervical chain are then too far from the anterior beam to receive an adequate dose.

For tumours above the epiglottis where there is macroscopic nodal disease in the neck, care should be taken to avoid having the field junction within the affected area. Where this is not a consideration, as, for example, an oral cavity lesion without nodes, the junction may be positioned high up. Because there is no critical disease in the mid-line, this allows central lead shielding to be used which protects not only the spinal cord but also the larynx and the upper aero-digestive tract (Fig. 6.5).

For disease in the larynx and hypopharynx, the position of the field junction needs to be below the site of the primary, and it is usually necessary to omit mid-line shielding.

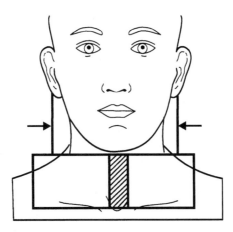

Fig. 6.5 High field junction for disease originating above the epiglottis, with central mid-line shielding to protect the spinal cord, larynx and hypopharynx.

A half-beam block technique may be used where parallel lateral fields are either very close to the eye anteriorly (Fig. 6.6) or very close to the spinal cord posteriorly. Alternatively, asymmetric collimators or customized blocks to shape fields or reduce transmission of the beam can be used to protect the spinal cord.

If the first phase of treatment does not cover the spinal cord, placement of a lead block is not necessary. It is also unnecessary if the anterior field has mid-line shielding for the spinal cord.

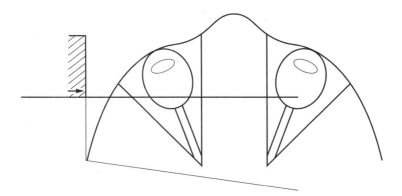

Fig. 6.6 Half-beam block technique to protect contralateral eye from beam divergence.

Patient care

Dental review is essential before irradiation, although many elderly patients are edentulous. Instructions for oral hygiene, including the use of mouthwashes, are essential to prevent tooth decay and to reduce the risk of subsequent bone necrosis. Dental extraction should be avoided unless the teeth are severely damaged.

Patients should be advised to stop smoking and avoid alcohol. Loss of appetite and impaired sense of taste in patients undergoing irradiation may lead to inadequate nutrition. This is made worse by mucosal reactions causing a sore mouth and difficulty in swallowing, which may be reduced by aspirin mucilage. Systemic analgesia may be needed. Liquidized foods, high-calorie supplements and increased fluids should be advised. Patients are weighed weekly during treatment and dietary advice is given. Nasogastric tube-feeding may be needed if mucosal reactions are severe, and elective PEG tube insertion may be useful for patients who have tumour-related dysphagia before radiotherapy. Specific speech and swallowing therapy may be very helpful for patients who are experiencing difficulty in resuming swallowing after radiotherapy.

If the airway is impaired, the patient is admitted to hospital for observation, but tracheostomy is avoided where possible. Acute laryngeal oedema may occur during irradiation of the larynx, but usually subsides rapidly if the patient is treated with bed rest, antibiotics and high-dose steroids. Patients with hypopharyngeal tumours are susceptible to chest infections because of regurgitation and inhalation of fluid. Regular examination of the chest should be performed in such cases.

Xerostomia is an inevitable result of irradiation of both parotid glands, which occurs, for example, in the treatment of nasopharyngeal tumours. The condition may be severe and can be helped by the use of artificial saliva and drinking with meals.

In cases where the eye cannot be shielded, e.g. during irradiation of some orbital and antral tumours, loss of secretions from the lacrimal gland causes a dry eye. This may be treated by the regular use of hypromellose eye drops. Painful corneal reactions are rare, since techniques are designed to spare the cornea, but when they occur they may be relieved by steroid eye drops.

Otitis externa is commonly seen when the ear is irradiated, as occurs during treatment for parotid and middle ear tumours. One per cent hydrocortisone cream may be useful in such cases. Serous otitis media may also occur.

Brachytherapy

Tumours of the oral cavity provide an ideal indication for brachytherapy in that they are usually relatively small, accessible and well localized, and yet have a substantial local recurrence rate with conventional external beam therapy alone. Brachytherapy should therefore be considered for all cases and, if not appropriate at the outset, should be reconsidered after 40 to 50 Gy fractionated external beam therapy. Tumours with nodal involvement are probably best managed by surgery and postoperative radiation. The neck should therefore be carefully imaged to exclude subclinical disease before proceeding with brachytherapy.

Patient care after interstitial implantation in the mouth is very similar to that for external beam therapy. In addition, platelet count and blood-clotting factors should be checked before implantation. Extra care may also be necessary in cases of haemorrhage or infection.

Because normal tissues appear to tolerate continuous low-dose-rate irradiation with brachytherapy better than external beam radiation, it is sometimes possible to consider salvage re-treatment with an implant. Salvage implants can be performed using conventional techniques, taking extra care to avoid hot spots and choosing lower than usual dose rates, which appear to be better tolerated. Even though the patient may have already received a radical dose of radiation, at least 60 Gy must be prescribed for salvage implantation to be effective in achieving local control.

Further reading

Million, R.R. and Cassisi, N.J. (eds) 1994: *Management of head and neck cancer: a multi-disciplinary approach*. Philadelphia, PA: J.P. Lippincott.

Saunders, M.I., Dische, S., Barrett, A., Parmar, M.K.B., Harvey, A. and Gibson, D. on behalf of the CHART Steering Committee 1996: Randomised multicentre trials of CHART vs. conventional radiotherapy in head and neck and non-small-cell lung cancer: an interim report. *British Journal of Cancer* **73**, 1455–62.

Wang, C.C. (ed.) 1997: *Radiation therapy for head and neck neoplasms: indications, techniques and results*. 3rd edn. New York: John Wiley & Sons.

CHAPTER 7

Larynx

Role of radiotherapy

The choice of treatment for carcinoma of the larynx depends on many factors apart from local control rate. These include the importance of voice preservation, fitness for surgery and reliability of follow-up.

Glottic tumours are treated initially by radical radiotherapy. For T_1 and T_2 tumours, this gives 5-year survival rates of 80 to 95 per cent depending on stage. Only 10 to 20 per cent of T_1 and 25 to 30 per cent of T_2 tumours recur locally and need salvage laryngectomy. For T_3 tumours, radical radiotherapy gives a similar survival rate to surgery, namely about 50 per cent, but 60 per cent of survivors retain the larynx. Careful follow-up is necessary, however, and recurrence may be difficult to detect. The majority of patients should have an examination under anaesthesia and biopsy 3 months after completion of radiotherapy in order to obtain histological confirmation of the response status.

T_1 and T_2 supraglottic tumours are rare, and may be treated by radiotherapy or horizontal partial laryngectomy if this expertise is available. For advanced lesions, local control rates are poor, and combined treatment is necessary. Patients with T_3 or T_4 (N_0, N_1) lesions are treated by laryngectomy with postoperative radiotherapy, since this may have a lower morbidity than pre-operative radiotherapy. An alternative approach for selected patients may be radical radiotherapy, followed if necessary by salvage laryngectomy.

For subglottic tumours, radiotherapy is the initial treatment unless tracheostomy is necessary to relieve obstruction, when laryngectomy followed by radiotherapy is undertaken.

Regional anatomy

The larynx is divided into three regions, namely the supraglottis, true glottis and subglottis (Fig. 7.1).

Since the true vocal cords have a poor lymphatic supply, lymph-node spread from glottic tumours is rare. In contrast, supraglottic tumours involve the upper deep cervical nodes at an early stage because of lymphatic spread upwards through the thyrohyoid membrane. Subglottic tumours spread via lymphatics through the cricothyroid membrane, to the pretracheal and paratracheal nodes in the superior mediastinum, and to the lower deep cervical nodes (see Fig. 7.2).

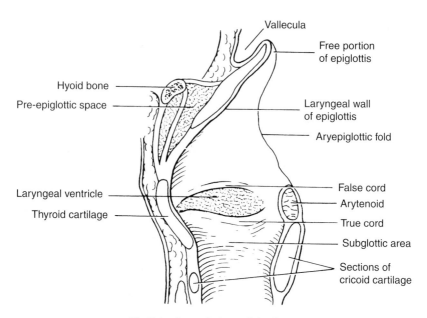

Fig 7.1   Lateral view of the larynx.

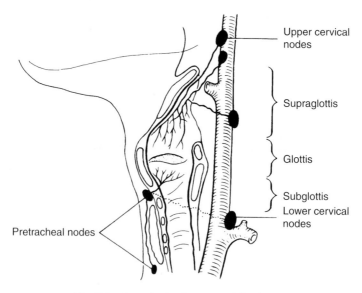

Fig. 7.2   Lymphatic drainage of the larynx.

Planning technique

ASSESSMENT OF PRIMARY DISEASE

The extent of laryngeal tumour is assessed by indirect laryngoscopy and palpation of the neck, to detect posterior fixation or lymphadenopathy. Direct laryngoscopy (EUA) gives a more detailed assessment of the tumour and permits histological confirmation. Other investigations include chest X-ray, lateral X-ray of neck (to detect soft tissue disease) and barium swallow if the patient has dysphagia, to exclude a second tumour of the hypopharynx or oesophagus. CT scanning may detect involvement of adjacent cartilage, and gives the relationship of the primary tumour (Fig. 7.3) to bony landmarks, as well as evaluating metastatic lymphadenopathy. MRI is useful for defining the extent of the primary tumour, and gives an accurate assessment of soft tissue disease.

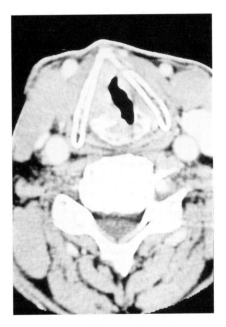

Fig. 7.3 CT image of tumour of the vocal cord (courtesy of Dr. B. Carey).

DEFINITION OF TARGET VOLUME

Glottis

The commonest tumour is that of the true vocal cord, which presents early with hoarseness. The risk of lymphatic spread is low, and prophylactic lymph-node irradiation is unnecessary.

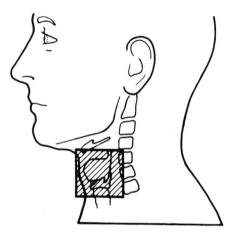

Fig. 7.4 Field margins for T_1 and T_2 glottic carcinoma.

The target volume for T_1 and T_2 tumours is centred on the vocal cord, which lies 1 cm below the palpable promontory of the thyroid cartilage. The whole of the thyroid and cricoid cartilages must be encompassed by a 4×5 or 5×5 cm field. Figure 7.4 shows the field margins, which include allowance for movement of the larynx with respiration as well as subclinical extension of disease. For T_2 tumours with extension to the supra/subglottis or impaired mobility, the volume is larger (6–7 cm in length), to include this extension with a margin. If radiotherapy is indicated postoperatively for $T_{3,4}$ tumours, the target volume is individualized to cover sites at risk of recurrence.

Supraglottis without lymphadenopathy (N_0)

The initial target volume includes the primary tumour and upper deep cervical nodes, which are involved in 70 per cent of patients at presentation. The upper border of this volume includes the tonsillar region with lead shielding to the oral cavity (Fig. 7.5). The upper deep cervical nodes are included in all patients by extending the volume posteriorly to lie just in front of the spinal cord. A second, reduced target volume encompasses the primary tumour alone.

Supraglottis with lymphadenopathy (N_1)

If there are palpable lymph nodes, the entire deep cervical chain and supraclavicular nodes should be irradiated bilaterally in continuity with the primary tumour.

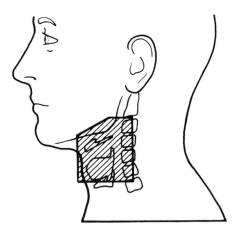

Fig. 7.5 Field margins for supraglottic carcinoma (N_0).

Subglottis

The target volume should include the primary site, the pre- and paratracheal lymphatics, the lower deep cervical nodes and the superior mediastinum. This is a difficult volume to treat in continuity because of varying body contour and the obstruction of beam entry by the shoulders.

LOCALIZATION

The patient is placed in a supine cast without a mouth-bite, with the neck straight to prevent the spinal cord from curving anteriorly. Palpable lymph nodes are marked with wire, and AP views of the lower neck and lateral films are taken in the simulator. The target volume and spinal cord are localized on to a transverse outline.

Field arrangements

Glottis

The whole larynx should be treated uniformly using opposing lateral fields. A 15° or 30° wedge is used to compensate for changes in the contour of the neck (Fig. 7.6). If the anterior commissure is involved, 15° wedges or open fields are used to increase the dose by 5 to 10 per cent anteriorly or bolus may be applied to the front of the larynx.

In an obese patient with a rounded neck, it is preferable to use two anterior oblique wedged fields to treat a smaller volume and spare skin laterally in the neck (Fig. 7.7). The gantry angle is chosen at 45–60° from the vertical to avoid the spinal cord. This technique is more complicated to use than lateral fields if

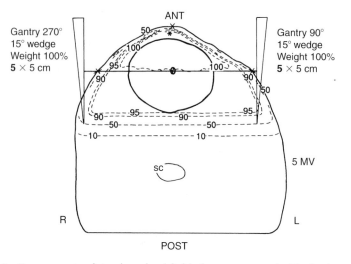

Fig. 7.6 Two opposing lateral wedged fields for treatment of a T₁ glottic tumour.
x = laser reference point.

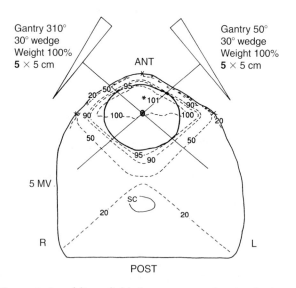

Fig. 7.7 Two anterior oblique fields for treatment of early glottic carcinoma.

the volume is not parallel to the couch top. The outline should then be taken at an angle to match the treatment plane, and a couch and gantry angle calculated to treat the sloping volume. Alternatively, a head twist can be added to a vertical outline and slight inhomogeneity accepted.

Advanced glottic tumours are treated using opposing lateral fields.

Supraglottis (N_0)

Opposing lateral fields are used to cover the target volume as shown in Fig. 7.8. The fields are wedged to compensate for the change in contour of the neck and give a homogeneous distribution.

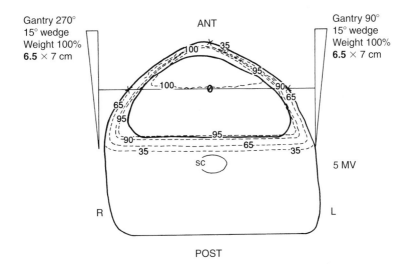

Fig. 7.8 Opposing lateral fields for treatment of supraglottic carcinoma.

Supraglottis (N_1)

The primary site and upper cervical nodes are treated using opposing lateral fields. The lower neck and supraclavicular nodes are included in a matched anterior field as discussed in Chapter 6, with the infraclavicular fossae shielded as shown in Fig. 6.2. Reduced lateral fields may be used to give a higher dose to the primary lesion and involved nodes where these do not overlie the spinal cord.

This technique cannot be used in cases where there are large node masses because cord tolerance would be exceeded. Treatment is therefore continued with small lateral fields anterior to the cord and direct lateral electron fields to the posterior volume. Fields are matched at the skin surface, while accepting that some overlap at depth is inevitable. Alternatively, a technique similar to that used for pyriform fossa lesions may be appropriate (see Fig. 8.5). Field arrangements must be chosen and the target volume reduced to limit the spinal cord dose to 44–6 Gy.

Subglottis

It is desirable (but difficult) to treat the larynx, upper trachea and lymph nodes in continuity. This is possible in some patients with a long neck, using two lateral fields angled inferiorly and an anterior field, extending down to cover the superior media-stinum, with lead blocks to shield the lung apices (Fig. 7.9). The anterior field is wedged longitudinally to correct for the supero-inferior curvature of the neck, and the lateral fields are wedged in the AP dimension to compensate for curvature of the neck as it narrows anteriorly.

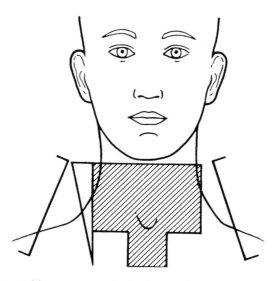

Fig. 7.9   Field arrangement for treatment of subglottic tumours using an anterior and two lateral fields.

To increase the dose to the inferior part of the volume, the lateral fields are angled inferiorly by a couch twist of about 30°. The posterior border of the lateral field is aligned in front of the spinal cord by using an appropriate head twist. It is difficult to achieve accurate calculation of isodose distributions using this technique.

Where this arrangement is not possible, two lateral fields are used to treat the upper part of the volume, and a single anterior field is used to treat the media-stinum, with the junction at least 1 cm below the primary tumour. Lateral fields need either double wedges or an AP wedge with a longitudinal compensator. The disadvantages of this are twofold, as there may be an unsatisfactory margin around the primary lesion because of the junction, and a relatively poor depth dose to the lower part of the volume from the single anterior field. Following laryngectomy, however, this field arrangement is satisfactory.

Implementation of plan

The patient is treated with either a cobalt unit or a linear accelerator. Opposing lateral fields are treated isocentrically and are aligned using opposing lasers.

Dose prescription

66 Gy in 33 fractions given in 6.5 weeks.

If radiotherapy is needed after primary surgery, treatment is individualized, but radical doses of 58–60 Gy are still needed.

Alternative fractionation

Where the target volume is small, an increase in daily fraction size is well tolerated and may be more convenient:

55 Gy in 20 fractions given in 28 days

or 50 Gy in 16 fractions given in 23 days.

Further reading

Mendenhall, W.M., Parson, J.T., Stringer, S.P., Cassisi, N.J. and Million, R.R. 1992: Stage T_3 squamous cell carcinoma of the glottic pharynx: a comparison of laryngectomy and irradiation. *International Journal of Radiation Oncology, Biology and Physics* **23**, 725–32.

Turesson, I., Sandberg, N., Mercke, C., Johanssen, K., Sandin, I. and Wallgren, A. 1991: Primary radiotherapy for glottic laryngeal carcinoma stage I and II. A retrospective study with special regard to failure patterns. *Acta Oncologica* **30**, 357–62.

CHAPTER 8

Hypopharynx

Role of radiotherapy

Most tumours in the pyriform fossa present with advanced local disease, and are best treated with radical surgery followed by radiotherapy to reduce the local recurrence rate. Early tumours on the lateral wall are associated with a higher incidence of involvement of the thyroid cartilage and, since this reduces radiocurability, they are also treated surgically. Early medial wall tumours may be treated with radical radiotherapy, reserving laryngectomy for recurrence. Radiotherapy is also used for patients who are unfit for surgery or who have T_4 or N_3 lesions which require palliation. Many patients are unsuitable for radical treatment, and the overall 5-year survival rate is only about 15 per cent.

For postcricoid tumours without lymphadenopathy or with a mobile unilateral node, the highest control rate is obtained with laryngopharyngectomy. Radical radiotherapy is given if the patient is unfit for surgery, or as palliation for advanced disease. Tumours of the posterior pharyngeal wall are the least common type, and radical radiotherapy is the treatment of choice.

Regional anatomy

The hypopharynx extends posterolaterally in relation to the larynx, from the aryepiglottic fold at the level of the hyoid bone to the lower level of the cricoid cartilage (see Fig. 7.1). It is divided into three sites, namely the pyriform fossa, the postcricoid region and the posterior pharyngeal wall (Fig. 8.1). The pyriform fossae are elongated gutters that extend down on both sides of the larynx, lying against the inner aspects of the thyroid cartilage (Fig. 8.2). The postcricoid region lies posterior to the larynx, and extends from the arytenoids to the lower border of the cricoid cartilage. The posterior pharyngeal wall extends from the level of the floor of the vallecula to the cricoid cartilage.

There is rich lymphatic drainage through the thyrohyoid membrane to the upper and lower deep cervical and supraclavicular nodes. Pyriform fossa tumours spread at an early stage to the upper deep cervical nodes, and up to 80 per cent of patients have palpable lymphadenopathy at presentation.

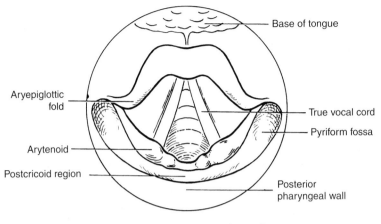

Fig. 8.1 Mirrow view of the hypopharynx.

Planning technique

ASSESSMENT OF PRIMARY DISEASE

Tumours of the pyriform fossae and posterior pharyngeal wall may be visible with a laryngeal mirror. Postcricoid tumours are rarely visible, but indirect laryngoscopy may reveal displacement of the larynx anteriorly, pooling of saliva in the hypopharynx, or oedema of the vocal cords. Endoscopy is essential to visualize the pharynx, larynx and trachea, to define the lower extent of disease, and for tumour biopsy. Palpation of the neck will reveal node involvement and loss of laryngeal crepitus due to tumour invasion of the larynx. Direct lateral extension from a pyriform fossa tumour may give rise to a mid-cervical soft tissue mass

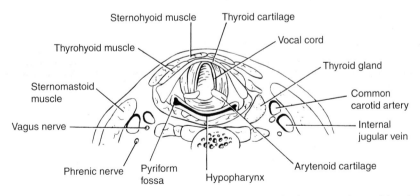

Fig. 8.2 Transverse section through the anterior neck showing relationship of pyriform fossae to the thyroid cartilage.

which moves with swallowing, unlike lymph nodes. Lateral soft-tissue X-rays of the neck may show widening of the prevertebral space with posterior pharyngeal wall tumours, anterior displacement of the larynx with postcricoid tumours, and destruction of the thyroid cartilage with tumours of the pyriform fossa. CT scanning may also delineate soft tissue masses and the involvement of cartilage.

DEFINITION OF TARGET VOLUME

Pyriform fossa (T_1/T_2, N_0 or minimal lymphadenopathy)

The initial target volume includes the primary tumour and the upper cervical lymph nodes from the angle of the jaw to the lower border of the cricoid cartilage. The superior and inferior borders are modified if necessary to cover tumour extension. The posterior border should lie in front of the spinal cord (Fig. 8.3). A reduced target volume includes only the primary tumour and any involved lymph nodes.

The patient is treated in a supine cast with the cervical spine straight in order to prevent anterior spinal cord curvature. Antero-posterior and lateral films are taken in the simulator, and the target volume and spinal cord are localized on to a transverse outline.

Opposing lateral fields are used, wedged anteriorly if necessary to compensate for the curvature of the neck. The submandibular gland is shielded in order to reduce the risk of a dry mouth.

Dose prescription

Initial target volume

50 Gy in 25 fractions given in 5 weeks.

Reduced target volume

16 Gy in 8 fractions given in 10 days.

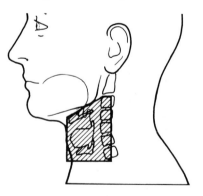

Fig. 8.3 Field margin for early pyriform fossa tumours.

Total dose

66 Gy in 33 fractions given in 6.5 weeks.

Pyriform fossa (T₃ tumours with extensive lymphadenopathy)

The target volume includes the primary tumour and lymphatic drainage of the involved side of the neck up to the base of the skull (Fig. 8.4). Patients are treated in a supine cast with the chin extended as far as possible to move the oral cavity and mandible out of the field. Node masses are marked with wire for simulation, and the primary tumour, lymph nodes and spinal cord are localized on to a transverse outline taken through the centre of the volume matching the inclined treatment plane.

Large lymph-node masses in the neck cannot be treated with opposing lateral fields because tolerance of the underlying spinal cord is limited to about 45 Gy in 4.5 weeks. A wedged lateral field and a contralateral anterior oblique field are used to treat the tumour and ipsilateral nodes while sparing the spinal cord. This arrangement is shown in Fig. 8.5, where the treatment plane is perpendicular to the couch. For an inclined treatment plane, the appropriate head twist and couch angle must be applied. A boost may be given to any residual node mass using electron therapy. When this isocentric technique is used, the contralateral neck nodes receive only a low dose, and if prophylactic treatment to these is intended, additional electron therapy should be given. An alternative approach, if the position of the nodes makes it appropriate, is to use opposed lateral fields for a first-phase treatment, and the arrangement described above for the second phase.

Dose prescription

66 Gy in 33 fractions given in 6.5 weeks.

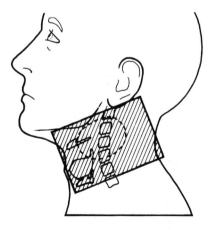

Fig. 8.4   Lateral field margins for T₃ pyriform fossa tumour with large node mass (dotted line) showing an inclined treatment plane.

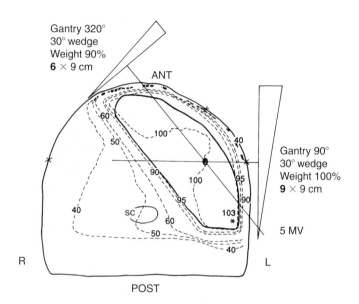

Gantry 320°
30° wedge
Weight 90%
6 × 9 cm

ANT

Gantry 90°
30° wedge
Weight 100%
9 × 9 cm

5 MV

R

L

POST

Fig. 8.5   Isodose distribution for treatment of T$_3$ pyriform fossa tumour with node
mass. sc = spinal cord; x = laser reference point.

Residual nodal disease

Additional 4–6 Gy given in 2–3 daily fractions.

Postcricoid region

Radical radiotherapy is only feasible in patients without node involvement,
because of the relationship of the regional nodes to the spinal cord. The target
volume includes the primary tumour and the adjacent lymphatics, covering any
inferior spread into the cervical oesophagus with a 2- to 3-cm margin (Fig. 8.6).
No prophylactic irradiation is given to the upper deep cervical nodes, since the
volume would be too extensive for a radical dose.

The patient is treated in a supine cast, keeping the cervical spine as straight as
possible. Antero-posterior and lateral simulator films are taken and the target
volume and spinal cord drawn on to the lateral film. Transverse and coronal outlines are taken through the centre of the target volume.

Two lateral double-wedged fields are used (Fig. 8.7), angled inferiorly to
increase the dose to the cervical oesophagus and superior mediastinal nodes. If
the patient has a short neck, an anterior mediastinal field may also be needed.
The isodose distribution in the coronal plane using angled lateral fields is shown
in Fig. 8.8. Each wedged lateral field is set at gantry 90° at an FSD of 100 cm
and centred on the entry point marked on the cast. An exit point and back-
pointing are used to ensure correct alignment. The gantry angle, head twist and
couch angle are altered according to the instructions on the plan. Alternatively,
in short-necked patients, two anterior oblique wedged fields may be used in an

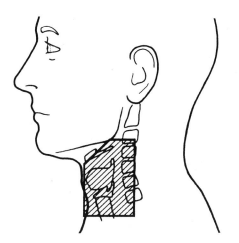

Fig. 8.6 Field margins for postcricoid tumour without lymphadenopathy.

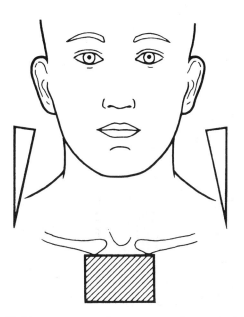

Fig. 8.7 Field arrangements for treatment of postcricoid tumour.

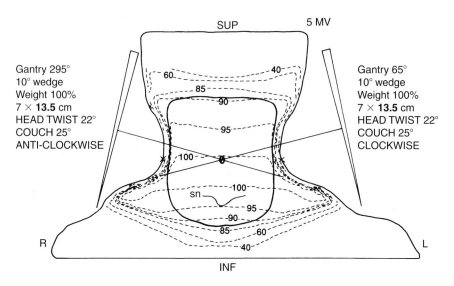

SUP   5 MV

Gantry 295°
10° wedge
Weight 100%
7 × **13.5** cm
HEAD TWIST 22°
COUCH 25°
ANTI-CLOCKWISE

Gantry 65°
10° wedge
Weight 100%
7 × **13.5** cm
HEAD TWIST 22°
COUCH 25°
CLOCKWISE

60   40
85
90
95
100
100
sn
95
90
85   60
40

R   L

INF

Fig. 8.8   Isodose distribution for treatment of postcricoid tumour using two lateral wedged fields angled inferiorly. sn = sternal notch; x = laser reference point.

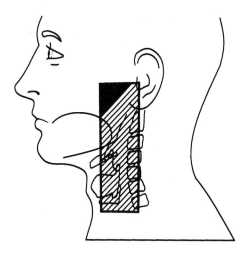

Fig. 8.9   Field margins for posterior pharyngeal wall tumour.

arrangement similar to that shown in Fig. 7.7, with appropriate head twist and compensators.

Dose prescription

66 Gy in 33 fractions given in 6.5 weeks.

Posterior pharyngeal wall

The target volume includes the whole hypopharynx and adjacent deep cervical lymph nodes bilaterally, including the retropharyngeal space which lies at the skull base and contains the lateral pharyngeal nodes, as shown in Fig. 8.9. A 2-cm margin is allowed above and below visible tumour, and the posterior border is placed anterior to the spinal cord. The patient is treated in a supine cast with the cervical spine straight.

The volume is localized using a lateral simulator film with the outline taken through the centre of the volume. Opposing lateral fields are used with a 15° wedge as compensator if necessary. If the patient has a short neck and the tumour extends into the cervical oesophagus, some inferior angulation of the beams may be necessary to cover the lowest part of the volume.

Dose prescription

66 Gy in 33 fractions given in 6.5 weeks.

If there is no palpable lymphadenopathy, the final 10 Gy may be given to a reduced volume encompassing the primary tumour alone. The cervical lymph nodes will then have received prophylactic irradiation to a dose of 55 Gy given in 5.5 weeks.

Further reading

Jones, A.S. 1992: The management of early hypopharyngeal cancer: primary radiotherapy and salvage surgery. *Clinical Otolaryngology* **17**, 545–9.

CHAPTER 9

Nasopharynx

Role of radiotherapy

Radical radiotherapy is the treatment of choice for all stages of carcinoma of the nasopharynx. Around 80 per cent of patients present with palpable cervical lymphadenopathy, and even if this is unilateral, bilateral cervical irradiation is necessary because of the pattern of lymphatic drainage. The local control rate after radical radiotherapy is about 30 per cent for all stages, persistence of the primary tumour being the main cause of failure. Chemoradiation may improve outcome. However, localized well-differentiated tumours without lymphadenopathy have a cure rate of more than 80 per cent because a high dose can be given to a small volume.

Regional anatomy

The nasopharynx is cuboidal in shape. Tumours occur most frequently in the lateral walls or roof, and arise less commonly from the posterior wall and floor. The nasopharynx is related superiorly to the body of the sphenoid and the basal part of the occipital bone. Direct superior extension of tumour leads to destruction of the skull base with involvement of cranial nerves III to VI lying in the cavernous sinus (Fig. 9.1). Inferiorly, tumour may erode the soft and hard palates with extension into the oral cavity and base of the tongue. Anteriorly, tumour spread may occur through the nasal fossa to the ethmoid sinuses, cribriform plate, anterior cranial fossa, maxillary antrum, pterygopalatine fossa and apex of the orbit. Posteriorly, extension may involve the retropharyngeal space which contains the retropharyngeal nodes of Rouvière, lying anterior to the lateral processes of the atlas. Nodal metastases at this site lead to compression of cranial nerves IX to XII in the carotid sheath.

The lateral walls contain the opening of the Eustachian tube and the fossa of Rosenmuller as shown in Fig. 9.2a. Lateral spread from the fossa of Rosenmuller into the parapharyngeal space occurs superiorly into the pterygoid muscles, parotid gland and muscles of mastication, and inferiorly to compress the carotid sheath (Fig. 9.2b).

Extensive lymphatics crossing the mid-line account for the high incidence of bilateral node involvement with early spread to the retropharyngeal, submastoid

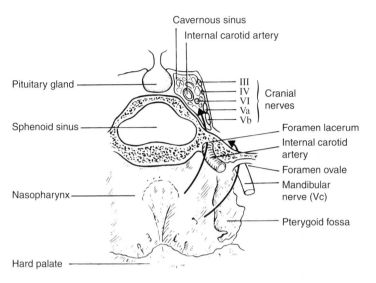

Fig. 9.1 Oblique section through the nasopharynx showing relationship to sphenoid bone and cavernous sinus. Paths of tumour spread arrowed. (Reproduced with permission from Moss, W.T., Brand, W.N. and Battifora, H., 1979: *Radiation Oncology*, 5th edn. St Louis, USA: C.V. Mosby Co.)

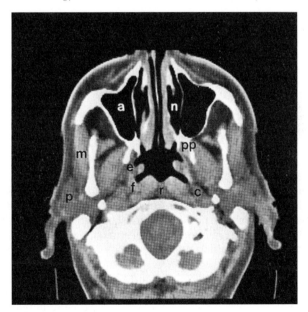

Fig. 9.2a CT scan showing the nasopharynx. a = antrum; pp = pterygoid plates; e = Eustachian tube; f = fossa of Rosenmuller; n = nasal fossa; r = retropharyngeal space with Rouvière's node; c = carotid sheath; m = masseter muscle; p = parotid.

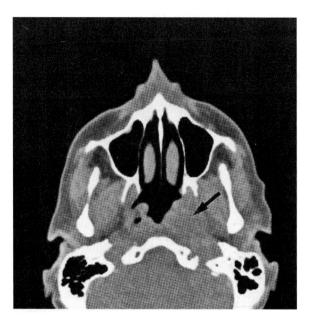

Fig. 9.2b CT scan showing tumour in fossa of Rosenmuller involving parapharyngeal space (arrowed).

and internal jugular nodes. Later on, involvement of the anterior and posterior cervical chains and supraclavicular fossa nodes may occur.

Planning technique

ASSESSMENT OF PRIMARY DISEASE

Patients most commonly present because of enlarged neck nodes, often in the posterior triangle. The physician must examine the nose for obstruction or discharge indicating local tumour extension into the nasal cavity, and must also examine the nasopharynx by posterior rhinoscopy, the pharynx and larynx for signs of local tumour or cranial nerve involvement, and the ears. Deafness due to obstruction of the Eustachian tube by primary tumour is a common presenting symptom, and hearing must be tested. Examination of all the cranial and upper cervical sympathetic nerves is important, to define involvement by local extension of the primary tumour. Direct endoscopy under anaesthesia is carried out in all cases. In patients with cervical lymphadenopathy in whom no tumour is seen, multiple biopsies of the nasopharynx are taken. Lateral X-rays of the neck, and special views of the petrous bones and base of the skull are taken. CT scanning may define soft-tissue disease and demonstrate bone erosion.

DEFINITION OF TARGET VOLUME

The target volume encompasses the primary tumour and potential routes of spread, and the entire lymphatic drainage system of the neck. Because of the proximity of the brainstem and optic chiasm to the primary lesion and that of the spinal cord to nodes, it is impossible to irradiate the entire volume in continuity to a radical dose. To cover undetectable microscopic disease, the volume must include the base of the skull, the floor of the middle cranial fossa, and the posterior half of the nasal fossa and orbit, the sphenoidal and posterior ethmoidal sinuses and the parapharyngeal space. The target volume includes the lateral pharyngeal, posterior cervical, deep cervical and supraclavicular lymph nodes, except for well-differentiated tumours without lymphadenopathy, where the lower cervical nodes are excluded. For these tumours, a second target volume includes the nasopharynx only.

LOCALIZATION

The patient is treated in a supine cast with the neck extended to elevate the chin, but keeping the spinal cord straight. Nodal masses in the neck, and the lateral orbital margins, are marked with wire before simulation. The treatment fields as defined below are marked on the perspex shell with the exact position of shielding, and simulator films are taken. The entry and exit points of each field are marked for alignment in the treatment unit.

Field arrangements

PATIENTS WITH LYMPHADENOPATHY

Treatment is initially given by large opposing lateral fields covering the entire target volume, including the spinal cord, to a dose not exceeding 40 Gy given in 4 weeks with daily fractionation. The brainstem, optic chiasm and anterior half of the orbit are shielded as illustrated in Fig. 9.3. This arrangement avoids a field junction over lymph-node disease in the neck. However, low cervical nodes may have to be treated with an anterior field because of the position of the shoulders. The junction should not overlie palpable disease.

The volume is then divided into an area covering the primary tumour, which is treated with two small opposing lateral fields, and the rest of the neck. The lateral fields encompass the nasopharynx, parapharyngeal space, base of the skull and posterior half of the orbit, including any extension anteriorly to the nasal fossa or inferiorly to the oropharynx. The position of the inferior border varies according to the technique used to treat the neck nodes. A half-beam blocking technique may be used for the lateral fields to reduce divergence. Where there is involvement of the nasal fossa, an additional anterior field may be needed to ensure an adequate dose to this area, with shielding to protect the lacrimal gland

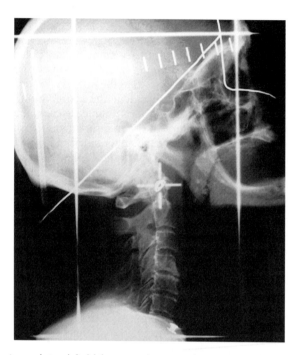

Fig. 9.3   Large lateral field for nasopharyngeal tumours with lead shielding to anterior orbit, brainstem and optic chiasma.

and globe. Doses to the optic nerves should be limited to 55 Gy unless there is invasion of the posterior orbit.

The neck nodes are best treated with two lateral fields using high-energy electrons chosen according to the depth of lymphadenopathy. The infero-posterior border of the small megavoltage lateral fields then lies in front of the spinal cord. Posterior deep cervical nodes usually regress sufficiently to permit the field junction to lie above the level of node involvement. If high-energy electrons are not available, an anterior field is used to treat the neck nodes, with central shielding to protect the spinal cord and larynx. (See discussion in Ch. 6.)

The lateral fields extend inferiorly and posteriorly, with spinal cord shielding introduced at 45 Gy. This allows a direct anterior field to be positioned below the mouth, using half-beam blocking at the junction with the lateral fields. If the posterior deep cervical nodes have not regressed sufficiently or the depth dose is inadequate, a small electron boost is given to residual disease.

PATIENTS WITHOUT LYMPHADENOPATHY

For a well-differentiated squamous cell carcinoma without lymphadenopathy, opposing lateral fields with an anterior neck field are used, and the lower cervical lymph nodes are not treated. It is often necessary to treat in two or three phases with reducing fields. Either of the above techniques is suitable. Anaplastic carcinomas presenting without lymphadenopathy are treated in the same way, but the entire neck is irradiated down to the clavicles.

An additional boost may be given to the primary site using two lateral wedged fields and an anterior field as shown in Fig. 9.4. Where the shape of the volume is complex and near to the brainstem, the boost can be given using three-dimensional conformal techniques, with CT planning and use of the multileaf collimator.

For patients with relatively limited recurrence at the primary site, salvage treatment may be delivered with brachytherapy. This can be done with a remote afterloading system at a high dose rate. After local anaesthesia, balloon catheters can be inflated in the nasopharynx and the position of afterloading catheters imaged on AP and lateral X-rays. From the latter the loading positions can be selected to deliver a boost dose of radiation to an isodose approximately 5 mm from the surface of the balloon. The use of CT images and optimized source placement can shape the isodose to cover known sites of residual disease while minimizing the dose to adjacent critical structures.

Implementation of plan

The patient is treated in a supine cast on which the treatment fields are marked. Lateral and anterior nasopharyngeal fields are treated isocentrically. Anterior

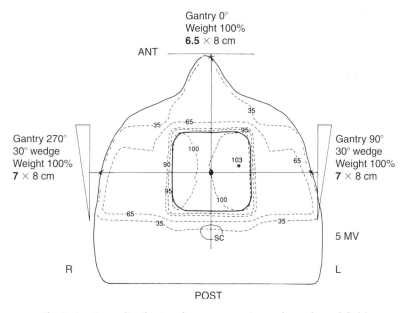

Fig. 9.4 Dose distribution from an anterior and two lateral fields.
sc = spinal cord, x = laser reference point.

megavoltage and lateral electron fields to the neck are set up at the machine FSD. Lasers are used to oppose lateral fields, and shielding is positioned to match the marks on the cast. Eye doses are measured with thermoluminescent dosemeters.

Dose prescription

Patients with lymphadenopathy

Large lateral fields

40 Gy in 20 fractions given in 3 weeks.

Nasopharyngeal fields

26 Gy in 13 fractions given in 2.5 weeks.

Neck fields

26 Gy in 13 fractions given in 2.5 weeks.

Total dose to the whole volume

66 Gy in 33 fractions given in 6.5 weeks.

Patients without lymphadenopathy

Nasopharyngeal and neck fields

56 Gy in 28 fractions given in 5.5 weeks.

Nasopharynx alone

10–14 Gy in 5–8 fractions given in 1 to 1.5 weeks.

Total dose to primary tumour

66–70 Gy in 33–36 fractions given in 6.5 to 7 weeks.

Further reading

Lee, A.W.M., Law, S.C.K., Foo, W. *et al.* 1993: Nasopharyngeal carcinoma: local control by megavoltage radiation. *British Journal of Radiology* **66**, 528–36.

CHAPTER 10

Oropharynx

Role of radiotherapy

Of the tumours that arise in the oropharynx, 60 per cent originate in the tonsil, 25 per cent in the base of the tongue and 10 per cent in the soft palate. Radiotherapy is used for all squamous cell carcinomas, giving overall 2-year control rates of 60, 30 and 50 per cent for each tumour site, respectively. Early $T_1 - T_2$ tumours are curable by radiotherapy alone so that the morbidity of surgery can be avoided. More advanced tumours are rarely cured by single-modality treatment, and are best managed by radical resection and postoperative radiotherapy. Non-Hodgkin's lymphomas arising in Waldeyer's ring are treated by a combination of chemotherapy and radiotherapy.

Sixty per cent of patients present with node involvement, but contralateral spread is uncommon (15 to 25 per cent). In patients without lymphadenopathy, elective irradiation of adjacent lymph nodes is carried out because of the high risk of microscopic involvement. Mobile unilateral lymph-node metastases are treated either by radiotherapy alone, or by block dissection followed by postoperative radiotherapy to reduce the local recurrence rate. Bilateral or fixed lymph nodes, which are unsuitable for surgery, are treated by radical radiotherapy with local removal of residual masses if the primary tumour is controlled.

Regional anatomy

The oropharynx extends from the soft palate to the hyoid bone. It comprises the tonsillar fossae laterally, the soft palate superiorly, the posterior third of the tongue, vallecula and free portion of the epiglottis anteriorly, and the posterior pharyngeal wall (Fig. 10.1). Lymphatics from the tonsillar region drain to the adjacent jugulo-digastric nodes. The remaining structures in the oropharynx drain bilaterally – the base of the tongue to the mid-cervical nodes (jugulo-omohyoid), and the soft palate and posterior wall to the retropharyngeal and upper deep cervical lymph nodes (see Fig. 11.1).

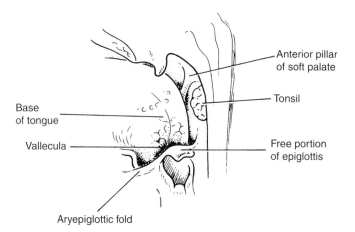

Anterior pillar
of soft palate

Tonsil

Base
of tongue

Free portion
of epiglottis

Vallecula

Aryepiglottic fold

Fig. 10.1 Anatomy of the oropharynx. (Adapted with permission from del Regato, J.A., Spjut, H.J. and Cox, J.D. 1984: *Ackerman and del Regato's Cancer*, 6th edn. St Louis, USA: C.V. Mosby Co.)

Planning technique

ASSESSMENT OF PRIMARY DISEASE

The primary tumour is usually visible either directly or with a mirror. The neck is examined for lymphadenopathy. Trismus may occur with deep infiltration of tumour into the parapharyngeal space. Tonsillar tumours spread from the posterior faucial pillar to the lateral pharyngeal wall, and from the anterior pillar to the soft palate and base of the tongue. The extent of disease is best assessed under general anaesthesia, which permits a full examination of the upper respiratory tract and biopsy of tumour for histology. Lateral soft-tissue X-rays of the neck may be useful for demonstrating soft-tissue masses.

DEFINITION OF TARGET VOLUME

Tonsil

Small primary tumours confined to the tonsillar fossa, anterior faucial pillar or retromolar fossa without lymph node involvement are irradiated to a small volume, including the primary site and ipsilateral submandibular and upper deep cervical lymph nodes. The fields extend from the top of the hard palate to the bottom of the hyoid bone (Fig. 10.2). The anterior margin lies through the middle third of the tongue and the posterior margin lies just in front of the spinal cord. The medial border is at the mid-line.

For all cases with lymph-node involvement or larger tumours involving the soft palate or posterior third of the tongue which have a propensity for bilateral

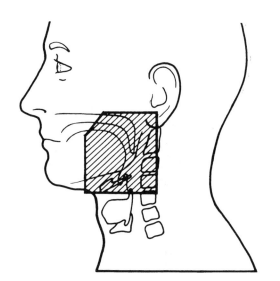

Fig. 10.2   Field margins for small tumours of the tonsillar fossa. Shielding is used as indicated for opposing lateral fields.

spread, the target volume includes the primary tumour and bilateral neck nodes in continuity.

Other sites

All other tumours arise near the mid-line and spread to lymph nodes on both sides of the neck. In patients without lymphadenopathy, the volume covers the primary site, the parapharyngeal, and the upper and mid-cervical lymph nodes bilaterally. Thus the volume lies slightly lower than that used for tonsillar lesions (Fig. 10.3). In a patient with lymphadenopathy, the lower half of the neck is also treated.

In patients with bulky bilateral lymph-node metastases, the volume may have to extend posteriorly to include most of the cervical spinal cord. For radical treatments, a two-phase technique is therefore needed.

Non-Hodgkin's lymphomas

If irradiation is required for patients with nodular Stage I_E disease of the tonsil, Waldeyer's ring and the lymph nodes on both sides of the neck are treated with lateral fields extending from the base of the skull to the lower neck as shown in Fig. 9.3.

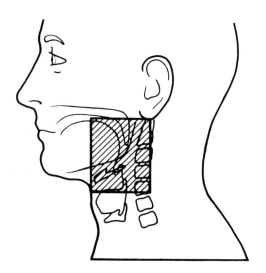

Fig. 10.3 Field margins to cover target volume for tumours of the posterior third of the tongue.

LOCALIZATION

Patients are treated in a supine cast with a straight neck and no mouth-bite. In the simulator, lymph-node masses are marked with wire and the target volume is defined on a lateral film. This volume and the spinal cord are drawn on to a transverse outline taken through the centre of the volume. When a unilateral wedged technique is used, the shell must be offset on the couch to the side of the lesion in order to make room for entry of the posterior oblique field.

Field arrangements

WEDGED PAIR TECHNIQUE

Small primary tumours of the tonsillar fossa are treated with anterior and posterior oblique wedged fields on the affected side. This technique spares the contralateral oral mucosa and parotid gland, and reduces acute mucositis and xerostomia. The gantry angle of the posterior field is chosen to minimize the dose to the spinal cord as shown in Fig. 10.4.

OPPOSING LATERAL FIELDS

All other lesions are treated with opposing lateral fields. For some tonsillar tumours, a 2:1 weighting is used to give a high dose to the primary site and

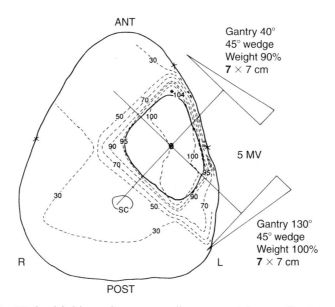

Fig. 10.4 Wedged fields used to treat small tumours of the tonsillar fossa.
sc = spinal cord.

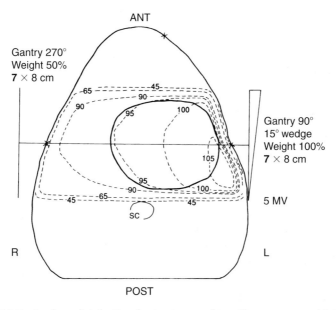

Fig. 10.5 Isodose distribution for treatment of tonsillar tumours, with 2:1
weighting of opposing lateral fields.

adjacent lymph nodes, and prophylactic irradiation to the contralateral tonsil and upper deep cervical nodes (Fig. 10.5). If there is invasion of the tongue or soft palate, equal weighting must be used to ensure an adequate dose to the primary site, and to cover lymphatic drainage bilaterally. Where there is involvement of the ipsilateral upper deep cervical nodes, the neck below the opposing lateral fields is irradiated using an anterior field with shielding to the larynx and spinal cord. Care must be taken to ensure that the junction does not overlie palpable disease. If there is residual tumour in the base of the tongue following external beam irradiation, an interstitial iridium implant may be considered using the plastic loop technique described in Chapter 11.

TWO-PHASE TECHNIQUE

Where bulky bilateral nodes lie posteriorly, treatment is given initially with opposing lateral fields which include the spinal cord to a dose of 40 Gy in 4 weeks, treating daily. Small opposing lateral fields lying anterior to the spinal cord are then used to give a radical dose to the primary tumour, and any residual posterior nodes are treated with electrons.

Implementation of plan

Patients are treated lying in a supine cast offset on the couch for the technique using oblique fields. Opposing lateral and oblique wedged fields are treated isocentrically using lasers to align entry and exit points on the cast. Anterior and lateral fields are matched with a half-beam blocking technique, and shielding is added to the larynx and spinal cord for the anterior field.

Dose prescription

66 Gy in 33 fractions given in 6.5 weeks.

Alternative fractionation for small target volume

55 Gy in 20 fractions given in 4 weeks.

Non-Hodgkin's lymphoma

40 Gy in 20 fractions given in 4 weeks.

Further reading

Bataini, J., Asselain, B., Jaulerry, C. *et al.* 1989: A multi-variant primary tumour control analysis in 465 patients treated by radical radiotherapy for cancer of the tonsillar region: clinical and treatment parameters as prognostic factors. *Radiotherapy and Oncology* **14**, 265–77.

Wong, C., Ang, K., Fletcher, G. *et al.* 1989: Definitive radiotherapy for squamous cell carcinoma of the tonsillar fossa. *International Journal of Radiation Oncology, Biology and Physics* **16**, 657–62.

CHAPTER 11

Oral cavity

Role of radiotherapy

Both radical radiotherapy and primary surgery are used to treat squamous cancers of the oral cavity, and they are increasingly being used in combination. Where radiotherapy is used alone, local control rates for T_1 tumours are approximately 80 per cent, with 60 to 75 per cent control for T_2 tumours. For large tumours, the control rate falls to considerably less than 50 per cent, and they are therefore treated by primary surgery and postoperative radiotherapy. Salvage of surgical failures by radiotherapy is usually unsuccessful. Primary surgery is indicated for tumours with bone involvement where there is a low cure rate with radiotherapy. Melanomas, adenocarcinomas and tumours surrounded by areas of pre-malignant change are treated with surgery. Salivary gland tumours are the commonest neoplasms in the hard palate, and these are treated surgically.

Malignant lymphadenopathy is usually an indication for combined surgery and radiation. Malignant nodes less than 2 cm in diameter can be controlled in 70 to 80 per cent of cases by radiation alone, but nodes larger than 4 cm in diameter are controlled in only 20 to 25 per cent of cases.

TONGUE

Surgery is indicated for small superficial tumours, those arising on the tip where implantation would be difficult, and for tumours associated with syphilitic glossitis. Functional results may be better after interstitial implantation where this is technically feasible, and this also allows treatment of a wider margin than surgery. T_1 and small T_2 tumours are treated with interstitial implantation alone to a radical dose using iridium hairpins. For larger T_2 and T_3 tumours, external beam therapy is given first to the primary and adjacent lymph nodes, followed by implantation to the primary tumour. Treatment for early tumours with mobile lymphadenopathy is surgical excision or interstitial implantation of the primary lesion, and removal of nodes by block dissection of the neck. If postoperative radiation to the neck is indicated, it may be difficult to shield the brachytherapy-implanted volume without shielding the adjacent jugulo-digastric nodes.

FLOOR OF THE MOUTH

Interstitial implantation may be used alone for T_1 and small T_2 tumours. However, when the tumour is attached to but not necessarily infiltrating the periosteum of the mandible, there is a risk of osteoradionecrosis if sources are positioned close to bone. Treatment with surgery may then be indicated, as it is when there is detectable bone involvement, or external beam irradiation may be given and surgery reserved for local failure. For the larger T_2 tumours, implantation is carried out following external beam therapy to the primary and adjacent lymph nodes. T_3 and T_4 tumours with attachment to or invasion of the mandible are treated surgically. In all cases of patients who are unfit for anaesthesia, external beam radiotherapy is given.

BUCCAL MUCOSA AND LOWER ALVEOLUS

T_1 and small T_2 tumours of the buccal mucosa are treated by radical implantation unless the lesion extends close to bone or into the retromolar trigone, when it is difficult to achieve satisfactory geometry and external beam irradiation is given. Larger tumours are treated by a combination of external beam irradiation and implantation. Where there is bone invasion, surgery is the treatment of choice because of poor blood supply and hypoxic tumour cells. If the patient is unfit for surgery, external beam therapy is given to the primary site and submandibular lymph nodes.

RETROMOLAR TRIGONE

These tumours arise in close proximity to bone, which is often involved, and they also tend to spread posteriorly and superiorly into the pterygoid fossa, which can cause trismus. It is not possible to achieve a satisfactory implant in this site and treatment is usually by surgery with postoperative radiation or radical radiotherapy alone. In N_0 cases, radiotherapy is given to the primary and ipsilateral upper deep cervical nodes only, because spread to contralateral lymph nodes is rare. Where there is palpable lymphadenopathy, all of the nodes on the affected side are treated.

Regional anatomy

The oral cavity includes the anterior two-thirds of the tongue, the floor of the mouth, the buccal mucosa, alveoli, hard palate and retromolar area.

The mobile anterior two-thirds of the tongue lies in the oral cavity, in contrast to the posterior third, which forms part of the anterior wall of the oropharynx. Tumours most commonly arise on the lateral border of the anterior tongue. The infiltrative type spreads through muscle to the floor of the mouth and mandible, and posteriorly to the anterior faucial pillar, but less commonly across the mid-line.

Lymphatic drainage from the anterior two-thirds of the tongue is to the submental, submandibular and upper, mid- and lower cervical lymph nodes (Fig. 11.1). Fifty per cent of patients have palpable lymphadenopathy at presentation, commonly involving the jugulo-digastric node. Tumours of the floor of the mouth spread to the submental, submandibular and upper deep cervical nodes, and 30 per cent of patients have submandibular lymphadenopathy at presentation. Tumours of the lower alveolus tend to spread into the mandible and to the submandibular nodes.

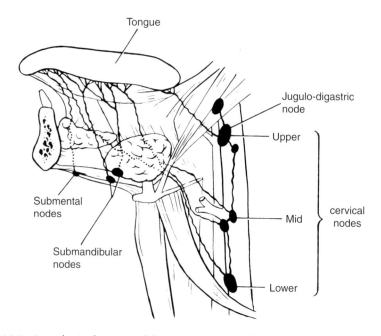

Fig. 11.1 Lymphatic drainage of the tongue. Copyright 1959. Novartis. Reprinted with permission from *The Ciba Collection of Medical Illustrations, Vol. 3, Part I,* illustrated by Frank H. Netter, M.D. All rights reserved.

Planning technique

ASSESSMENT OF PRIMARY DISEASE

The primary tumour should be easily visible on direct inspection during a full ENT examination, but palpation is essential to define the dimensions of the tumour. Bimanual examination should be performed to detect submental infiltration and submandibular lymph nodes. Limitation of protrusion of the tongue out of the mouth is an indication of deep infiltration. Examination under general anaesthesia is useful for delineating tumour extent, particularly posterior spread to the oropharynx, and for biopsy. MRI is useful for evaluation of the primary tumour. The neck is palpated to exclude lymphadenopathy. X-ray of the mandible is important, especially in tumours of the lower alveolus where there is a high risk of bone involvement. Careful examina-tion of the teeth should be carried out, and any damaged teeth should be treated conservatively where possible.

LOCALIZATION

Patients are treated in a supine cast with a mouth-bite. When oblique fields are used, the head rest is offset to allow entry of the posterior field. Palpable lymphadenopathy is marked with wire, and AP and lateral films are taken on the simulator. The primary site, lymph nodes, spinal cord and mid-line are marked on the transverse outline through the centre of the volume.

Tongue

External beam therapy

T_2 tumours of the tongue, which are too extensive for implantation and unsuitable for combined surgery and radiation, are treated with external beam therapy. The target volume includes the primary tumour with a 2-cm margin and the ipsilateral submandibular and upper deep cervical nodes, as shown in Fig. 11.2.

If a patient with mobile nodes is unfit for surgery, irradiation is given to all of the ipsilateral neck nodes. For large T_2 and T_3 tumours, and for those which have spread across the mid-line, the lymphatic drainage of both sides of the neck is treated.

Early lateral tumours of the tongue are treated using anterior and lateral wedged fields to give a homogeneous dose to the primary site and adjacent lymph nodes, with sparing of the contralateral oral cavity and spinal cord

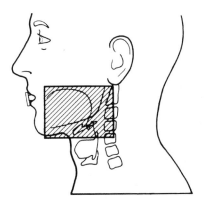

Fig. 11.2   Lateral field margins for localized carcinoma of the tongue.

(Fig. 11.3). This technique produces less acute mucositis and xerostomia than opposing lateral fields, which may be necessary for more extensive tumours.

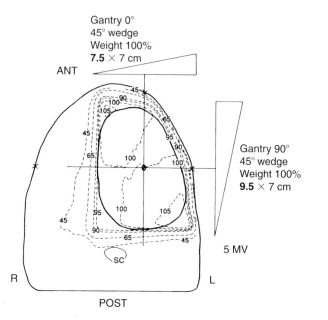

Fig. 11.3   Anterior and lateral fields used to treat early lateral tumours of the tongue and floor of the mouth. sc = spinal cord; x = laser reference point.

Brachytherapy

Small tumours of the tongue can be implanted using the hairpin technique (Fig. 11.4). The separation between the limbs of the hairpin is only 12 mm, so thicker tumours must be implanted using the plastic loop technique.

Hairpin technique
Once the target volume has been defined, 2 to 4 hairpins are used to form a double-plane implant along the lateral border of the tongue (Fig. 11.5). A single hairpin can sometimes be used to increase the dose in order to encompass small peripheral extensions of tumour.

Single-plane implantation for superficial tumours of the lateral border of the tongue is not recommended, as this results in an inadequate dose to the deeper parts of the tongue, where there may be undetected tumour infiltration.

The inactive phase of the implant is performed by inserting stainless steel slotted hairpin guides into the tongue under general anaesthesia in the operating theatre. It is best to position the most anterior and posterior hairpins first in order to identify the limits of the target volume, and then to decide on the number of hairpins that are required to lie between them, aiming at a separation of 12–15 mm between each hairpin. When implanting near the front of the tongue,

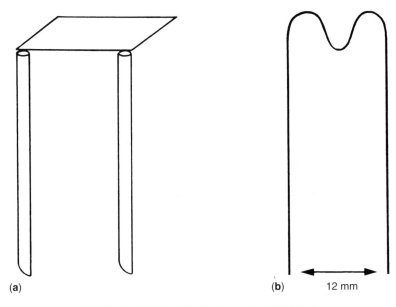

Fig. 11.4   (a) Slotted hairpin guides. (b) Hairpin.

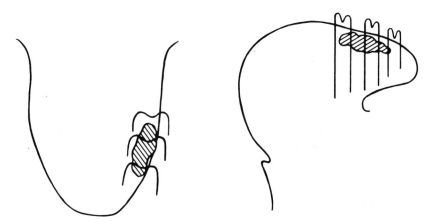

Fig. 11.5   Three hairpins forming a double-plane implant for a tumour of the lateral border of the tongue.

it is important to remember that the mandible will reflect the tip of the needles backwards, and this must be predicted when choosing the angle of the implant to avoid convergence at depth. The parallelism of the hairpin guides must be checked either by an image intensifier in the operating theatre or by an X-ray. Once the position is satisfactory, a suture is passed under the cross-piece of each guide. The hairpins are supplied with limbs 6 cm in length. These usually have to be cut to between 3 and 5 cm depending on the volume to be implanted. It must be remembered that whereas the top of the implant is effectively crossed by the bridge of the hairpin, the bottom ends are uncrossed and need to be longer than the target volume in order to compensate for this and ensure an adequate dose at depth.

The implant is loaded by pushing the active hairpin down the guide and then withdrawing the latter while the bridge of the hairpin is held down in the tongue. The suture is then tied over the bridge of the hairpin to keep it in the tongue for the duration of the implant. Once the implant has been completed, orthogonal check radiographs are taken for dosimetry.

Plastic tube loop technique

Where the target volume is too thick to be encompassed by a hairpin implant, it is necessary to form a loop of radioactive wire over the tumour. The separation between the branches of the loop can be varied up to a maximum of 18 mm.

The inactive phase of the implant consists of forming a loop of plastic tubing into which the active wire is afterloaded. The loops are used to form a two-plane implant, usually in the same orientation as that used for hairpins. A pair of stainless steel needles are first pushed into the mouth from the skin below, and are positioned to lie on either side of the lesion (Fig. 11.6a). A nylon cord is then passed up one needle and down the other to form a loop (Fig. 11.6b). After withdrawal of the needle, plastic tubing is threaded over the nylon cord and clamped at one end. It is then pulled into the mouth by the nylon cord to reform a loop of hollow plastic tubing (Fig. 11.6c). Depending on the size of the target volume, three or four loops are similarly constructed and their position is checked for parallelism.

Inert fuse wire is passed up each loop so that the position can be seen on orthogonal check radiographs for dosimetry. The active wire is afterloaded into the previously implanted plastic tubing and secured with nylon balls and lead discs at each end.

Remote afterloading machines can be used to replace manual afterloading, but it is difficult to reproduce the hairpin or loop distribution because the afterloading source cannot usually negotiate around the top of a tight loop. Techniques using straight-line sources overcome this problem, but it is necessary either to position the top sources 4–5 cm above the surface mucosa, or to weight the top few source dwell positions in order to compensate for the lack of a crossing source at the top of the implant.

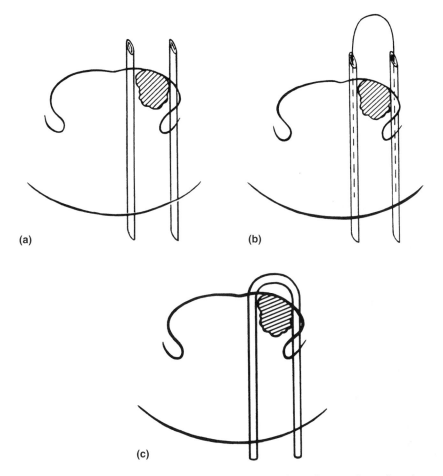

Fig. 11.6 Plastic tube loop technique. (a) Insertion of stainless steel needles. (b) Passage of nylon cord through needles. (c) Loop of hollow plastic tubing in place.

Floor of mouth

External beam therapy

Anterior T_1 and small T_2 floor of mouth lesions which are not considered suit-able for implantation are treated by small-volume external beam therapy using two anterior wedged fields as shown in Fig. 11.7. This allows a 1.5- to 2-cm margin, and spares much of the oral mucosa and parotid glands. For other T_2 tumours the target volume includes the primary tumour, submental, sub-mandibular and upper deep cervical nodes as shown in Fig. 11.8. If there is

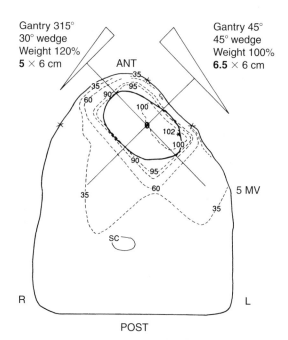

Gantry 315°
30° wedge
Weight 120%
5 × 6 cm

ANT

Gantry 45°
45° wedge
Weight 100%
6.5 × 6 cm

5 MV

R

L

POST

Fig. 11.7 Anterior wedged oblique fields to treat small anterior floor of mouth tumour.

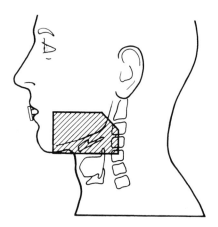

Fig. 11.8 Lateral field margins for T_2N_0 carcinoma of the floor of the mouth, with shielding of part of the parotid gland.

palpable lymphadenopathy, lymph nodes on both sides of the neck are included because drainage is bilateral and treatment is then given with parallel opposed lateral fields.

Brachytherapy

The techniques used for implantation of tumours of the floor of the mouth are the hairpin and plastic tube loop techniques as described for tumours of the tongue. The choice of technique depends on the size and thickness of the target volume and its accessibility in the mouth.

Buccal mucosa and lower alveolus

External beam therapy

The target volume for tumours of the buccal mucosa includes the primary tumour and ipsilateral submandibular nodes. A small anterior field and an ipsi-lateral field as shown in Fig. 11.9 are used to minimize irradiation of the lip.

For tumours of the lower alveolus, the target volume includes the mandible on the affected side and the submental and submandibular lymph nodes. This vol-ume lies laterally in the oral cavity, and a lateral wedged field and oblique ante-rior field as shown in Fig. 11.10 may be used to allow maximum sparing of the oral mucosa and lip.

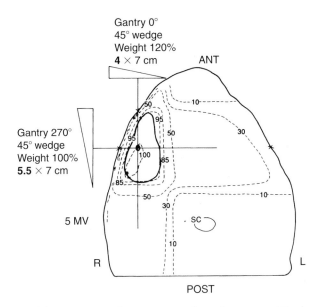

Fig. 11.9   Field arrangement for treatment of small tumour of the buccal mucosa.

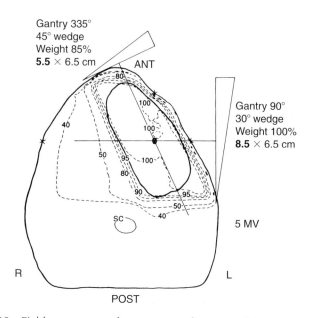

Gantry 335°
45° wedge
Weight 85%
5.5 × 6.5 cm

ANT

Gantry 90°
30° wedge
Weight 100%
8.5 × 6.5 cm

5 MV

R

L

POST

Fig. 11.10   Field arrangement for treatment of tumour of the lower alveolus.

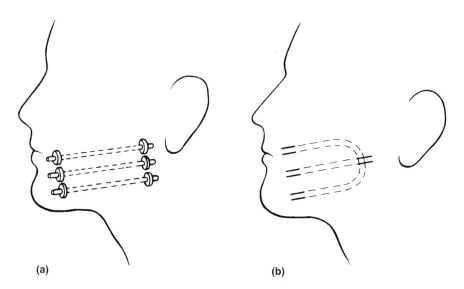

(a)

(b)

Fig. 11.11   Plastic tubes inserted for treatment of tumour of (a) buccal mucosa
and (b) retromolar trigone.

Brachytherapy

Small tumours of the buccal mucosa that are suitable for implantation can usually be encompassed in a single plane, but it may sometimes be necessary to use
two planes. A straight plastic tube technique can be used. Stainless steel needles
are inserted through the skin of the cheek and run submucosally in the buccal
mucosa before exiting through the cheek once more. Three or four parallel stainless steel guides are inserted and then replaced with plastic tubing ready for
afterloading with the active iridium wire (Fig. 11.11a).

If the lesion extends close to the retromolar trigone it may be necessary to
form an intra-oral loop so that the posterior margin of the tumour can be covered
(Fig. 11.11b).

Retromolar trigone

External beam therapy

For tumours of the retromolar trigone, the primary tumour and ipsilateral upper
deep cervical lymph nodes are included in the target volume. Anterior and
posterior oblique wedged fields are used as shown in Fig. 11.12 to spare the
contralateral parotid gland and mucosa as much as possible. If there is palpable
lymphadenopathy, an anterior field is added, with a suitable junction, to treat the
rest of the ipsilateral cervical node chain.

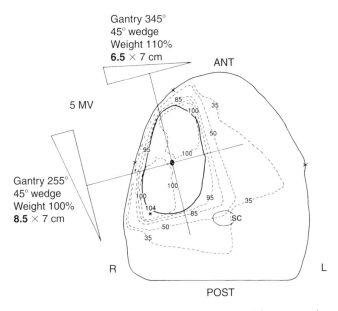

Fig. 11.12   Field arrangement for treatment of tumour of the retromolar trigone.

T_3 and T_4 tumours with lymphadenopathy

For extensive T_3 and T_4 tumours with involved lymph nodes, parallel opposed lateral fields may be necessary to encompass the disease. This causes considerable mucositis and may result in a dry mouth. An anterior field is matched below the opposing lateral fields if treatment of the whole neck is required (see Chapter 6).

Implementation of plan

Patients are treated with a megavoltage machine using an isocentric technique. The pin depth is measured from the plan and the FSD set accordingly. An optical back-pointer is used to align the cast using entry and exit points, and the gantry is angled according to the plan. The anterior neck field is matched on the skin, and central shielding is used to protect the larynx, spinal cord and lung apices (Fig. 11.13). Where only the ipsilateral nodes are treated, the medial border of the anterior field lies over the mid-line and the gantry is angled at 15° to avoid the spinal cord.

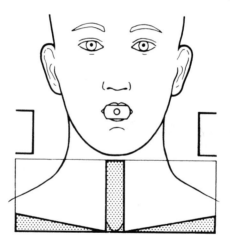

Fig. 11.13 Anterior neck field matched below opposing lateral fields for T_3N_1 tumour of the floor of the mouth.

Dose prescription

External beam therapy

Radical treatment

66 Gy in 33 fractions given in 6.5 weeks.

Alternative fractionation regimen

55 Gy in 20 fractions given in 4 weeks.

Pre-implantation

40–50 Gy in 20–25 fractions given in 4 to 5 weeks.

Brachytherapy

Radical treatment

65 Gy to the 85 per cent reference isodose using the Paris system.

Boost treatment

25–30 Gy to the 85 per cent reference isodose using the Paris system.

Further reading

Bachaud, J.M., Delanne, S.M., Allouache, N. *et al.* 1994: Radiotherapy of stage I and II carcinomas of the mobile tongue and/or floor of the mouth. *Radiotherapy and Oncology* **31**, 199–206.

Wang, C. 1989: Radiotherapeutic management and results of T_1N_0, T_2N_0 carcinoma of the oral tongue: evaluation of boost techniques. *International Journal of Radiation Oncology, Biology and Physics* **17**, 287–91.

CHAPTER 12

Ear

Role of radiotherapy

The natural history, prognosis and management of squamous cell carcinoma of the middle ear and external auditory canal are similar. Radical treatment, by either surgery or radiotherapy, gives low overall 5-year survival rates of approximately 25 per cent. The best chance of achieving local control is by radical surgery with postoperative radiation. However, this usually results in complete facial nerve palsy. Where tumour is not controlled by radiotherapy, persistent pain may be a problem.

Regional anatomy

The external auditory canal is 2.5 cm long and consists of an outer cartilaginous portion and an inner bony segment. The middle ear lies between the tympanic membrane and the inner bony and membranous labyrinth. It contains the ossicles and semicircular canals, and communicates posteriorly with the mastoid air cells.

The lymphatic drainage of the external ear is to the pre-auricular and parotid lymph nodes anteriorly, and to the postauricular and upper deep cervical nodes posteriorly.

Carcinoma of the external auditory canal spreads to the auricle and middle ear with early bone invasion. Squamous cell carcinoma of the middle ear spreads outwards to the canal and medially to the inner ear and facial nerve. Spread also occurs anteriorly into the parotid gland, superiorly into the middle cranial fossa, inferiorly to the jugular bulb and posteriorly to the mastoid bone (Fig. 12.1).

Planning technique

ASSESSMENT OF PRIMARY DISEASE

Clinical examination of the ear, parotid and mastoid region, including palpation of lymph nodes, is essential. The postnasal space should be inspected for anteromedial spread, and the cranial nerves carefully assessed. Tomograms of the skull

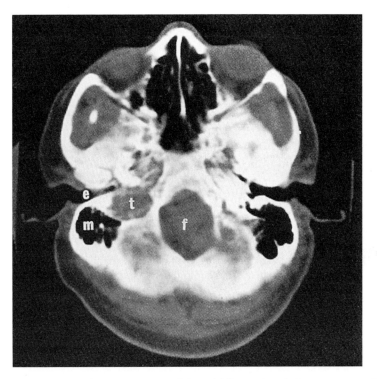

Fig. 12.1 CT scan showing tumour of the middle ear in relation to surrounding structures. e = external auditory canal; m = mastoid process; f = foramen magnum; t = tumour. (Courtesy of Dr C. Parsons.)

and mastoid region may show bone destruction, and CT scanning may demonstrate invasion of the base of the skull. Examination under general anaesthesia is performed with biopsy to establish a histological diagnosis.

DEFINITION OF TARGET VOLUME

The anterior and posterior limits of the volume are defined by the pre- and postauricular nodes and the mastoid process. The upper border lies below the eye and the lower border extends to the tip of the mastoid. In transverse section, the volume is triangular with the apex just anterior to the brainstem.

LOCALIZATION

The patient is treated supine because, in a lateral cast, lateral curvature of the cervical spine may bring the spinal cord within the high-dose volume inferiorly. The cast is made with the neck well extended to obtain a vertical line through

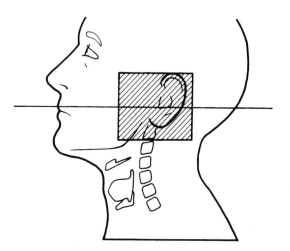

Fig. 12.2 Lateral view of the target volume showing the treatment plane perpendicular to the couch top.

the top of the pinna and the floor of the orbit. This avoids dose to the eye and keeps the treatment plane perpendicular to the couch (Fig. 12.2). Lateral and AP simulator films are taken, and the volume and spinal cord or brainstem are localized onto an outline taken through the centre of the volume. Alternatively, CT planning is used.

Field arrangements

Anterior and posterior oblique wedged fields are used to cover the triangular volume (Fig. 12.3). The posterior oblique field exits below the eyes, and the dose to the contralateral eye may be checked using lithium fluoride thermoluminescent dosimetry. If, despite careful positioning, the treatment plane is inclined, appropriate couch and head angles must be calculated.

Implementation of plan

The patient lies in a supine cast offset on the couch to the affected side. The fields are treated isocentrically, aligning entry and exit points with lasers. The gantry angle, head twist and couch angle, where appropriate, are adjusted according to the plan. Where there is no superficial extension of the tumour, the cast may be cut out to reduce skin reaction to the external ear.

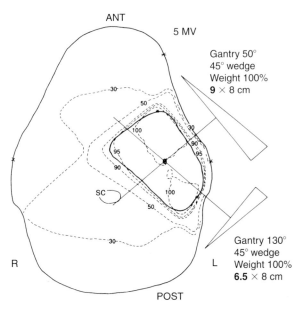

ANT

5 MV

Gantry 50°
45° wedge
Weight 100%
9 × 8 cm

Gantry 130°
45° wedge
Weight 100%
6.5 × 8 cm

R

L

POST

Fig. 12.3   Field arrangement for treatment of the middle ear tumour using anterior and posterior oblique wedged fields. x = laser reference point.

Three-dimensional conformal therapy

Because of the often complex volume and close proximity of several critical normal tissues, tumours of the middle ear provide a good indication for three-dimensional conformal planning. Beam's-eye-view techniques can ensure adequate coverage while avoiding adjacent normal tissue.

Dose prescription

66 Gy in 33 fractions given in 6.5 weeks.

Alternative fractionation regimen

55 Gy in 20 fractions given in 4 weeks.

Further reading

Korzeniowski, S. and Pszon, J. 1990: The results of radiotherapy of cancer of the middle ear. *International Journal of Radiation Oncology, Biology and Physics* **18**, 631–3.

CHAPTER 13

Parotid

Role of radiotherapy

Tumours of the salivary glands occur in many different anatomical sites with a variety of histological types. Between 80 and 90 per cent of tumours arise in the parotid, and approximately 9 per cent in the submandibular gland. This discussion will be confined to treatment of the parotid gland, since tumours at other sites are rare and treatment is individualized.

About 75 per cent of parotid tumours are benign mixed pleomorphic adenomas. Parotidectomy with preservation of the facial nerve is the treatment of choice. Radiotherapy may be given postoperatively if there has been incomplete excision or spillage of tumour at operation, and also after re-excision of locally recurrent tumours. In young patients the risk associated with radiation for benign disease must be balanced against the probability of local recurrence.

Malignant parotid tumours are treated primarily by surgical excision. They can be divided into low-grade tumours such as adenoid cystic carcinoma and acinic cell carcinoma, and high-grade tumours such as poorly differentiated adenocarcinoma. Low-grade tumours which have been completely excised with an adequate margin may not need any further treatment, but in practice the majority are treated with a combination of surgery and radiation. The indications for postoperative radiotherapy are:

- positive or very close excision margins;
- high-grade histology;
- positive nodes;
- skin or bone involvement;
- extensive perineural spread;
- recurrence after previous surgery.

The use of radiotherapy alone for inoperable or recurrent malignant tumours is essentially palliative, but in 20 to 30 per cent long-term local control may be achieved, and a high dose of radiation is therefore recommended.

Regional anatomy

The superficial part of the parotid gland lies between the masseter muscle anteriorly and the mastoid process posteriorly. The deep part of the gland lies posterior to the ramus of the mandible and extends medially in front of the sty-loid process to lie adjacent to the parapharyngeal space and the lateral pterygoid muscle (Fig. 13.1). The facial nerve follows a complex course within the parotid gland with the two structures becoming interwoven. The nerve lies on the deep posterior aspect of the gland adjacent to the styloid process, and splits within the parotid gland into a plexus with five main branches.

The lymphatics of the parotid gland drain into the pre-auricular and deep intra-glandular group of parotid lymph nodes, and from there to the upper deep cervical nodes.

Planning technique

ASSESSMENT OF PRIMARY DISEASE

Clinical examination of the parotid region and neck will reveal the superficial extent of the tumour and any associated lymphadenopathy. Facial nerve palsy may be seen with extensive local disease, and trismus indicates deep invasion of the parapharyngeal space and lateral pterygoid muscle. Examination of the pharynx may reveal a unilateral swelling if there is gross involvement of the deep part of the gland. This may also be detected by CT scanning as shown in Fig. 13.2.

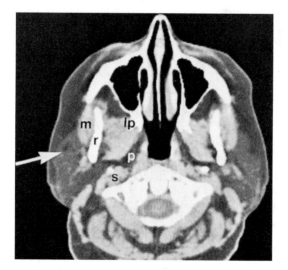

Fig. 13.1   CT section showing relationships of the normal parotid gland (arrowed).
m = masseter muscle; r = ramus of mandible; s = styloid process;
p = parapharyngeal space; lp = lateral pterygoid plate.

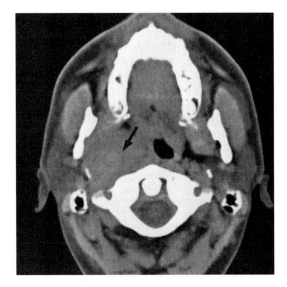

Fig. 13.2   CT section showing tumour in the deep part of the parotid gland (arrowed).

DEFINITION OF TARGET VOLUME

The entire parotid bed is irradiated in a volume extending longitudinally from 1 cm above the zygomatic arch to 1 cm below the angle of the mandible (Fig. 13.3). The superior border lies at the lower orbital margin and the inferior border

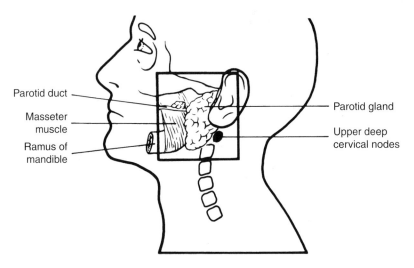

Parotid duct

Masseter muscle

Ramus of mandible

Parotid gland

Upper deep cervical nodes

Fig. 13.3   Target volume for treatment of a parotid tumour, in relation to underlying anatomy.

includes the lower part of the gland and the upper deep cervical nodes. Anteriorly, the volume covers the masseter muscle to include the parotid duct, and the posterior border passes through the mastoid process. Medially, the volume extends to 2 cm from the mid-line for benign lesions, but for malignant tumours the whole parapharyngeal space must be included. Laterally, the volume covers the operation scar and any palpable disease.

Adenoid cystic tumours have a local recurrence rate of about 60 per cent and a high incidence of perineural invasion, particularly along the facial nerve. The target volume for these tumours is therefore extended superiorly to include the base of the skull and the entire course of the facial nerve within the petrous temporal bone.

For malignant tumours without palpable lymphadenopathy, the parotid and upper deep cervical lymph nodes are included in the target volume. For undifferentiated or squamous cell tumours, where the risk of lymphatic spread is high, or where there is palpable lymphadenopathy, the entire ipsilateral lymphatic drainage of the neck is treated.

LOCALIZATION

The patient lies in a supine cast which is offset on the couch to the side of the lesion. If a lateral cast is used, it is essential to ensure accurate positioning of mid-line structures such as the spinal cord. No mouth-bite is needed, and the head should be extended as much as possible so that the superior border of the volume lying below the eye is perpendicular to the couch top. This ensures a vertical treatment plane so that neither head twist nor couch angulation are needed (Fig. 13.4).

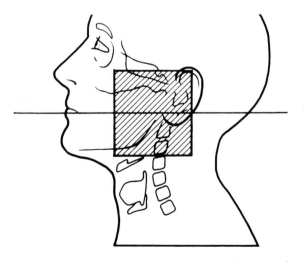

Fig. 13.4 Lateral projection of target volume for parotid tumour, showing vertical treatment plane.

If the patient is unable to extend his or her neck, or the volume includes the base of the skull, an inclined treatment plane may have to be used.

The operation scar and any palpable disease are marked with wire on the simulator, and AP and lateral films are taken. The target volume is localized on the films and transferred to a transverse outline taken through the centre of the volume. CT planning improves the localization of the spinal cord, brainstem, nasopharynx and parapharyngeal space, and in some cases delineates the tumour and defines the depth of the target volume.

Field arrangements

Anterior and posterior oblique wedged fields are used to obtain a homogeneous distribution and avoid the opposite parotid gland (Fig. 13.5). The superior border is chosen so that the posterior field exits below the opposite eye. The gantry angle of the posterior field lies along the petrous bone to minimize dose to the brainstem and spinal cord, which should not exceed 40 Gy in 4 weeks. Where there is a risk of skin involvement, the dose may be increased superficially by using wax bolus in addition to the perspex cast.

Where the entire ipsilateral neck is to be irradiated, an anterior field covering the lower neck is matched to the oblique fields, taking care that the junction does not overlie palpable disease. The medial border of the anterior field lies over the mid-line, with the gantry angled at 15° away from the spinal cord. Where

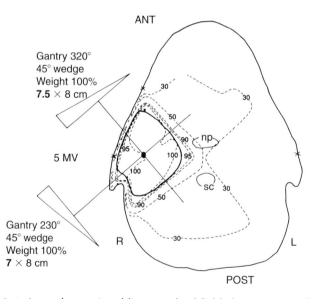

Fig. 13.5 Anterior and posterior oblique wedged fields for treatment of a parotid tumour. sc = spinal cord; np = nasopharynx; x = laser reference point.

appropriate, 10-MeV electrons may be used to boost the dose to superficial tissues. Alternatively, and more simply, a single lateral electron field may be used to cover the whole volume using an appropriate electron energy chosen to encompass the target volume within the 90 per cent isodose (Fig. 13.6).

Implementation of plan

The oblique wedged field technique is set up isocentrically using lasers to align entry and exit points on the opposite side of the cast and appropriate gantry angles as indicated on the plan. Head twist and couch angle are added where the treatment plane is inclined. The electron field is treated at the machine FSD. Thermoluminescent dosimetry is used to check that the dose to the lens is below 6 Gy to avoid contact.

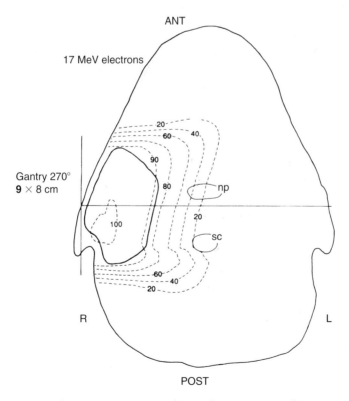

Fig. 13.6 Treatment of parotid tumour using electrons.

Three-dimensional conformal therapy

The parotid is a good site in which to consider three-dimensional conformal therapy because of the complexity of the shape of the volume and the proximity of critical normal tissues.

Patients should be scanned in the treatment position within a fixation shell (Plate 13.1a); 5-mm CT slices should be taken through the volume of interest, and the planning target volume and critical normal tissues marked on each slice (Plate 13.1b). The data are used to generate shaped shielding blocks or instructions for multileaf collimation to optimize target coverage while protecting normal tissue. Beam's-eye-view techniques are used to confirm field positions (Plate 13.1c).

Dose prescription

Macroscopic malignant disease

66 Gy in 33 fractions given in 6.5 weeks.

Microscopic malignant disease

60 Gy in 30 fractions given in 6 weeks.

Post-operative pleomorphic adenoma

55 Gy in 27 fractions given in 5.5 weeks.

Further reading

Fu, K.K., Leibel, S.A., Levine, M.L., Friedlander, L.M., Boles, R. and Philips, L. 1977: Carcinoma of the major and minor salivary glands. Analysis of treatment results and sites and causes of failure. *Cancer* **40**, 882–9.

Keus, R., Loach, P., de Boer, R. and Lebesque, J. 1991: The effect of customised beam shaping on normal tissue complications in radiation therapy of parotid gland tumours. *Radiotherapy and Oncology* **21**, 211–17.

CHAPTER 14

Maxillary antrum

Role of radiotherapy

Patients with carcinoma of the maxillary antrum commonly present with advanced local disease, although lymphatic spread occurs late and only about 15 per cent involve lymph nodes at presentation. The 5-year survival rates vary from 25 to 40 per cent depending on the size and site of the tumour and on histology. Early, well-differentiated tumours originating in the lower part of the antrum and extending only anteriorly or inferiorly have the best prognosis. Local control is best achieved by a combination of radiotherapy and maxillectomy, which can be accomplished with acceptable morbidity following high-dose irradiation to the upper jaw. However, advanced age, poor general condition or extensive tumour may make surgery impossible.

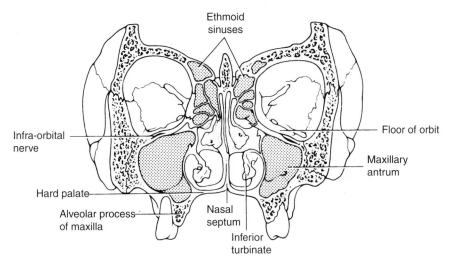

Fig. 14.1 Relationships of the maxillary antrum.

Regional anatomy

The maxillary antrum is related superiorly to the floor of the orbit and the infra-orbital nerve (Fig. 14.1). It is separated from the nasal cavity by its medial wall, and the anterior wall lies beneath the cheek. The floor of the antrum is formed by the alveolar process of the maxilla and the hard palate. Posteriorly it is adjacent to the pterygoid plates and the pterygopalatine fossa (Fig. 14.2a).

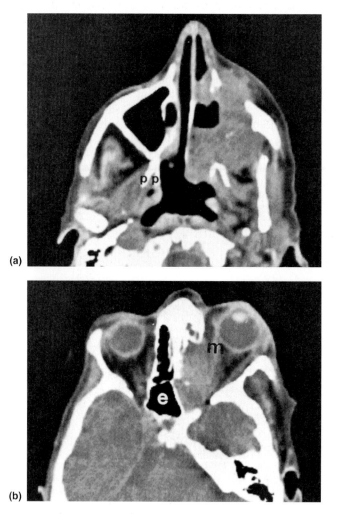

(a)

(b)

Fig. 14.2 (a) CT scan showing extension to the cheek, nasal cavity and pterygoid region from a tumour of the left maxillary antrum. pp = pterygoid plates. (b) CT scan showing involvement of the ethmoid sinuses and orbit by tumour of the left maxillary antrum. e = ethmoid sinus; m = medial rectus muscle.

Planning technique

ASSESSMENT OF PRIMARY DISEASE

Examination should include palpation of the gingivo-buccal gutter, palate and gums to detect tumour spread inferiorly. Involvement of the orbit may cause unilateral proptosis, abnormalities of ocular movements and impaired vision. The nasal cavity should be examined for extension medially, and the cheek should be assessed for swelling and loss of sensation due to infra-orbital nerve involvement. Trismus indicates posterior spread to the pterygoid fossa. Cervical lymph-node involvement must be excluded. Opacification of the paranasal sinuses may be seen on plain X-ray. Tomograms may detect bone destruction. CT scanning shows soft-tissue masses and extension into the ethmoid sinuses, orbit and pterygopalatine fossa (Fig. 14.2). Under general anaesthesia, biopsy is taken and drainage established by an intra-nasal antrostomy or Caldwell–Luc incision if maxillectomy is not performed.

DEFINITION OF TARGET VOLUME

The target volume is chosen to cover potential routes of spread, since local extension may be difficult to detect. The upper border of the anterior field (chosen to encompass the target volume with a margin) lies at the supra orbital ridge, extending medially to the contralateral inner canthus to include both ethmoid sinuses and the nasal cavity (Fig. 14.3). The inferior, lateral and anterior field margins cover the hard palate, gingivo-buccal sulcus and cheek. Posteriorly

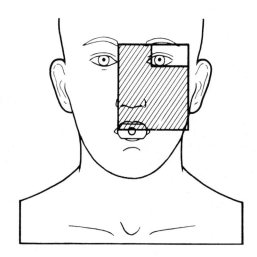

Fig. 14.3   Margins of the anterior field with lead shielding to the cornea, lens and lacrimal gland.

the volume must include the pterygoid fossa and lateral retropharyngeal node (Fig. 14.4).

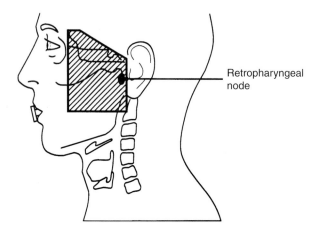

Retropharyngeal node

Fig. 14.4   Margins of the lateral field with shielding to the optic chiasm and hypothalamus.

LOCALIZATION

The patient lies in a supine cast with the head in a neutral position. A mouth-bite is used to depress the tongue and lower lip away from the target volume.

Field arrangements

Anterior and lateral wedged fields are used to cover the target volume. The lateral field is placed so that its anterior margin lies immediately behind the lateral bony margin of the orbit, to avoid the anterior chamber of the ipsilateral eye. It is angled 5–10° posteriorly so that the exit beam avoids the opposite eye (see Fig. 1.18b). The optic chiasm and hypothalamus are shielded from the lateral field unless the skull base is involved. The dose to the contralateral eye is measured with lithium fluoride placed on the outer canthus. Where there is no gross involvement of the orbit, the cornea, lens and lacrimal gland are shielded from the anterior field. If there is disease in the orbit, the eye cannot be shielded, and the cornea is spared by cutting out the cast and treating with the eye open. If there is involvement of the cheek or anterior nasal cavity, an open anterior field may be used to increase the dose to these areas.

To achieve a homogeneous dose throughout the volume, the anterior field is weighted by at least 2:1. The cast is cut out anteriorly to reduce skin reaction over the cheek, unless there is direct tumour involvement, when the cast is used

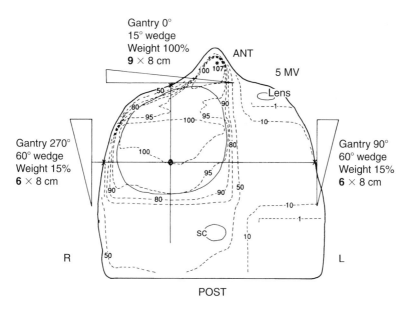

Fig. 14.5 Dose distribution from anterior and two lateral wedged fields with unequal weighting.

as bolus. It may be necessary to add an additional contralateral wedged field (Fig. 14.5) to avoid under-dosing the postero-medial part of the volume when this contains tumour.

Implementation of plan

The patient is treated in a supine cast with a mouth-bite. Anterior and lateral wedged fields are set up isocentrically. The patient is aligned using longitudinal and lateral lasers matched with marks on the cast. A coronal laser is aligned with the transverse outline through the centre of the volume marked on the cast. Films are taken on the first day of treatment to check the position of the shielding.

Dose prescription

66 Gy in 33 fractions given in 6.5 weeks.

Alternative fractionation regimen

55 Gy in 20 fractions given in 4 weeks.

Further reading

Haylock, B.J., John, D.J. and Paterson, I.C.M. 1991: The treatment of squamous cell carcinoma of the paranasal sinuses. *Clinical Oncology* **3**, 17–21.

Jiang, G.L., Ang, K., Peter, L.G., Wendt, C.D., Oswald, M.J. and Goepfert, H. 1991: Maxillary sinus carcinomas: natural history and results of post-operative radiotherapy. *Radiotherapy and Oncology* **21**, 193–200.

Nagata, Y., Okajima, K., Murata, R. *et al.* 1994: Three-dimensional treatment planning for maxillary cancer using a CT simulator. *International Journal of Radiation Oncology, Biology and Physics* **30**, 979–83.

CHAPTER 15

Orbit

Role of radiotherapy

Radiotherapy has an important role to play in the treatment of the wide variety of tumours which arise in the orbit and intra-ocular structures. For retinoblastoma, lesions between 4 and 13 mm may be treated with radioactive plaques, whereas larger single or multiple tumours are treated with external beam radiotherapy. Postoperative treatment is given after enucleation if disease extends into the orbital contents. For rhabdomyosarcoma, radiation may be needed to ensure local control if chemotherapy does not produce complete regression. For lymphomas, local control is always achieved with radiotherapy, but chemotherapy is given for tumours with aggressive histology in order to prevent systemic relapse. Surgery is used for carcinoma of the lacrimal gland, melanoma and sarcomas of the orbit, with postoperative radiotherapy if excision is incomplete. Some uveal melanomas may be suitable for treatment with radioactive plaques or protons. The prognosis for these very rare tumours is generally poor. Palliative radiotherapy is useful for painful orbital metastases, and to prevent loss of vision from choroidal metastases.

Radiation to the posterior orbit can be helpful in patients with dysthyroid eye disease, and can help to prevent blindness from macular degeneration associated with neovascular membrane formation.

Regional anatomy

The globe, rectus muscles, optic nerve and connective tissue lie in a pyramidal space within the bony walls of the orbit, as shown in Fig. 15.1. True lymphatics are only present in the eyelids, conjunctiva and lacrimal gland, draining primarily to the pre-auricular and submaxillary nodes.

Planning technique

ASSESSMENT OF PRIMARY DISEASE

Both orbits are examined for palpable tumour and signs of proptosis or displacement of the globe. The appearance of the fundi, visual acuity, visual fields

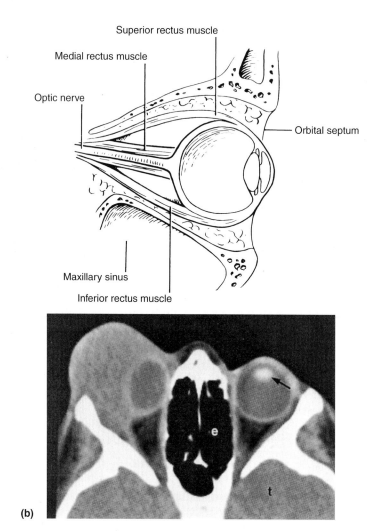

Fig. 15.1 (a) Sagittal section of orbit. (b) Transverse CT scan showing rhabdomyosarcoma of the right orbit and normal anatomy of the left orbit including lens (arrowed). e = ethmoid; t = temporal lobe.

and eye movements are assessed. Cranial nerve function is tested and the nose and nasopharynx are examined for tumour extension. The neck is palpated to exclude lymphatic involvement, particularly of the pre-auricular and upper deep cervical nodes. Plain X-rays are used to show bony erosion. Ultrasound may be useful, but CT scanning delineates the soft-tissue extension of orbital tumours more clearly. Biopsy is essential to provide a histological diagnosis, except for orbital metastases from a known primary tumour (and retinoblastoma where biopsy increases the risk of tumour seeding).

DEFINITION OF TARGET VOLUME

The target volume depends on the exact position of the tumour within the orbit, its local extensions and patterns of spread. Irradiation of the cornea and lens must be avoided wherever possible. Doses of more than 50 Gy to the cornea will cause painful acute reactions and subsequent blindness. Irradiation of the lacrimal and secretory glands to doses above 30 Gy causes a dry eye. Cataract may be produced by doses of more than 6 Gy to the lens, and optic nerve damage may result if doses to the optic chiasma exceed 55 Gy. These limits are for doses given with conventional 2-Gy daily fractionation. Doses to the pituitary gland should be minimized.

LOCALIZATION

Patients are treated in a supine cast with the chin vertical. The outer margins of the lateral orbital walls or bony canthus are marked on the cast, the target volume is chosen and a transverse outline is taken through the centre of the volume. The margins of the bony orbit and the position of the lens and pituitary fossa (the bony landmark for the optic chiasma) are drawn on to the outline using CT scan data and AP and lateral simulator films (Fig. 15.2).

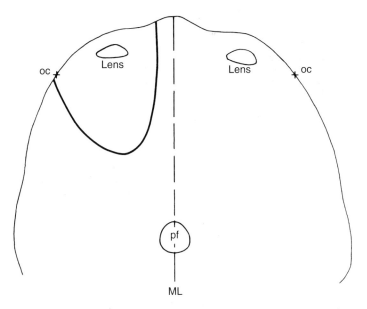

Fig. 15.2 Localization of the target volume, lens and pituitary fossa. pf = pituitary fossa; ML = mid-line; oc = outer bony canthus.

Field arrangements

Techniques depend on the position of the tumour in relation to sensitive normal structures.

SUPERFICIAL TUMOURS

Small, anterior lymphomatous lesions can be treated with a single anterior field using 150–300 kV X-rays chosen according to tumour depth. A thin cylindrical shield is placed in the beam to protect the cornea. This is possible with a diaphragm system of field definition, but not if applicators are used. Electron therapy is not usually employed because of lateral scatter to the contralateral eye, but this can be reduced by a 3- to 4-mm lead face mask which covers that eye.

EXTRACONAL TUMOURS WITH AN INTACT EYE

Most lymphomas, pseudotumours, rhabdomyosarcomas and lacrimal gland tumours arise extraconally and are treated with wedged anterior and lateral fields. The lateral field is positioned with its anterior border at the outer bony canthus of the affected eye so that it lies behind the cornea and lens. It is angled 5–10° posteriorly to avoid irradiation of the opposite lens by the exit beam. To

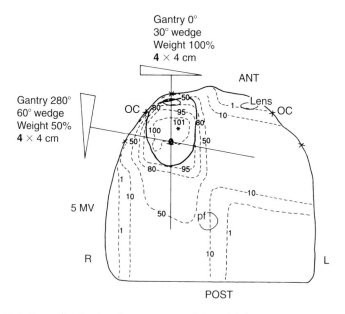

Fig. 15.3 Dose distribution for treatment of the orbit from an anterior and a lateral field weighted 2:1.

ensure adequate dosage to the antero-medial part of the volume, the anterior to lateral field weighting is at least 2:1 (Fig. 15.3).

The cornea and lens are shielded during irradiation of the anterior field by a narrow lead cylinder as shown in Fig. 15.4. This reduces the dose to the

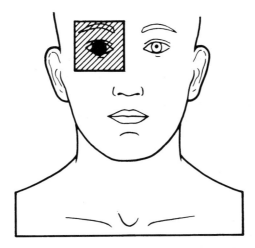

Fig. 15.4 Anterior field with shadow cast by corneal shield.

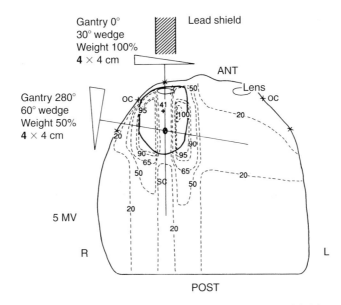

Fig. 15.5 Dose distribution from anterior and lateral wedged fields with lead shielding to the cornea.

posterior orbit behind the globe (Fig. 15.5), and is only used in cases where there is no risk of involvement within the muscle cone. This dose reduction is more marked with a linear accelerator than with a cobalt unit, because of the difference in penumbra.

After enucleation or exenteration, care must be taken to preserve vision in the remaining eye by avoiding radiation damage to the optic chiasm and contra-lateral optic nerve. The lateral field can be positioned further anteriorly to give a more homogeneous distribution, as shown in Fig. 15.6.

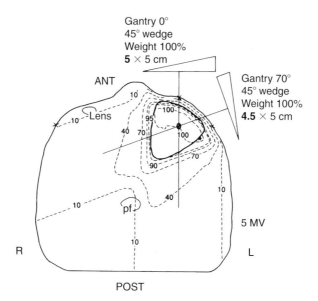

Fig. 15.6   Field arrangement following enucleation or exenteration of the orbit.

TUMOURS WITH DISPLACEMENT OF THE GLOBE

The technique described in Fig. 15.3 may not be suitable for patients with gross proptosis or lateral displacement of the globe from tumours situated antero-medially, e.g. those arising from the lacrimal sac or medial canthus. It is also inappropriate if there is involvement of the muscle cone posteriorly. Superior and inferior oblique wedged fields in the sagittal plane are used, as shown in Fig. 15.7. The cornea may be shielded from either field depending on the posi-tion of the tumour. If corneal shielding is inadvisable, the cast is cut out and the patient is instructed to keep the eye open during treatment to ensure maximum skin-sparing effect, and to reduce the risk of corneal complications. The lens lies at a depth of approximately 7 mm and is not spared, so future cataract is likely. However, vision can usually be restored by lens extraction.

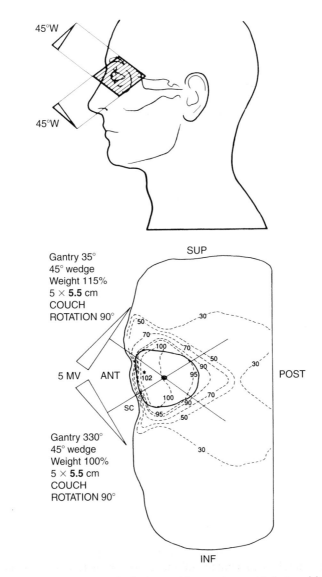

(a)

(b)

Fig. 15.7 (a) Treatment in a sagittal plane with superior and inferior oblique wedged fields. (b) Dose distribution for the same arrangement.

POSTERIOR TUMOURS

For intraconal lymphoma, retinoblastoma, choroidal metastases and pseudo-tumour or malignant exophthalmos, where disease is limited to the posterior orbit, a single lateral field or a pair of lateral fields may be used. These are placed so that the anterior margin does not extend beyond the outer bony canthus, and they are angled 5–10° posteriorly to avoid the opposite lens, as shown in Fig. 15.8.

In patients with less radiosensitive intraconal tumours, such as sarcomas or melanomas, where a higher tumour dose is needed, treatment is given in the coronal plane to avoid high-dose irradiation of the brain. Superior and inferior oblique wedged fields are used and angled to avoid the contralateral eye and optic nerve, as shown in Fig. 15.9.

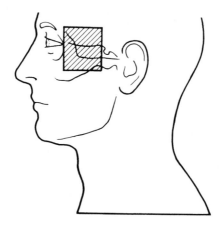

Fig. 15.8 Position of lateral field for treatment of the posterior orbit.

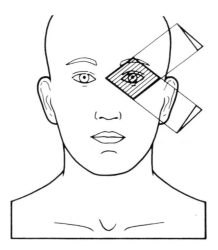

Fig. 15.9 Treatment in the coronal plane using superior and inferior oblique wedged fields.

DYSTHYROID EYE DISEASE

It is usually necessary to treat both eyes with parallel opposed lateral fields as shown in Fig. 15.8. The exit dose to the contralateral lens can be reduced either by a half-beam block or by posterior angulation of the fields by 5–10°.

MACULAR DEGENERATION

A lateral 4 × 4 cm field with the anterior margin at the outer bony canthus, as shown in Fig. 15.8, is used with either posterior angulation or a half-beam block. Smaller fields can be used, but are not readily available. The dose is prescribed to the macula, which is 3 to 4 cm from the skin surface over the temple, and is most accurately located by performing a CT scan with the patient in a perspex cast.

Implementation of plan

The patient is treated in a supine cast, with lateral fields set up at the machine FSD and other techniques isocentrically. When corneal shielding is used, the patient should look at the beam, and the shadow cast by the lead cylinder is checked on the cornea. The dose to the anterior chamber of the opposite eye is measured using lithium fluoride thermoluminescent dosimetry.

Dose prescription

Retinoblastoma

Plaque

40 Gy given to apex.

External beam

40 Gy in 20 fractions given in 4 weeks.

Rhabdomyosarcoma

45 Gy in 25 fractions given in 5 weeks.

Lymphoma

30 Gy in 15 fractions given in 3 weeks (low grade).

40 Gy in 20 fractions given in 4 weeks (high grade).

Pseudotumour

24 Gy in 12 fractions given in 2.5 weeks.

Melanoma

Plaques

70–100 Gy.

External beam

50 Gy in 25 fractions given in 5 weeks.

Protons

70 Gy in 5 fractions given in 1 week.

Carcinoma of the lacrimal gland

60 Gy in 30 fractions given in 6 weeks

or 50 Gy in 20 fractions given in 4 weeks.

Dysthyroid eye disease

20 Gy in 10 fractions given in 2 weeks.

Macular degeneration

12–18 Gy in 6–9 fractions daily given in 2 weeks.

Further reading

Bessell, E.M., Henk, J.M., Wright, J.E. and Whitelock, R.A.F. 1988: Orbital and conjunctival lymphoma treatment and prognosis. *Radiotherapy and Oncology* **13**, 237–44.

Chakravarthy, U., Houston, R.F. and Archer, D.B. 1993: Treatment of age-related sub-foveal neovascular membranes by teletherapy: a pilot study. *British Journal of Ophthalmology* **77**, 265–73.

Hungerford, J.L. and Plowman, P.N. 1995: Ocular and adnexal tumours. In Price, P. and Sikora, K. (eds), *Treatment of cancer,* 3rd edn. London: Chapman and Hall, 249–70.

CHAPTER 16

Skin and lip

SKIN

Role of radiotherapy

In many instances, skin lesions can be equally effectively managed by surgery or radiotherapy, with high cure rates of 90 to 95 per cent, and other factors such as patient preference and convenience may tend to influence choice of treatment.

Indications for surgery include the following:

- small lesions amenable to simple excision and direct closure – this is quick, safe and usually gives a good cosmetic result and the highest cure rate;
- younger patients (<50–60 years) where the potential for deterioration of a radiation scar with time (>5–10 years) may detract significantly from the long-term cosmetic result;
- larger lesions involving cartilage, tendon, joint or bone, where the risk of radionecrosis is higher, and bulky lesions that are readily amenable to surgery without loss of function, and which would have a lower cure rate with radiotherapy;
- lesions where there is uncertainty about disease extent or histology even after biopsy;
- lesions that recur after radiotherapy.

Relative indications for radiotherapy include the following:

- older patients, if long-term atrophy caused by radiotherapy may not be considered relevant;
- large superficial lesions where extensive surgical repair is required for a relatively minor clinical problem and would give a poorer cosmetic result than radiotherapy;
- multiple (especially superficial) lesions where surgery would be onerous for the patient;
- patients who refuse surgery, are unfit or are on anti-coagulation therapy;
- larger lesions where surgery would cause major loss of function such as paralysis, numbness, mouth dribbling and eyelid ectropion, or extensive lesions where mutilation such as nasectomy, ear amputation and eye enucleation may be avoided;

• recurrent lesions after surgery, incomplete surgical excision, perineural invasion and poor-prognosis nodal metastatic spread.

The use of superficial X-ray therapy (SXRT) for small lesions can give excellent cosmetic results, and may be ideal in small concave contours such as inner canthus and ala nasi. Radiation changes may be more noticeable on flat or larger convex contours such as the forehead. Curative radiotherapy causes permanent epilation, and in scalp, eyebrow and eyelash regions this can be an important consideration. Around the eye lacrimal gland dryness, upper eyelid conjuctival keratinization and nasolacrimal duct stenosis can be complications of radiotherapy, and consequently it should be avoided in this area unless an alternative treatment would produce even more problems. Some sites, such as the lower leg and back, present particular problems for all treatment modalities. Lower leg lesions are usually better managed with surgery, but this may be unacceptable for older patients.

Small-diameter lesions (0.5–2 cm and less than 5 mm thick) are best treated with superficial X-ray therapy. Lesions that are more than 4 cm in diameter and which are not near the eyes or complicated air spaces (e.g. nasal cavity, sinuses, mastoid air cells) should be considered for electron beam therapy. Eye shielding is difficult with electron beam therapy because of lateral scatter of radiation. Complex or tangential contours and inhomogeneity of tissues can lead to unsatisfactory dose distributions. However, electron beam therapy is often ideal for large, flat, relatively superficial treatment volumes on the trunk, limbs and scalp. Bolus material (such as wax or perspex) is used to increase the skin surface dose to 100 per cent or to compensate for an irregular contour such as the nose. Electron therapy can be used to give a greater depth dose with appropriate energy for large or thick lesions or those with a high risk of deep penetration between tissue planes, such as the postauricular area.

Interstitial implantation is indicated in special circumstances. Local control and cosmetic results are excellent and treatment can be completed within 5 or 6 days, although hospital admission is necessary. The major indication is for tumours which lie in a curved plane (e.g. in the nasolabial fold or on a finger), and where stand-off of the applicator hinders superficial therapy.

Recurrent skin tumours are treated with surgical excision. Moh's technique of micrographically controlled surgery is particularly useful in this situation and for large morphoeic tumours.

Planning technique

ASSESSMENT OF DISEASE

Biopsy is always essential for obtaining a histological diagnosis. The limits of the skin tumour should be established by careful palpation and examination under a strong light. A magnifying glass may help to define the edges of 'morphoeic' lesions. The depth of the tumour must be assessed, particularly at sites such as the inner canthus where deep tumour infiltration along the medial border of the orbit may occur. Deep penetration of tumour may also occur at the nasolabial fold, ala nasi, tragus and postauricular area, and adequate margins at depth are essential for these sites, which have the highest risk of recurrence. Regional lymph-node areas must be examined in order to exclude involvement, which may occur with squamous cell carcinomas.

DEFINITION OF TARGET VOLUME

A margin must be allowed around the tumour to encompass subclinical extension into surrounding tissues. This depends on tumour size, morphology, histology and aggressiveness, and on evidence of perineural infiltration. If the tumour is less than 0.5 cm in diameter, cystic or superficial with a well-defined edge, margins of 5–8 mm are satisfactory, but for large lesions margins of 1 cm or more may be needed. An additional margin must be allowed for electron therapy because of the shape of the isodose curves. The depth of the lesion is estimated and the same margin allowed to define the depth of the base of the target volume. CT scanning may be useful in planning treatment of large lesions.

TREATMENT TECHNIQUE

The margin around the lesion is drawn on the skin by the radiotherapist, the depth of the tumour is estimated, and an appropriate beam energy is chosen.

Mould room

Sheets of lead with the area for treatment cut out are used to protect the surrounding skin (Fig. 16.1). For volumes of regular shape, standard lead cut-outs may be used, or the applicator may be applied directly to the skin surface. The thickness of the lead depends on the energy of the beam used: 1.5 mm is adequate for 90–150 kV and 4 mm is used for electrons up to 10 MeV. Individualized cut-outs may be required, and cosmetic results may be improved by using serrated edges and rotating the cut-out slightly each day. Secondary electrons produced by X-ray absorption in the lead may be absorbed with plastic on the inner surface of the cut-out. For electron therapy, wax is added to the lead mask over the cut-out area to provide build-up of dose at the skin.

Shielding

When lesions of the eyelids and inner or outer canthus are treated, a lead shield must be used to protect the eye. An internal lead eye shield, shaped like a large contact lens, is commonly used to protect the conjunctiva, cornea and lens (Fig. 16.2a). These shields are available in various sizes and are shaped differently for the left and right eyes.

Alternatively, a spade-shaped eye shield may be used, which is placed under the upper or lower eyelid. This type of shield also protects the conjunctiva, cornea and lens, as illustrated in Fig. 16.2b, and is easier to use.

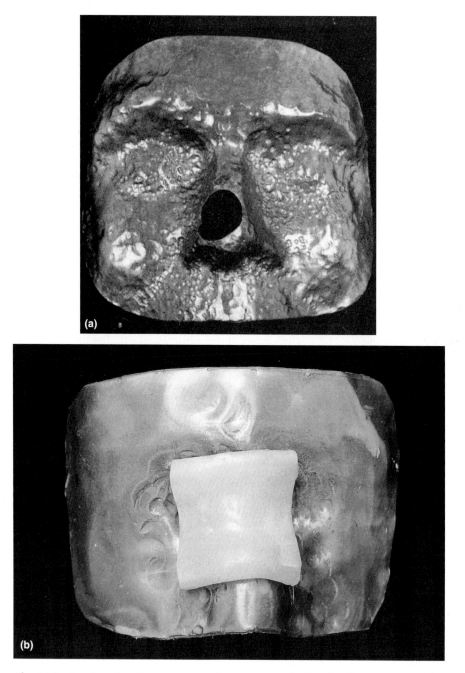

Fig. 16.1 Lead mask with area cut out for treatment of a basal cell carcinoma of the nose (a) for superficial X-ray therapy and (b) with wax bolus for electron treatment.

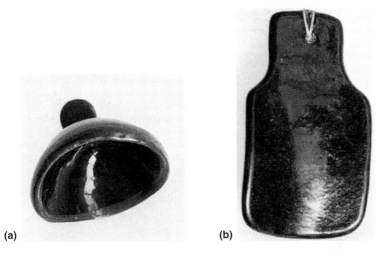

(a)   (b)

Fig. 16.2   (a) Internal lead eye shield. (b) Spade-shaped eye shield.

The eye shields are inserted using local anaesthetic eye drops and sterile lubricant to prevent discomfort and abrasion of the cornea. A completely sterile technique is essential. The patient is instructed to wear an eye pad for 2 h after insertion of the shield, until the effect of the local anaesthetic is reversed and the corneal reflex is restored.

When lesions of the ala nasi are treated, an intranasal lead shield is needed to protect the mucosa and cartilage of the nasal septum from irradiation. The shield is wrapped in a finger cot before it is inserted into the nostril.

Treatment machine

SUPERFICIAL X-RAY THERAPY

Most superficial lesions are treated with 80–150 kV X-rays with appropriate filtration which defines the beam characteristics. Percentage depth doses for different field diameters and energies are obtained from tables drawn up for each therapy unit, and an appropriate energy is selected to encompass the target volume with the 90 per cent isodose (Table 16.1).

ELECTRON THERAPY

For electron therapy, field sizes smaller than 4 cm should not be used because the advantage of beam flatness is lost. The chart shown in Fig. 1.19 gives the physical characteristics of some electron beams. The energy of electron therapy (4–15 MeV) is chosen so that the target volume is encompassed by the 90 per

Table 16.1 Sample percentage depth dose data for 80 kV (HVL = 2.0 mm aluminium)

15-cm SSD

Applicator (cm)	1.0	1.5	2.0	2.5	3.0	3.5	4.0	4.5	5.0
Equivalent diameter (cm)*	1.0	1.5	2.0	2.5	3.0	3.5	4.0	4.5	5.0
BSF†	1.06	1.09	1.11	1.12	1.14	1.15	1.16	1.17	1.18

Depth (cm)									
0	100	100	100	100	100	100	100	100	100
0.5	76	78	80	81	82	83	84	84	85
1.0	58	61	64	66	68	69	71	71	72
2.0	37	40	42	44	46	48	49	50	51
3.0	24	26	28	30	32	33	34	35	36
4.0	16	18	19	21	22	23	23	24	25
5.0	11	12	13	14	15	16	17	17	18
6.0	8	9	10	10	11	12	12	13	13
7.0	6	6	7	7	8	8	9	9	10
8.0	4	5	5	5	6	6	7	7	7
9.0	3	3	4	4	4	5	5	5	6
10.0	2	2	3	3	3	4	4	4	4

25-cm SSD

Applicator (cm)	6.0	8.0	10.0	12.0	15.0	8 × 10	10 × 15
Equivalent diameter (cm)*	6.0	8.0	10.0	12.0	15.0	9.9	13.3
BSF†	1.20	1.22	1.24	1.25	1.26	1.24	1.26

Depth (cm)							
0	100	100	100	100	100	100	100
0.5	87	88	89	90	90	89	90
1.0	76	78	79	80	81	79	80
2.0	57	59	60	61	62	60	61
3.0	42	44	45	46	48	45	47
4.0	30	32	34	35	37	34	36
5.0	22	25	26	28	29	26	28
6.0	17	19	21	22	23	21	22
7.0	13	15	16	17	19	16	18
8.0	10	12	13	14	15	13	14
9.0	8	9	10	11	12	10	11
10.0	6	7	8	8	9	8	9

*Equivalent diameter of cut-out treatment area.
†BSF, back scatter factor.

cent isodose with a sharp fall in dose beyond, as shown in Fig. 1.20. This characteristic of the electron beam spares underlying tissues. The effective treatment depth expressed in centimetres is about one-third of the beam energy in MeV, depending on field size. Bolus is used for an irregular contour and to increase the skin surface dose to 100 per cent. This must be taken into account when calculating the depth of the target volume from the surface and choosing an electron energy.

Implementation of plan

The patient lies on the treatment couch wearing the lead mask or cut-out, against which an applicator of the appropriate diameter is positioned to cover the area to be treated. Because of curving body contours, it may not be possible to appose the applicator of the machine to the mask. The SSD will be increased or decreased by the amount of 'stand-off' between the applicator and the lesion (Fig. 16.3). For superficial X-ray therapy, allowance must therefore be made for the change in output with variation in SSD according to the inverse square law.

Tables for superficial X-ray therapy are available which give multiplication factors to correct for different amounts of both positive and negative 'stand-off' (Table 16.2).

SAMPLE CALCULATION FOR SUPERFICIAL X-RAY THERAPY

For an applicator 3 cm in diameter, lead cut-out 2 cm in diameter, positive stand-off of 0.5 cm treating at 80 kV (HVL = 2.0 mm aluminium) and 15-cm SSD with a daily fraction size of 4.5 Gy.

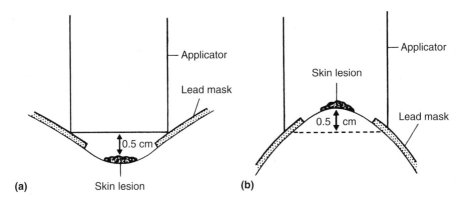

Fig 16.3   (a) Positive stand-off of 0.5 cm between lesion and applicator. (b) Negative stand-off of 0.5 cm.

Table 16.2 Multiplication correction factors for stand-off

Stand-off distance (cm)	15-cm SSD applicator	25-cm SSD applicator
−1.5	1.23	1.13
−1.0	1.15	1.09
−0.5	1.07	1.04
0.0	1.00	1.00
0.5	0.94	0.96
1.0	0.88	0.92
1.5	0.83	0.89
2.0	0.78	0.86
2.5	0.73	0.83
3.0	0.69	0.80
3.5	0.66	0.77
4.0	0.62	0.74
4.5	0.59	0.72
5.0	0.56	0.69

Table 16.3 Sample table for calculation of surface dose rate for a given applicator size and treatment time in minutes (energy = 80 kV, HVL = 2.0 mm aluminium, filtration = 1.7 mm)

Applicator size (cm)	Surface dose rate (Gy/min)	Treatment time (min) for varying doses (Gy)							
		1	4	5	6	6.25	6.3	8	9
15-cm SSD applicators									
1.0 circle	2.46	0.41	1.62	2.03	2.44	2.54	2.56	3.25	3.66
1.5 circle	2.56	0.39	1.56	1.95	2.34	2.44	2.46	3.13	3.52
2.0 circle	2.64	0.38	1.51	1.89	2.27	2.36	2.38	3.03	3.40
2.5 circle	2.75	0.36	1.46	1.82	2.19	2.28	2.29	2.91	3.28
3.0 circle	2.81	0.36	1.42	1.78	2.14	2.22	2.24	2.85	3.20
3.5 circle	2.84	0.35	1.41	1.76	2.12	2.20	2.22	2.82	3.17
4.0 circle	2.87	0.35	1.39	1.74	2.09	2.18	2.19	2.79	3.13
4.5 circle	2.91	0.34	1.37	1.72	2.06	2.14	2.16	2.75	3.09
5.0 circle	2.93	0.34	1.37	1.71	2.05	2.14	2.15	2.73	3.07
25-cm SSD applicators									
6.0 circle	1.03	0.97	3.89	4.87	5.84	6.08	6.13	7.79	8.76
8.0 circle	1.06	0.95	3.78	4.73	5.67	5.91	5.96	7.56	8.51
10.0 circle	1.09	0.92	3.68	4.60	5.51	5.74	5.79	7.35	8.27
12.0 circle	1.10	0.90	3.62	4.52	5.43	5.65	5.70	7.24	8.14
15.0 circle	1.11	0.90	3.59	4.48	5.38	5.61	5.65	7.18	8.07

Formula

Using data from tables which incorporate back scatter factor (BSF) for size of applicator and treatment area and surface dose rates and treatment times, the treatment time can be calculated (Table 16.3).

Beam data	Surface dose rate (SDR)	= 2.64 Gy/min	(Table 16.3)
	% DD	= 100%	(Table 16.1)
	BSF (3 cm)	= 1.14	(Table 16.1)
	BSF (2 cm)	= 1.11	(Table 16.1)
	Stand-off correction factor (SOF)	= 0.94	(Table 16.2)

Calculation

$$\text{Output (Gy/min)} = \text{SDR} \times \frac{\text{BSF (cut-out)}}{\text{BSF (applicator)}} \times \text{SOF} \times \frac{\% \text{ DD}}{100}$$

$$\text{Output (Gy/min)} = 2.64 \times \frac{1.11}{1.14} \times 0.94 \times \frac{100\%}{100}$$

$$\text{Treatment time per fraction} = \frac{4.5}{2.57} = 1.75 \text{ min}$$
$$= 1 \text{ min } 45 \text{ sec}$$

When there is no stand-off and no cut-out, the treatment time in minutes can be read directly from tables (Table 16.3).

For electron therapy, a correction is made for stand-off between the applicator and skin surface by using the inverse square law and an effective SSD (read from tables for varying electron energy and applicator size).

Dose prescription

The daily dose and fractionation scheme depend on the site and size of the lesion, the histology and the age of the patient. Doses are specified at D_{max} which, for electrons, may be obtained at the skin surface by the addition of wax build-up. To ensure that the base of the lesion is adequately treated, energies are chosen which will include the target volume within the 90 to 95 per cent isodose.

Many different regimens have been shown to be effective and are in widespread use. The treatment regimen should be chosen to produce optimum cure rates with least normal tissue damage. Factors such as patient age and convenience may then also be taken into account.

Basal cell or squamous cell carcinoma

1. Lesions of diameter less than 3 cm

Superficial X-ray therapy

      40–45 Gy in 10–12 fractions given in 2 to 2.5 weeks

  or 36 Gy in 8 fractions given in 17 days

  or 30–32 Gy in 4 fractions given in 2 to 4 weeks

  or 18–22 Gy in a single fraction.

Fewer fractions or alternate-day regimens are used for elderly patients for whom travelling is difficult.

2. Large lesions (more than 3 cm in diameter) or special situations (nose, pinna, lower leg or poorly vascularized skin)

Electron therapy

      50 Gy in 20 fractions given in 28 days (optimum cosmesis)

  or 45 Gy in 9–15 fractions given in 21 days.

3. Large (greater than 5 cm) usually squamous cell carcinomas

Electron therapy or megavoltage irradiation

      60 Gy in 30 fractions given in 6 weeks

  or 50 Gy in 20 fractions given in 4 weeks.

Patient care

Scabs over the lesion may need to be removed before treatment to ensure adequate depth dose. Skin should be kept dry, and shaving or the application of make-up and chemicals to the area should be avoided. Acute erythema is treated with aqueous cream or soft paraffin. If the skin becomes broken, paraffin gauze or hydrogel is applied with a dry dressing. Vaseline can be used inside the nostril to help prevent scabbing and nose bleeds. Patients should be advised to avoid exposure to cold winds and sun, to use ultraviolet sun barrier cream, and to wear a hat.

Brachytherapy

For tumours in a curved plane, a small interstitial implant may give a more homogeneous dose. The majority of tumours can be encompassed by a single-plane implant using the plastic tube technique. The target volume must be identified on the skin and the number and position of the sources planned. When using the Paris system, the thickness of the treated volume is approximately 50 per cent of the separation between the sources, and this must be taken into account when planning the source geometry. Hollow stainless steel guides are placed underneath the skin, lying parallel and covering the target volume. These guides are replaced by hollow plastic tubing which must be sufficiently long to allow active wire to be loaded so that it extends 5–10 mm distal to the limits of the target volume for adequate dose distribution. Solder wire is put into the tubes and radiographs are taken for dosimetry. The active iridium wire can then be inserted into the tubes and fixed in place with lead crimps.

For implants around the face, a miniaturization of the plastic tube technique has been developed using a prolene suture beneath the skin. This suture is threaded down a pre-loaded inner plastic tubing which is clamped to the proximal end and then drawn through to lie underneath the skin.

Dose prescription

65 Gy to the 85 per cent reference isodose using the Paris system.

LIP

Role of radiotherapy

Carcinomas of the lip most commonly arise on the vermilion border of the lower lip, they are invariably squamous cell or carcinoma *in situ,* and they are diagnosed early as T_1 and T_2 tumours. Wedge excision of small lesions of the lower vermilion gives excellent results. Radical radiotherapy is the treatment of choice for larger lesions, either with interstitial implantation or with external beam electron therapy. Interstitial therapy gives excellent cosmetic and functional results with a short overall treatment time, and it achieves local control rates of 95 to 98 per cent. It is particularly suitable for young patients, but necessitates hospitalization. Because of the good blood supply to the lip, it is possible to use implants for radical salvage treatment after failure of previous external irradiation. Surgical removal of lesions is effective, but rarely results in such good cosmesis.

Regional anatomy

The outer skin of the lip has a good vascular supply and heals better than commissure areas. Tumours of the lip spread superficially and only at a late stage may infiltrate deeply or invade the mandible and involve cervical nodes (particularly the submandibular). Carcinomas of the commissure and inner mucosa behave like buccal lesions and have a poor prognosis. Lymph-node metastases occur late, with only 8 per cent involvement at presentation.

Planning technique

ASSESSMENT OF DISEASE

The borders of the lesion are assessed by examination with a bright light and palpation of both surfaces of the lip. A margin greater than 1 cm is required for the target volume if the lesion is infiltrative or has poorly defined borders. Commissure lesions tend to extend along the buccal mucosa, and the inner mucosa of the lips and oral cavity must be examined carefully. The neck is palpated for lymph-node metastases, particularly in the submental, submandibular and deep cervical node areas.

BRACHYTHERAPY

The majority of tumours can be treated with a template technique using rigid needles implanted horizontally along the axis of the lip. The target volume should include the tumour plus a 1-cm margin around it, and the active length of implanted wires will need to be greater than this to take into account non-crossing of ends. This means that in most patients almost the whole length of the lip is implanted. For superficial tumours a single plane may be sufficient, but for more deeply infiltrating lesions, three or more sources may be necessary (Fig. 16.4a). The distribution of sources in the central plane may be either that of an equilateral triangle (Fig. 16.4b) or a square, with further sources added if necessary to follow extension of the tumour down the lip. The separation between sources is usually 10–15 mm, and the source length is usually 5–8 cm.

ELECTRON BEAM THERAPY

The tumour volume is determined by inspection and palpation, and a 1.5- to 2-cm margin is included in the target volume to allow for reduced dosage at the edge of the electron beam. Field sizes of less than 4 cm in diameter should not be used because of loss of beam flatness, and in the case of very small lesions, interstitial implantation should be considered.

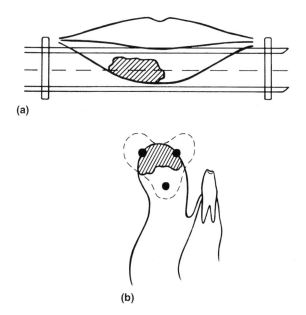

(a)

(b)

Fig. 16.4 Three-source implant for carcinoma of the lip. (a) Anterior view. (b) Sagittal view showing arrangement of sources in an equilateral triangle.

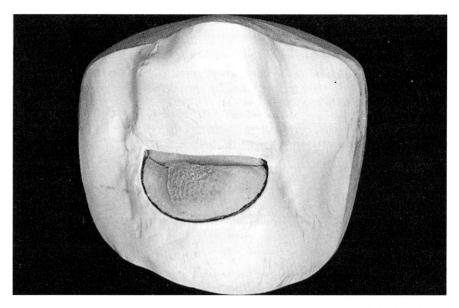

Fig. 16.5 Lead mask used for treating carcinoma of the lower lip with electrons.

A lead mask is constructed in the mould room using lead of 3–4 mm thickness (6–10 MeV electrons) with a cut-out delineating the treatment area (Fig. 16.5). An intra-oral lead shield is used to protect the gums and teeth from the exit beam of irradiation, and is inserted behind the lip and lined with wax to absorb secondary electrons. A single anterior electron field is used, with the energy chosen in the range 6–10 MeV according to the thickness of the lesion to encompass the target volume with the 90 per cent isodose in all planes, using 5–7 mm build-up if necessary to increase the surface dose.

Dose prescription

BRACHYTHERAPY

65 Gy to the 85 per cent reference isodose according to the Paris system.

ELECTRON THERAPY

65 Gy in 32 fractions given in 6.5 weeks.

Alternative fractionation regimen

50–55 Gy in 20 fractions given in 4 weeks.

Patient care

Mucositis of the inner lip or buccal mucosa may be troublesome. The lips should be kept well moisturized with white soft paraffin. If the skin becomes broken, hydrogel is used with a dry dressing. The lip must be protected from sunburn and tobacco irritation following treatment.

Secondary skin metastases

Simple field arrangements may be used to control locally troublesome skin metastases which are fungating, bleeding or painful. Beam quality and energy are chosen according to the size, site and thickness of the lesion.

SUPERFICIAL X-RAY THERAPY OR ELECTRON THERAPY

8 Gy given as a single fraction

or 20 Gy in 5 fractions given in 1 week.

Kaposi's sarcoma

Nodular localized disease can be treated with single doses of radiotherapy to good effect. Widespread lower limb skin involvement is treated with a 'waterbath' megavoltage photon technique. Mucosal lesions (such as mouth and conjunctiva) are best treated with fractionated courses to avoid radiation reactions, which appear to be more severe in patients with HIV-associated Kaposi's sarcoma.

ELECTRON THERAPY

8 Gy given as a single fraction.

This dose can be repeated if necessary and multiple lesions treated.

SUPERFICIAL X-RAY THERAPY

15 Gy in 3 fractions in 5 days.

'Classic' non-AIDS-related disease may require higher doses such as 16 Gy in 4 fractions given over 8 days.

Mucosal lesions

20 Gy in 10 fractions given over 2 weeks.

Primary lymphoma of skin (mycosis fungoides)

Psoralens plus ultraviolet A (PUVA) therapy is used for plaques, and whole-body electron therapy can be used for widespread infiltrative lesions. Focal nodular lesions causing symptoms can be treated with localized electron therapy with effective relief of symptoms.

SUPERFICIAL X-RAY THERAPY OR ELECTRON THERAPY DEPENDING ON THICKNESS OF LESION

8 Gy in 2 fractions given in 2 days.

12 Gy in 3 fractions given in 3 days (for thick lesions).

Keloid lesions

Following surgical excison of keloid scars, radiotherapy treatment may be given with superficial X-ray therapy (80 kV) to attempt to prevent the reformation of scar tissue.

9-Gy single fraction given within 24–72 h of surgery.

Malignant melanoma

Primary surgery is the treatment of choice for malignant melanomas of the skin. Radiotherapy may be used for lentigo malignant melanoma (pre-malignant change) in the same doses as those described for malignant skin tumours. Palliative radiotherapy may be given for bone or brain secondaries.

Further reading

Ashby, M.A., Smith, J., Ainslie, J. and McEwan, L. 1989: Treatment of non-melanoma skin cancer at a large Australian center. *Cancer* **63**, 1863–71.

British Institute of Radiology 1996: Central axis depth dose data for use in radiotherapy. *British Journal of Radiology*, Supplement 25. London: British Institute of Radiology.

Russell-Jones, R. and Spittle, M.F. 1996: Management of cutaneous lymphoma. *Baillieres Clinical Haematology* **9**, 743–67.

CHAPTER 17

Thyroid

Role of radiotherapy

The choice of treatment for thyroid tumours depends on the stage and histology of the lesion.

WELL-DIFFERENTIATED PAPILLARY AND FOLLICULAR CARCINOMA

For localized carcinoma, total or near total thyroidectomy is desirable, since these tumours may be multifocal or diffusely infiltrating. If there is palpable lymphadenopathy, or if nodes are discovered during surgery, a modified block dissection of the neck is carried out, leaving the sternomastoid muscle, jugular vein and spinal accessory nerve.

In young female patients (<35 years) with small (<1 cm $T_1N_0M_0$) well-differentiated papillary tumours, the prognosis after subtotal thyroidectomy followed by thyroxine treatment alone is excellent. Ablative doses of radioactive iodine are given to all other patients after surgery. Three months later, a tracer dose of ^{131}I is given and the whole body is scanned. If metastases are demonstrated, further therapeutic doses are given. External beam radiation is rarely required except when local extension prevents complete surgical removal. However, in older patients with poorly differentiated tumours, surgery tends to be less complete, iodine uptake may be inefficient and external beam radiation is more often required.

ANAPLASTIC CARCINOMA

These tumours are typically inoperable and are treated by high-dose external beam radiation for palliation. Iodine-131 is not concentrated in these tumours. Attempts are being made to improve the poor prognosis by chemotherapy given either alone or in combination with radiotherapy, and by changes in radiotherapy fractionation schedules.

MEDULLARY CARCINOMA

Near total or total thyroidectomy is again the operation of choice, combined with block dissection of the neck if nodes are present. As these tumours do not concentrate radio-iodine, external beam radiation is recommended postoperatively. For advanced tumours, primary radiotherapy may make subsequent excision possible. Somatostatin receptor scintigraphy may be useful for detecting occult metastases, but if these are found the outcome is poor. Early diagnosis and aggressive surgery of the primary tumour with radiotherapy are the most important factors for cure.

NON-HODGKIN'S LYMPHOMA

Most patients present with bulky localized disease (stage IE or IIE) which may be difficult to distinguish from anaplastic carcinoma without immunocytochemistry. Local radiotherapy will produce cure rates of approximately 40 per cent at 5 years in this group of patients, who are often elderly. For patients with stage IIE disease who are fit, primary chemotherapy followed by local radiotherapy has been shown to give improved 5-year survival rates of 70 per cent.

METASTATIC DISEASE

External beam radiotherapy may be given to patients with disseminated disease for relief of local symptoms from the primary tumour or painful bony metastases. Because of the slow response to treatment with ^{131}I in metastases from follicular thyroid carcinoma, additional treatment with surgery or external beam radiation may be needed in acute situations such as fracture or threatened compression of the spinal cord.

Regional anatomy

The two lobes of the thyroid gland are connected by a thin isthmus which lies immediately in front of the trachea (Fig. 17.1).

Lymphatics drain to the para- and pretracheal lymph nodes and inferiorly into the mediastinum. There is also drainage to the deep cervical chain, which communicates with the supraclavicular region laterally and the submandibular region superiorly (Fig. 17.2).

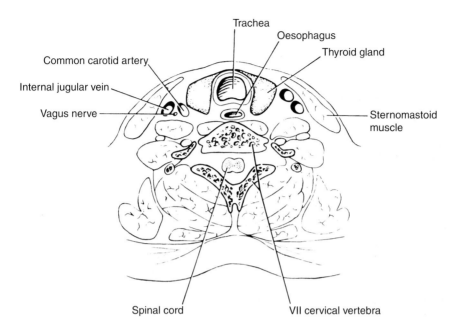

Fig. 17.1 Relationships of the normal thyroid gland shown in transverse section.

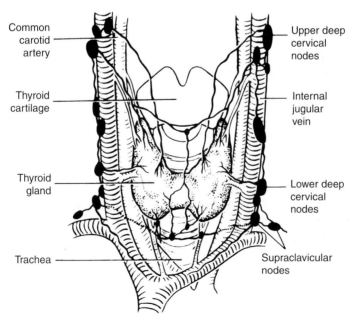

Fig. 17.2 Lymphatic drainage of the thyroid gland.

Planning technique

ASSESSMENT OF PRIMARY DISEASE

Symptoms such as hoarseness, dysphagia and stridor indicate tumour spread outside the thyroid gland to structures such as the recurrent laryngeal nerve, oesophagus and trachea. The neck is palpated to determine local extension of the primary tumour and to detect lymphadenopathy. Indirect laryngoscopy should be performed to exclude recurrent laryngeal nerve palsy. Lateral soft-tissue X-rays of the neck may show calcification or a soft-tissue mass. Ultrasonography or CT scanning may be used to assess the extent of primary disease and lymphadenopathy.

DEFINITION OF TARGET VOLUME

The target volume varies according to the histological type and stage of the tumour, and whether there is lymph-node involvement. The shape of the volume, which curves around the spinal cord, presents a problem for planning if spinal cord tolerance is not to be exceeded. If the entire lymphatic drainage of the thyroid gland is to be included, the volume extends from the tip of the mastoid bone superiorly to the tracheal bifurcation.

LOCALIZATION

Two-dimensional planning

A perspex cast that covers the neck and upper chest from the base of the skull to the mid-thoracic level is made with the patient in the supine position and the chin extended. Any palpable disease in the neck is marked with wire, and AP and lateral films are obtained on the simulator. Transverse outlines are taken at single or multiple levels according to the variation in patient contour within the target volume.

Three-dimensional conformal therapy

CT scans are taken of the patient in the treatment position wearing the immobilization perspex cast. The target volume of the primary tumour and the second volume encompassing lymphadenopathy can be localized in three dimensions, with outlining of the spinal cord throughout its length. Optimization of a plan using non-coplanar beams and three-dimensional dose calculations can be sought, with multileaf collimators used to shape the target volume around the spinal cord. When available, the use of intensity-modulated beams will be particularly useful in this situation, to ensure a homogeneous dose to the curved thyroid target volume while keeping the dose to the spinal cord within tolerance levels.

Well-differentiated carcinoma

WITHOUT LYMPHADENOPATHY

When irradiation is given after incomplete excision, the volume may be confined to the thyroid bed and adjacent lymph nodes bilaterally. The upper and lower margins are the tip of the mastoid bone and sternal notch, respectively. This localized volume can be treated isocentrically using anterior oblique wedged fields as shown in Fig. 17.3.

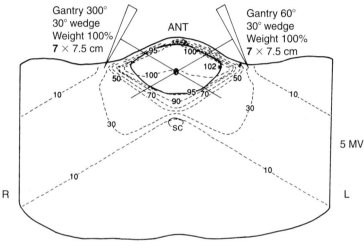

Fig. 17.3 Anterior oblique wedged fields used to treat localized tumour of the thyroid. sc = spinal cord.

WITH LYMPHADENOPATHY

Where carcinoma has spread to the lymph nodes laterally or posterolaterally, the volume envelops the spinal cord whose tolerance therefore limits the tumour dose, which can be given from lateral opposing fields.

The absorption characteristics of a 20-MeV electron beam field give an ideal distribution for treatment of this volume. The addition of build-up material such as wax to the perspex shell in the mid-line anteriorly will alter the position of isodoses, as shown in Fig. 17.4. This reduces the dose to the spinal cord, but gives a 100 per cent dose to the skin relative to the target volume which is defined by the 85 to 90 per cent isodoses. Wax is also placed around the neck to ensure accurate dosimetry at the lateral margins. An alternative technique is to use two anterior fields centred laterally to the spinal cord, each rotating through an arc of 100–120°, as shown in Fig. 17.5.

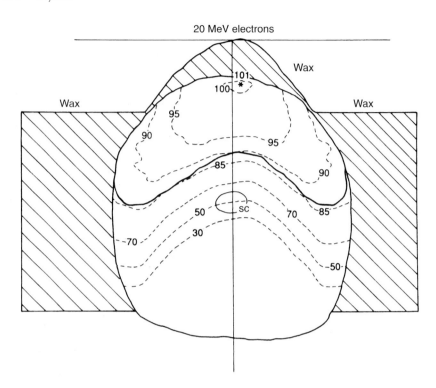

Fig. 17.4 Isodose distribution from an anterior 20 MeV electron beam with additional bolus.

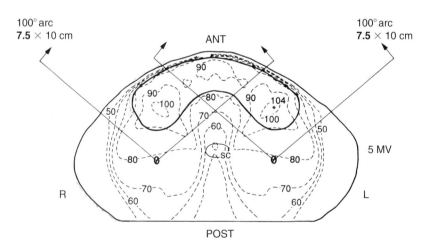

Fig. 17.5 Technique using two anterior fields with a 100° arc.

TUMOUR EXTENSION INTO THE SUPERIOR MEDIASTINUM

For well-differentiated carcinomas with superior mediastinal extension, and for many medullary carcinomas, the target volume must extend inferiorly to include the paratracheal lymph nodes and superior mediastinum. The superior and inferior margins are the tip of the mastoid bone and carina. The lateral margins include the deep cervical nodes bilaterally. In the AP dimension, the field covers the thyroid bed anteriorly, with the posterior margin lying along the front of the spinal cord. The volume slopes, being superficial in the neck and lying in the mid-plane in the mediastinum. This results in inhomogeneity of the dose in the target volume, which may be improved by using a specially designed compensator or a wedge in the supero-inferior dimension. Two anterior oblique wedged fields are then used, arranged to diverge inferiorly as described for the post-cricoid region in Chapter 8.

If good compensation is achieved, the doses at the dose specification points at each level should not vary by more than 5 per cent, and the dose can then be prescribed at the central level.

Anaplastic and poorly differentiated tumours

The target volume for these patients must include the thyroid bed and all lymph nodes in both sides of the neck in continuity with the superior mediastinum, where spread commonly occurs, causing tracheal and oesophageal obstruction.

For palliative irradiation, large anterior and posterior opposing fields are used to cover the neck and mediastinum, with shielding to the lungs as shown in Fig. 17.6. Because of the slope in target volume and body contour, compensation in the supero-inferior direction may be needed as described above. After 40 Gy have been given in 4 weeks, spinal cord shielding is added to the posterior field and treatment continued to a dose of 54 Gy. This may be adequate for palliation, or treatment may be continued to a reduced volume using anterior oblique wedged fields to deliver a higher dose.

Non-Hodgkin's lymphoma

The target volume encompasses the thyroid bed and lymphatic drainage of both sides of the neck, from the mastoid process down to the carina, including the supra- and infra-clavicular and mediastinal lymph nodes. Anterior and posterior opposing fields are used. Shielding is used to protect the oral cavity and lungs, but not the larynx. The spinal cord may be shielded from the posterior field at 20 Gy unless there is bulky mid-line tumour. If a higher dose is required in selected cases, lateral fields may be used for additional treatment. Small antero-lateral fields may be used to give a higher dose to the thyroid gland alone in selected patients.

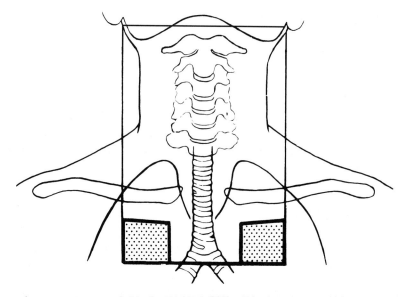

Fig. 17.6 Anterior and posterior fields used to treat anaplastic tumours.

Dose prescription

WELL-DIFFERENTIATED TUMOURS

60 Gy in 30 fractions given in 6 weeks.

Alternative fractionation regimen

50 Gy in 20 fractions given in 4 weeks.

ANAPLASTIC TUMOURS

Initial volume

54 Gy in 27 fractions given in 5.5 weeks.

Reduced volume

10 Gy in 5 fractions given in 1 week.

Total dose of 64 Gy in 32 fractions given in 6.5 weeks in selected patients.

NON-HODGKIN'S LYMPHOMA

35–40 Gy in 20 fractions given in 4 weeks.

Patient care

Mucositis may be treated with mucaine or soluble aspirin. A high fluid intake is encouraged. The skin should be kept dry and 1 per cent hydrocortisone cream used to treat erythematous reactions.

Further reading

O'Connell, M.E.A., A'Hern, R.P. and Harmer, C.L. 1994: Results of external beam radiotherapy in differentiated thyroid carcinoma: a retrospective study from the Royal Marsden Hospital. *European Journal of Cancer* **30A**, 733–9.

Tubiana, M., Haddad, E., Schlumberger, M. *et al*. 1985: External radiotherapy in thyroid cancers. *Cancer* **55**, 2062.

CHAPTER 18

Bronchus

Role of radiotherapy

SMALL-CELL LUNG CANCER (SCLC)

Limited disease (LD)

In patients with good prognostic factors (good performance status, localized disease and normal biochemistry), the 2-year survival rate is approximately 15 per cent, whereas in patients with poor prognostic factors, the 6-month survival rate is 40 to 50 per cent, but 2-year survival is unlikely.

Combination chemotherapy significantly increases survival and quality of life, and is started as soon as possible after diagnosis. Consolidation radiotherapy in patients who achieve a complete response to chemotherapy increases local control and survival rates (by about 5 per cent at 3 years), and is most beneficial in patients with good prognostic factors.

About 50 per cent of patients with SCLC develop brain metastases at some time during their disease, and 10 per cent of these are present at the time of diagnosis. Prophylactic cranial irradiation (PCI) halves the risk of developing brain metastases. It should be offered to those achieving complete remission of primary limited disease with chemotherapy, and in this group it may produce some improvement in survival.

Extensive disease (metastases beyond the mediastinum and supraclavicular nodes)

Complete remissions may be obtained with chemotherapy in 65 to 85 per cent of patients, but are usually short-lived. Radiotherapy does not improve survival, although local control may be improved. The median survival time is 9 months. Local radiotherapy is recommended for palliation.

NON-SMALL-CELL LUNG CANCER (NSCLC)

For non-small-cell lung cancer, postoperative radiotherapy following complete resection of $T_{1-2}N_0$ tumours does not improve local control or survival.

In patients with N_2 tumours or residual disease, postoperative radiotherapy may reduce the incidence of loco-regional relapse but does not improve survival.

In patients for whom surgery is contraindicated for medical reasons, radical radiotherapy can cure a small proportion of cases (< 20 per cent), especially those with small tumours (< 3 cm) treated with high doses (60 Gy or more).

Mediastinal node irradiation is unnecessary for peripheral lesions, and is of uncertain value for central lesions.

Most patients with stage III disease have unresectable bulky T_3 tumours or N_2 or N_3 disease, and have a 5-year survival of approximately 5 per cent. Treatment intent is therefore usually palliative. However, patients with stage IIIa disease have a better median survival of 12 months and a 5-year survival of 15 per cent; if they are of good performance status they may be treated with radical radiotherapy if their lesion is considered inoperable. This group may also benefit from induction chemotherapy before radiotherapy.

PCI is not indicated in non-small-cell lung cancer, where the risk of brain metastases is lower than for SCLC.

PALLIATIVE RADIOTHERAPY

For tumours of any histological type, palliative radiotherapy may give useful symptomatic relief of dyspnoea, dysphagia, haemoptysis or pain related to local disease. Brain and bone metastases are also effectively palliated with single fractions or short courses of radiotherapy.

The treatment of tumours of the superior sulcus (Pancoast tumours) remains unsatisfactory. Operability should be assessed and the same criteria used as for other lung carcinomas to decide whether postoperative radiotherapy should be given. If tumours are inoperable, high-dose palliative radiotherapy may be appropriate depending on the patient's performance status.

BRACHYTHERAPY

No clear advantage in terms of palliation or survival has been demonstrated for endobronchial brachytherapy compared with external beam treatment, or for the combination of treatment.

Regional anatomy

Tumours commonly arise in the major bronchi and spread directly to the surrounding lung, pleura, chest wall and mediastinal structures. Lymphatic spread occurs to the ipsilateral hilar nodes and bilaterally to paratracheal and subcarinal lymph nodes in the mediastinum (Fig. 18.1). Blood-borne dissemination is common and has occurred in the majority of patients by the time of presentation.

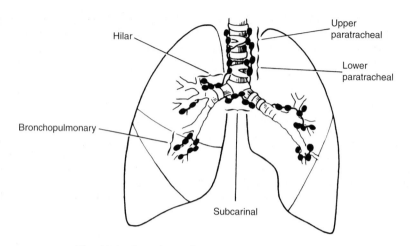

Fig. 18.1   Lymphatic drainage of the bronchial tree.

Planning technique

ASSESSMENT OF PRIMARY DISEASE

Clinical examination may reveal signs of collapse, consolidation, effusion, recurrent laryngeal nerve palsy or extrathoracic spread. Chest radiography (PA and lateral views) confirms the clinical findings and demonstrates the site and size of the primary tumour and grossly involved regional lymph nodes. CT shows the primary tumour (Fig. 18.2) and mediastinal nodes in greater detail. It may be difficult to define the tumour edges very accurately. MRI is used to show chest-wall invasion and involvement of the neurovascular bundle in the superior sulcus (Pancoast tumour). Positron emission tomography (PET) may be sufficiently sensitive to detect nodal disease. Pulmonary function must be assessed before deciding whether radical radiotherapy is appropriate.

DEFINITION OF TARGET VOLUME

Radical treatment

Target volumes for treatment with curative intent should be confined to tumours measuring less than 8 cm in diameter.

Two-phase treatment

This is used for the postoperative treatment of stage $T_{1-2}N_{0-1}$ incompletely resected tumours, patients with N_2 disease and some good-prognosis stage-IIIa patients, or for patients with operable disease who are not fit for surgery.

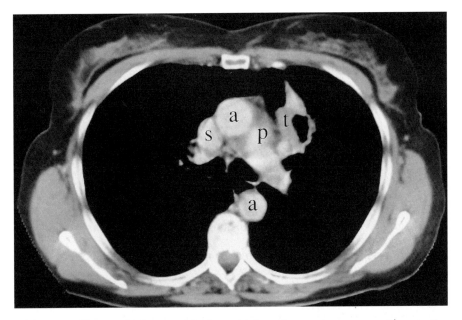

Fig. 18.2   CT scan of left upper lobe bronchial carcinoma. t = tumour with necrotic centre; a = aorta; p = pulmonary trunk; s = superior vena cava.

The clinical target volume should include the primary tumour, hilum and mediastinum, including subcarinal nodes. Margins are added to obtain the planning target volume (PTV), which should take into account organ movements, which are influenced by a number of factors, including the tumour site, lung capacity, immobilization, etc. Current recommendations suggest 1-cm margins in the transverse diameter and 1.5–2-cm margins in the vertical direction. The effect of respiratory movement may be minimized by using some type of gated or breath-holding technique with pulsed therapy. In the second phase of treatment, only the primary tumour and ipsilateral hilar nodes are included in the target volume, with margins added for movement.

Single-phase treatment

This is usually used for NSCLC peripheral $T_{1-2}N_0$ tumours, for patients in complete remission after chemotherapy for SCLC, or for patients unsuitable for surgery with small T_1 lesions. A 1-cm margin is added around the GTV as defined on the CT planning scan.

Superior sulcus tumours

The treatment fields will usually include the tumour, supraclavicular and adjacent mediastinal and hilar nodes, and the vertebral bodies to encompass tumour infiltration of neural exit foramina.

Palliative treatment

The volume includes the primary tumour with margins of approximately 2 cm and adjacent lymph nodes.

CT LOCALIZATION

The patient lies supine in an alpha cradle or vacuum bag with their arms fixed above their head to prevent obstruction of oblique treatment beams. A planning CT scan is performed with the patient in the treatment position, and the target volume is determined after scanning through the tumour with 0.5-cm slices at 0.5-cm intervals.

If conformal therapy is to be used, the rest of the thorax should be scanned with 0.5-cm-thick slices at 1-cm intervals, from the bottom of the larynx to the second lumbar vertebra to include all lung for three-dimensional calculations and dose–volume histograms.

The CT scan defines the local extent of the tumour, but may not clearly distinguish tumour from areas of atelectasis.

Normal organs of interest, such as heart, lung, oesophagus and spinal cord, should be outlined as completely as possible. If conformal therapy is being used, a beam's-eye view is used to assist choice of direction and size of beam and any beam-shaping needed. A pixel-by-pixel correction for lung is made, or a lung correction factor is used.

CONVENTIONAL LOCALIZATION

This is appropriate for palliative treatment or occasionally for a first phase of radical treatment. Palliative radiotherapy is usually given using anterior and posterior opposing fields with the patient supine and the arms adducted. AP simulator films are taken and field margins chosen to cover the target volume. The centre of this field is tattooed on the patient and the IPD is measured at this point (Fig. 18.3). If a plan is required, a lateral simulator film is taken and used to locate tumour, spinal cord and lungs on to a transverse outline taken through the centre of the proposed target volume. A correction factor of 0.2–0.3 is used to adjust for reduced attenuation in the lungs. In patients with opacification of the whole hemithorax, fields should cover the mediastinum and primary tumour defined by CT scanning or bronchoscopy.

Field arrangements

RADICAL TREATMENT – PHASE I

The first option is to use two parallel opposing AP/PA fields. This technique is simple, it enables treatment to start quickly and it delivers a lower dose to the lung than other techniques. However, the spinal cord is included within the high-

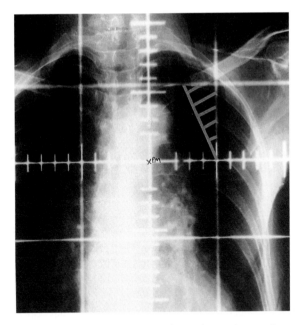

Fig. 18.3   Simulator film showing margins of anterior and posterior opposing fields for palliative treatment of left upper lobe tumour (with shielding).

dose volume. This arrangement gives an inhomogeneous distribution, with areas of high dose lying outside the tumour volume as shown in Fig. 18.4. Alternatively, a three- or four-field technique may be used.

Peripheral lesions may be treated as shown in Fig. 18.5a. This arrangement of fields is designed to spare the spinal cord and to give a homogeneous distribution, and to reduce the spinal cord dose to a maximum of 10 per cent. The lateral field is weighted down to 50 per cent to reduce irradiation to the opposite lung. Alternatively, a three-field arrangement as shown in Fig. 18.5b may be used. This produces a diamond-shaped distribution which gives a low dose to the opposite lung. Opposing oblique fields have 30° wedges. An additional anterior oblique field has a gantry angle of 45–55° to avoid the opposite lung, with a 50 per cent reduction in weighting to decrease the spinal cord dose to below 25 per cent.

RADICAL TREATMENT – PHASE II OR SINGLE PHASE

Phase II or single-phase treatments are usually delivered with a three-field technique chosen to minimize lung and spinal cord doses. This is facilitated by the use of three-dimensional planning and conformal therapy (Plate 18.1a, b, c, d).

If high-dose palliative radiotherapy is considered appropriate for patients with Pancoast tumour, field arrangements should be chosen to minimize the spinal cord dose. If anterior and posterior opposing fields are used, spinal cord shielding may be appropriate for the final fractions of treatment.

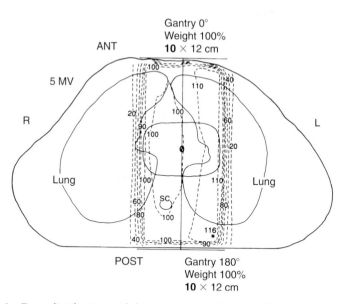

Fig. 18.4   Dose distribution with lung correction from parallel opposing fields to the mediastinum. sc = spinal cord.

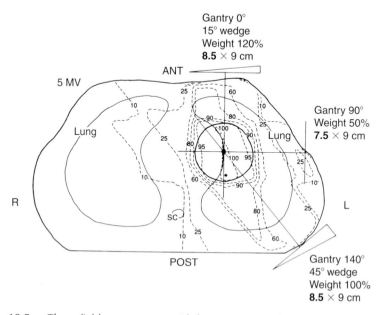

Fig. 18.5a   Three-field arrangement with lung correction for treatment of lung lesion to give minimum dose to the spinal cord (sc).

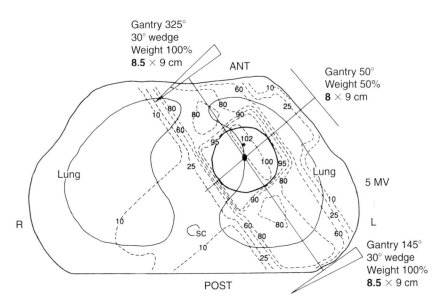

Fig. 18.5b   Three-field arrangement with lung correction for treatment of lung lesion to give minimum dose to the contralateral lung.

Implementation of plan

Most field arrangements are treated isocentrically with a linear accelerator, or cobalt 60 may be used for palliative treatment. For conventional treatment, the position of the spinal cord on anterior or posterior oblique fields must be checked at the upper and lower limits because the cord may curve into the volume, particularly in a patient with kyphosis. This requires shielding to be placed in the corner of the field. For conformal therapy, appropriate portal imaging and *in-vivo* dosimetry are used to ensure accurate delivery of the shaped treatment volume by comparison with simulator films and digitally reconstructed radiographs.

It is sometimes useful to check the plan on the simulator screen to ensure that the tumour is covered throughout the respiratory cycle.

Dose prescription

SCLC

Radical treatment after chemotherapy

45–50 Gy in 22–25 fractions given in 4.5 to 5 weeks.

Prophylactic cranial irradiation

30 Gy in 10 fractions given in 2 weeks
or 20 Gy in 5 fractions given in 1 week.

NSCLC

Radical postoperative treatment

50 Gy in 25 fractions given in 5 weeks.

Radiotherapy alone

Single-phase treatment

60–64 Gy in 30–32 fractions given in 6 to 6.5 weeks.

Two-phase treatment

Primary tumour and mediastinum

40–44 Gy in 20–22 fractions given in 4 to 4.5 weeks.

Primary tumour alone

20–24 Gy in 10–12 fractions given in 2 to 2.5 weeks.

Palliative treatment

10 Gy given in a single fraction

or 17 Gy in two fractions given in 8 days.

High-dose palliation for selected patients

39 Gy in 13 fractions given in 3 weeks.

Patient care

Side-effects of treatment include radiation oesphagitis, which is treated with mucaine or soluble aspirin and a soft diet. Adequate nutrition should be maintained with additional high-calorie or protein supplements where indicated. Patients with superior vena caval obstruction receive high-dose dexamethasone during initial radiotherapy.

Intraluminal brachytherapy

High-activity iridium can be used for intraluminal brachytherapy delivered by a high-dose-rate Microselectron or similar machine with afterloaded catheters 2–3 mm in diameter. The proximal and distal limits of the tumours are determined by bronchoscopy (Figs 18.6a and b) and recorded on radiographs with a measuring grid. A guide wire loaded into an afterloading catheter is used to determine the tumour length (Fig. 18.6c), and a margin of 1 cm is allowed at either end. Following removal of the guide wire, a small iridium source is then driven along the treatment length using a 'step-and-dwell' technique in order to achieve a high localized dose (Fig. 18.6d).

Palliative treatment may be given after intraluminal obstruction by tumour has been cleared by laser at bronchoscopy, and may also be useful in patients who have previously been treated with external beam radiotherapy. Fatal haemoptysis is a reported complication of this approach.

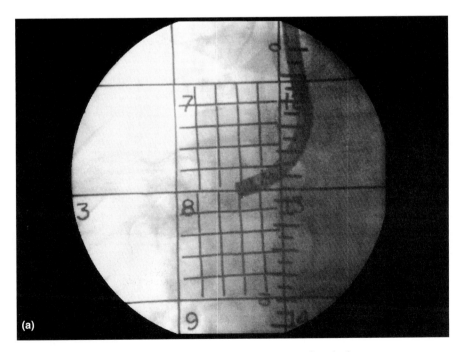

Fig. 18.6   (a) Tip of bronchoscope at proximal end of tumour.

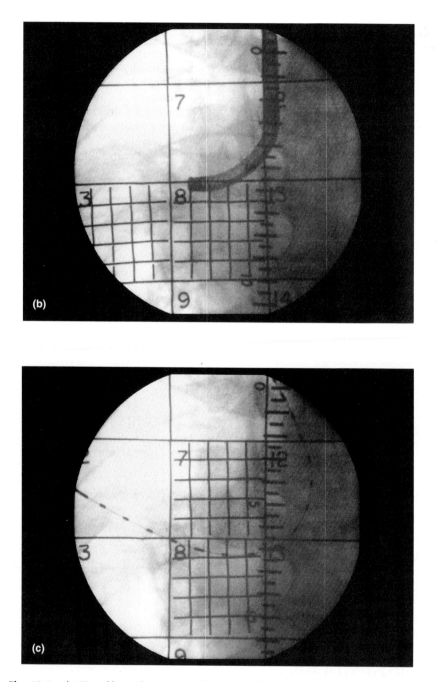

Fig. 18.6 (b) Tip of bronchoscope at distal end of tumour. (c) Guide wire with slots for iridium source and measuring grid used to determine treatment length.

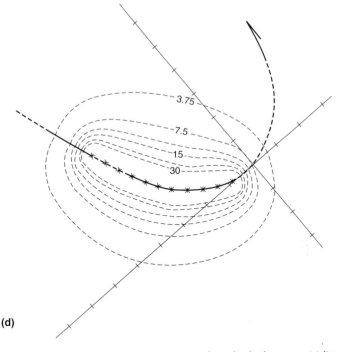

(d)

Fig. 18.6   (d) Isodose distribution from high-dose-rate iridium source.
(Courtesy of Dr H. Payne.)

Dose prescription

10 Gy at 1 cm given in one fraction (for palliation of recurrent disease)
or 15 Gy at 1 cm given in two fractions (with external beam therapy).

Further reading

Perez, C.A. 1986: Impact of tumour control on survival in carcinoma of the lung treated
with radiation. *International Journal of Radiation Oncology, Biology and Physics* **12**,
539–47.
Pignon, J.P., Arriagada, R. and Ihde, D.C. 1992: A meta-analysis of thoracic radiotherapy for small cell lung cancer. *New England Journal of Medicine* **327**, 1618–24.
Royal College of Radiologists Clinical Oncology Information Network 1998: *Lung
Cancer Working Group Report*. London: Royal College of Radiologists.

CHAPTER 19

Oesophagus

Role of radiotherapy

The majority of patients with squamous cell carcinoma of the oesophagus have extensive disease at presentation, with lymph node involvement in 70 per cent of cases and distant metastases in 30 per cent. Only about 25 per cent of patients have localized tumours less than 5 cm in length (T_1/T_2, N_0/N_1, M_0) which are suitable for primary surgical resection as first-line treatment. Adenocarcinomas are increasing in incidence, and commonly occur in the lower third, extend into the stomach and are treated surgically. However, oesophageal adenocarcinomas arising in Barrett's epithelium or at the gastric cardia spreading submucosally along the oesophagus are treated in a similar way to squamous cell tumours.

Radiotherapy is commonly used for primary tumours of the oesophagus that are deemed unsuitable for surgery. The 5-year survival rates are 5 to 10 per cent. Patients selected for surgery tend to have small tumours, minimal symptoms and good performance status, so comparison of the results of surgery with those obtained from radiation alone or chemoradiation are impossible because of selection bias.

The use of pre-operative or post-operative adjuvant radiotherapy has not yet resulted in improved survival benefit, partly because improvements in local control are currently offset by increased perioperative morbidity. Optimal radiation doses and timing between pre-operative radiation and surgery are currently being studied.

Where surgery is not indicated, chemotherapy and radiotherapy in combination have produced a significant increase in local control and survival compared with radiation alone, and are the radical treatment of choice. A 35 per cent survival rate at 2 years has been reported, but up to 40 per cent of tumours recur locally, indicating the need for clinical trials to assess the value of combining this approach with subsequent surgery.

Palliative radiotherapy to the primary tumour for obstructive symptoms produces relief of dysphagia in up to 80 per cent of patients. Tracheo-oesophageal fistula is a relative contraindication to radiation because of the risk of mediastinitis and haemorrhage from major vessels. Symptomatic patients, including those with a fistula, may be considered for stenting.

Endoluminal radiotherapy (with a low or high dose rate) can be used alone for palliation, or in combination with laser ablation or external beam radiation. The advantages of this technique in terms of better local control or longer duration of response are difficult to determine on the basis of available data, and trials of its value compared with external beam radiation are awaited.

Regional anatomy

The oesophagus extends 15–40 cm from the upper incisor teeth.

Early spread of carcinoma of the oesophagus occurs longitudinally in submucosal tissues and in the extensive lymphatic network. Spread through the muscle wall occurs later and, since there is no serosal covering, it leads to mediastinal involvement of adjacent organs such as the trachea, bronchi, recurrent laryngeal nerve, pericardium and phrenic nerve.

Lymph-node involvement is difficult to detect clinically. Upper-third lesions drain to retropharyngeal, paratracheal, deep cervical and supraclavicular nodes, while middle- and lower-third lesions drain to subcarinal, posterior mediastinal and abdominal nodes (Fig. 19.1).

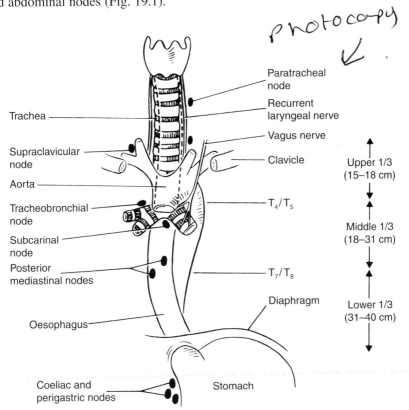

Fig. 19.1 Relationships of the oesophagus and lymph node drainage (distance in cm is measured from the upper incisor teeth).

Planning technique

ASSESSMENT OF PRIMARY DISEASE

The site and extent of the tumour are determined by barium swallow and oesophagoscopy, which also identifies intramural metastases. The diagnosis is confirmed by brush cytology and histological biopsy. Bronchoscopy may reveal tracheo-bronchial involvement by upper- or middle-third tumours, and vocal cord paralysis due to recurrent laryngeal nerve palsy may be found on laryngoscopy. Chest X-ray may show widening of the mediastinum or an elevated diaphragm due to phrenic nerve palsy. CT scanning is used to detect extra-oesophageal extension laterally, involvement of the airways or para-aortic regional nodes (particularly around the coeliac axis) and hepatic metastases. Endoluminal ultrasound may have a role in staging of the primary tumour prior to surgery or irradiation.

DEFINITION OF TARGET VOLUME

The length of the target volume is chosen to allow a 5-cm margin superior and inferior to the tumour limits as defined by oesophagoscopy and barium swallow, in order to cover potential submucosal spread. A reduction in length to allow a 2-cm margin may be made for a second phase of treatment. Extra-oesophageal spread laterally is defined by CT scan and barium swallow, and a 1.5- to 2.5-cm margin is used to include all soft-tissue disease in the oesophageal wall. The spinal cord, lungs and heart are defined as critical normal structures.

For palliative radiotherapy, a smaller margin around the tumour may be used to reduce morbidity.

LOCALIZATION

Patient position

For treatment of the upper third of the oesophagus, the patient lies supine with the cervical spine straight and parallel to the couch top, and a perspex cast is made to immobilize the neck, jaw and upper thorax. For middle- and lower-third oesophageal lesions, the patient lies supine with their arms above their head to facilitate entry into the CT scanner and to prevent obstruction of treatment beams by the arms. The shoulders are supported so that the vertebral column and intrathoracic oesophagus are parallel to the couch top, giving a horizontal target volume where possible. If the patient is kyphotic or frail this may not be possible, and the target volume will be at an angle to the horizontal.

Conventional localization

With the patient in the treatment position, antero-posterior simulator films are taken after the patient has swallowed barium in order to localize the length and width of the target volume. The mid-point of the length is tattooed on the skin as shown in Fig. 19.2. Lateral films are taken to determine the depth of the target volume (Fig. 19.3).

Three transverse outlines are taken at the upper, middle and lower levels of the target volume as defined above. The mid-line and plane through the tattoo (usually mid-line) are marked on each outline and the IPD is recorded at each level. The depth and width of the target volume are transferred on to the outline. The position of the spinal cord should be marked at each level. It may lie within the target volume at the superior level if there is kyphosis. The lungs can be localized using a simulator-CT facility at all three levels for inhomogeneity corrections.

For palliative treatment the patient is treated supine with their arms by their side, using anterior and posterior opposing fields. The field margins are simulated after the patient has swallowed barium. A central tattoo is marked on the patient's skin and the IPD is measured to enable dose calculations to be made.

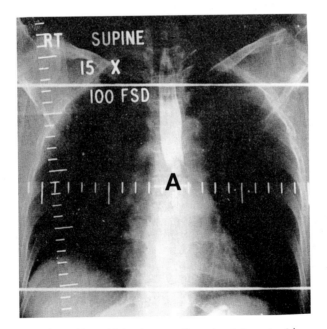

Fig. 19.2 AP simulator film with barium swallow. A = tattoo at mid-point of
15-cm-long target volume.

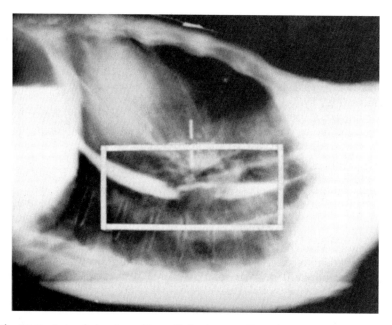

Fig. 19.3 Lateral simulator film with barium swallow showing target volume.

CT localization

The patient is positioned in a perspex shell for upper-third lesions or supine with their arms above their head for middle- and lower-third lesions. Tattoos are made anteriorly over the sterum and laterally in the mid-axillary line for alignment using laser lights, to prevent rotation and ensure reproducibility. CT scans are taken, with oral contrast to outline the oesophagus and stomach, throughout the chest and upper abdomen. The target volume and spinal cord, heart and lungs are outlined on each CT slice for three-dimensional localization, or on selected slices for two-dimensional planning.

CT localization defines the local extent of tumour more clearly than conventional simulation, and permits shaping of the target volume. The spinal cord can be recorded throughout its entire length and the lungs accurately localized for inhomogeneity corrections to be made. CT planning scans should include additional images taken during quiet respiration, to check that the PTV takes account of any movement of tumour during respiration.

Field arrangements

TWO-DIMENSIONAL PLANNING

The aim is to treat the volume homogeneously, avoiding the spinal cord and minimizing the dose to the lungs. Two factors contribute to inhomogeneity in dose distribution and present considerable problems for planning and treatment. Variation in body contour and the changing position of the oesophagus through-out its length may necessitate the use of an inclined plane for treatment. However, outlines of body contour are taken vertically and not in the inclined plane, treatment beams are not coplanar, and dosimetry is therefore complex. The alignment of oblique fields in an inclined plane is difficult to visualize and requires angulation of the treatment head and couch.

Anterior and posterior fields

Radical treatment of middle- and lower-third oesophageal tumours may be given using either a three-field technique throughout or with anterior and posterior opposing fields used for a first phase. A two-phase treatment minimizes the dose to peripheral lung tissue and ensures inclusion of the posterior mediastinum. However, there is no sparing of the spinal cord, and care must be taken not to exceed cord tolerance during the second phase of treatment. Anterior and posterior fields are defined on an AP simulator film and marked on the patient's skin.

Three-field technique

In order to check that localization has been correct, the three transverse outlines are superimposed on each other using the couch top as a baseline. If the volume

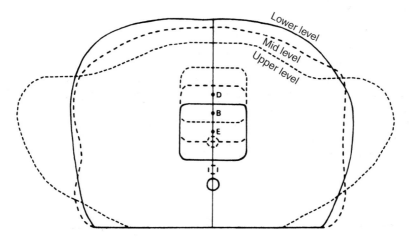

Fig. 19.4   Three superimposed outlines showing an angled target volume and the position of the spinal cord (sc) on all three levels. The distance DB = BE.

is parallel to the baseline, the centres at the three levels can be superimposed. If the volume is angled from the baseline, the centres of the volume at each level (D, B, E) cannot be superimposed, but on a transverse outline they will appear equidistant from each other (Fig. 19.4). This is derived from the geometrical arrangement shown in Fig. 19.5 where, for an angled volume, equal triangles confirm that the vertical distance of E and D from centre B is the same (X).

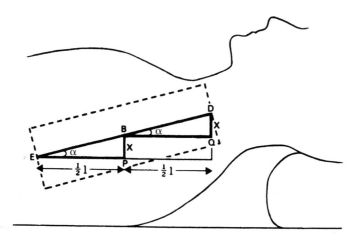

Fig. 19.5   Geometry of an inclined target volume.

The target volume is initially planned on a mid-level outline. For the middle and lower thirds of the oesophagus, an anterior and two posterior oblique fields are used. The gantry angle of the oblique fields is usually 115–120°. Larger gantry angles decrease the lung dose but increase the dose to the spinal cord. Before planning, the physicist needs to know the maximum acceptable cord and lung doses.

Using the same field arrangement, new isocentres must be constructed for the upper and lower levels to allow for the oblique fields. For a lateral field, the points D and E lie at the same distance as the isocentre B (e.g. 100 cm) on the central axis (Fig. 19.6).

For an oblique field with the isocentre at B (mid-level), the positions of the 'isocentres' for the upper and lower levels are shifted to A and C, respectively (Fig. 19.7). Point D now lies, for example, at 101 cm and point E lies at 99 cm.

New 'isocentres' are also drawn up for the other oblique field and the upper and lower levels are planned using these corrected 'isocentres' (Figs 19.8a, b and c).

Correction is also made for reduced attenuation of the beam in the lungs using a correction factor or density numbers if 2D planning is used. If the variation in mid-point dose to the tumour at the three levels is more than 10 per cent, a compensator is needed. A longitudinal wedge of, for example, 15° may be placed in the anterior field, usually with the thick end placed superiorly. Alternatively, an individual aluminium-alloy compensator may be designed. Doses at the

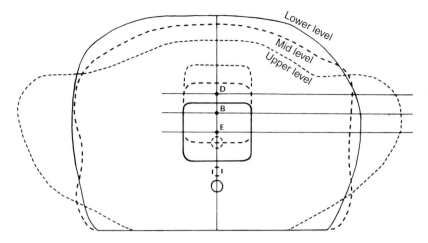

Fig. 19.6 For a lateral field, points D and E lie at the same distance as the isocentre B. DE = 4 cm.

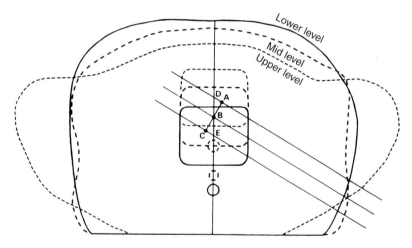

Fig. 19.7 For an oblique field, the isocentres for upper and lower levels are shifted to points A and C. AC = 3.5 cm.

dose specification points at each level should then vary by not more than 5 per cent, and the dose can be specified at the central level. The anterior field is not angled to match the inclined treatment plane, as the minimal difference in dosimetry is considered to be insignificant.

For the upper third of the oesophagus, an anterior open field and two anterior oblique wedged fields are used, usually with 30–45° wedges (Figs 19.9a, b and c). The gantry is angled to 50–60° because at an angle greater than 65° the beam would pass through the head of the humerus. The isocentres are corrected for

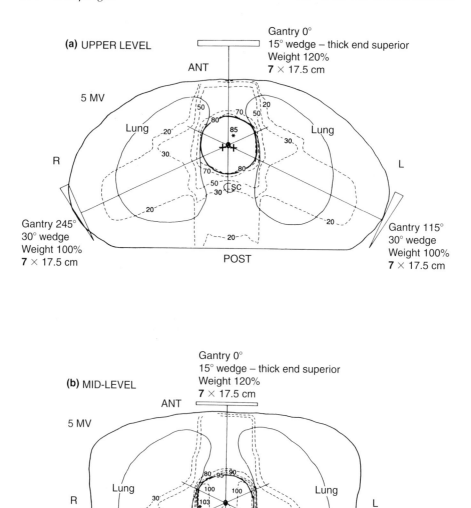

(a) UPPER LEVEL

Gantry 0°
15° wedge – thick end superior
Weight 120%
7 × 17.5 cm

ANT

5 MV

Lung

Lung

R

L

SC

Gantry 245°
30° wedge
Weight 100%
7 × 17.5 cm

POST

Gantry 115°
30° wedge
Weight 100%
7 × 17.5 cm

Gantry 0°
15° wedge – thick end superior
Weight 120%
7 × 17.5 cm

(b) MID-LEVEL

ANT

5 MV

Lung

Lung

R

L

SC

Gantry 245°
30° wedge
Weight 100%
7 × 17.5 cm

POST

Gantry 115°
30° wedge
Weight 100%
7 × 17.5 cm

Fig. 19.8 Distribution with lung correction at (a) the upper level and (b) the mid-level of the volume for middle or lower third oesophageal cancer. + = corrected isocentres; sc = spinal cord.

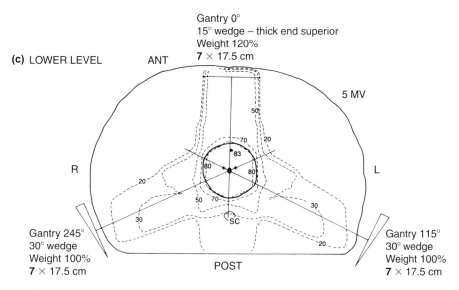

Fig. 19.8c   Distribution with lung correction at the lower level of the volume for middle or lower third oesophageal cancer. + = corrected isocentres; sc = spinal cord.

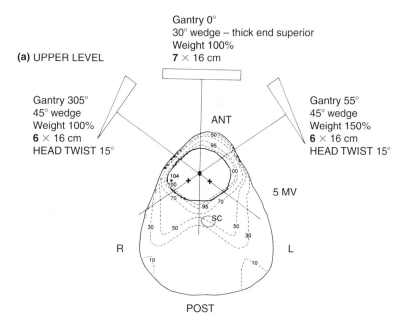

Fig. 19.9a   Distribution with lung correction at the upper level (drawn to double scale) of the volume for a cervical oesophageal cancer. + = corrected isocentres.

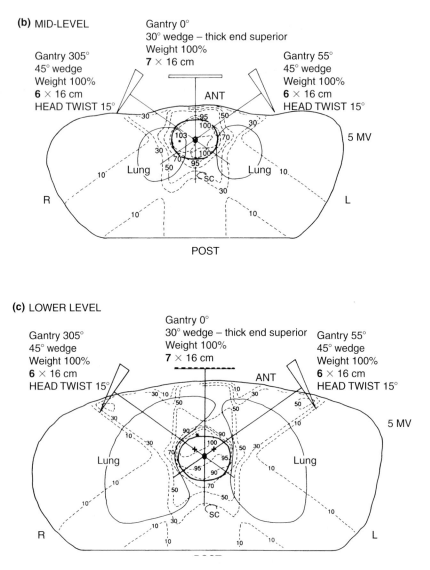

Fig. 19.9 Distribution with lung correction at (b) the mid-level and (c) the lower level of the volume for a cervical oesophageal cancer. + = corrected isocentres.

the upper and lower levels and the head twist is calculated as described below. Compensation for neck curvature in the supero-inferior direction can be provided by a longitudinal wedge in the anterior field or an individual aluminium-alloy compensator.

Calculation of head twist

If the volume is angled to the horizontal, a head twist is applied to the posterior oblique fields. If the fields were lateral (gantry angle 90°), then the head twist would be the angle t which the volume makes with the horizontal (Fig. 19.10). This can be measured from the lateral simulator film. It can also be calculated from the formula $\tan t = {}^h\!/_1$, where h is the vertical distance between the upper isocentre D and the lower isocentre E (Fig. 19.6), and 1 equals length.

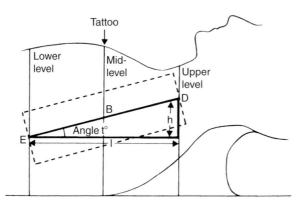

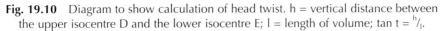

Fig. 19.10 Diagram to show calculation of head twist. h = vertical distance between the upper isocentre D and the lower isocentre E; 1 = length of volume; $\tan t = {}^h\!/_1$.

Because the fields are oblique, the head twist is reduced and is given by $\tan t$ = vertical distance between the new isocentres A and C divided by 1, where the distance AC can be measured on the superimposed outlines as shown in Fig. 19.7.

THREE-DIMENSIONAL CT PLANNING

Three-dimensional localization of the target volume, spinal cord, heart and lungs should be accompanied by a provisional dose prescription to the target volume and definition of the maximum doses permitted to the spinal cord (45–50 Gy), heart and lungs (see Chapter 4). An anterior and two posterior oblique fields can be used, and each beam shaped to conform to the target volume using alloy blocks or multileaf collimation. Pixel-by-pixel heterogeneity corrections are made to correct for reduced attenuation in the lungs in three dimensions. Non-coplanar beams and intensity-modulated beams may be used to produce an optimized dose distribution. Three-dimensional treatment planning provides greater scope for new beam arrangements and conformity of the isodose distribution to the unusual shape of the target volume, while taking into account all of the variations in body contours, tissue density and target-volume position.

Implementation of plan

The patient is aligned longitudinally using anterior and lateral lasers. The anterior field centre is marked on the cast or is found in relation to the skin tattoo. The pin depth is checked on the plan and the FSD set accordingly. The anterior field is treated with a compensating longitudinal wedge or aluminium-alloy compensator where appropriate. The machine is rotated at the set pin depth to the correct gantry angle for oblique fields, and the necessary head twist is applied. In some cases, shielding may be needed to protect the spinal cord at the upper or lower limits of the oblique field as determined when the plan is checked in the simulator. All fields are treated isocentrically each day.

Careful verification of the treatment is needed using portal films or on-line images. With conformal therapy, the positioning of the shielding must be carefully checked to avoid missing tumour at the margins of the target volume.

Dose prescription

PALLIATIVE TREATMENT

20 Gy in 5 fractions given in 1 week.

RADICAL TREATMENT

Initial target volume

40–45 Gy in 20–25 fractions given in 4 to 5 weeks.

Reduced target volume

Additional dose to a volume encompassing the tumour with a 1- to 2-cm margin.

15–25 Gy in 8–13 fractions given in 10 to 17 days.

Total dose with lung correction

60–66 Gy in 30–33 fractions given in 6 to 6.5 weeks.

Total doses are reduced when concomitant chemotherapy is used.

Patient care

Oesophagitis is inevitable and is treated with soluble aspirin or mucaine. Signs of oral or oesophageal candida should be sought and treated appropriately with antifungal medication. Careful monitoring of the patient's diet and weight is necessary. Supplements of protein and high-calorie drinks may be required, or intravenous nutrition if there is complete obstruction. Anaemia should be corrected.

Intraluminal brachytherapy

High-dose-rate afterloading machines similar to those used for intraluminal therapy of bronchial carcinoma are suitable for treatment of oesophageal cancer.

Following oesophageal dilatation, an afterloading catheter is passed through the obstructing tumour into the stomach. Where possible, it is convenient to pass a 12- or 14-gauge nasogastric tube and to use this as the vector for the afterloading catheters.

After positioning the catheter, the patient is screened to determine the length to be treated, and the distance from the end of the catheter to the beginning of the target volume, which is taken as the reference point for loading. It is normal practice to use active lengths of up to 15 cm.

Dose prescription

As for bronchial carcinoma, the dose is specified at 1 cm from the centre of the axis of the source. For simple palliative treatments, a single dose of 15 Gy is given at 1 cm. Intraluminal treatment can also be used to deliver a localized boost in association with external beam therapy. In these cases 7.5 Gy may be given at the start of treatment, and a further 7.5 Gy given at the end.

Further reading

Gaspar, L. 1994: Radiation therapy for oesophageal cancer. *Seminars in Radiation Oncology* **4**, 192–201.

CHAPTER 20

Breast

Role of radiotherapy

Radiotherapy is given for primary carcinoma of the breast to reduce the risk of loco-regional recurrence, and it has also been shown in recent studies to improve survival in patients after mastectomy.

The role of radiotherapy after conservative surgery for DCIS is under investigation. There is some evidence that it decreases the incidence of both DCIS recurrence and development of invasive disease.

Clinical $T_1T_2N_0$ lesions may be treated by wide local excision followed by radiotherapy to the breast, or by simple mastectomy, depending on the site and size of the tumour, the histological type, the grade and extent of *in-situ* change, and the size of the breast. Consideration of the cosmetic result and patient preference may determine the choice of treatment. Contraindications to conservative surgery and radiotherapy include multifocal breast tumours, extensive DCIS and patients with severe pre-existing cardiac or lung disease. After mastectomy, radiation to the chest wall is recommended for patients at high risk of local recurrence, i.e. if the primary tumour is more than 5 cm in diameter, of high-grade malignancy, involves the skin or axillary nodes, is incompletely excised, or there is tumour close to the excision margin. For inoperable T_3 and T_4 tumours, primary hormone therapy or chemotherapy may be given before loco-regional radiotherapy and possible subsequent surgery depending on systemic staging. T_{4d} inflammatory carcinomas are treated with primary chemotherapy and radiotherapy.

Patients with operable tumours 3–4 cm or more in diameter have a higher local recurrence rate with conservative surgery and radiotherapy, and may therefore be offered primary chemotherapy. This strategy aims to produce sufficient tumour regression to avoid mastectomy in many patients, and data on its effect on local control and survival are awaited.

Lymph-node irradiation is unnecessary if an axillary dissection up to the lower border of the pectoralis minor (level 1) is negative, since involvement of other nodes is unlikely. If axillary nodes are involved, radiation may be given to the axilla and supraclavicular fossa. If a formal axillary clearance has been performed, subsequent axillary radiotherapy is associated with considerable morbidity but supraclavicular node irradiation alone may be given. For central or medial quadrant tumours, irradiation to the internal mammary nodes may be considered, but isolated local recurrence is rare and routine radiotherapy is not recommended. The role of sentinel-node biopsy is currently under investigation, and may allow a policy of axillary dissection only in patients with a positive node biopsy.

Interstitial implants may be used:

- to give a boost to the site of excision following lumpectomy and external beam radiation as part of primary breast conservation therapy;
- to give a boost to residual tumour after external beam radiation for bulky inoperable disease;
- for salvage therapy for local recurrence.

With breast conservation, interstitial implantation may be considered to improve local control in patients with the following high-risk factors for recurrence:

- incomplete tumour excision;
- extensive intra-duct carcinoma in addition to invasive disease;
- patients under the age of 40 years;
- grade III tumours;
- tumours greater than 3 cm in diameter.

When a patient presents with bilateral tumours, treatment must be individualized according to the site and size of the lesions. Mastectomy may be appropriate in patients with large breasts because of the target volume which would be involved if radiotherapy were given.

Radiotherapy has a major role in the palliation of locally advanced fungating tumours and symptomatic metastases in sites such as bone, brain and skin.

Primary lymphoma of the breast is usually associated with diffuse histology and is treated by chemotherapy. Where local treatment is required for residual disease, this may be given to the breast by tangential fields as described below.

Regional anatomy

Breast cancer spreads locally by direct infiltration of the surrounding parenchyma, and may extend to underlying muscle and overlying skin, including the nipple. A dense network of lymphatics in the skin may facilitate widespread cutaneous permeation by tumour.

Lymphatics drain laterally to the axilla, medially to internal mammary nodes, and superiorly to the supraclavicular fossa (Fig. 20.1). Lymphatic vessels from the whole breast drain to the internal mammary nodes, which communicate with the contralateral chain superiorly. The internal mammary nodes lie on the internal surface of the anterior chest wall closely applied to the internal mammary artery. Although the anatomical drainage pattern is complex, involvement by tumour is most commonly found in the axillary nodes.

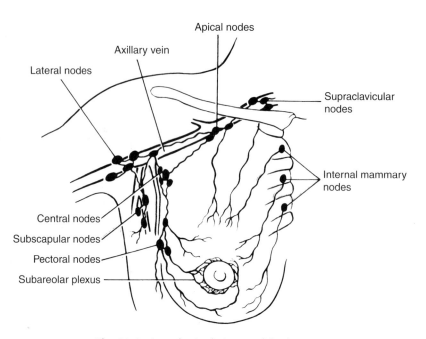

Fig. 20.1 Lymphatic drainage of the breast.

Planning technique

ASSESSMENT OF PRIMARY DISEASE

It is important for the radiotherapist to examine the patient pre-operatively. Breast examination includes inspection for nipple or skin retraction, discharge, ulceration or asymmetry, and palpation for site and size of the lump and fixation to adjacent structures. Glandular drainage areas are also assessed and TNM staging recorded on an accurate diagram. A photograph may be useful to show the exact position of the lesion. Mammography is performed to demonstrate the tumour and to detect multifocal or *in-situ* disease and bilateral involvement. Ultrasound is used to measure the lesion and guide fine-needle aspirate (FNA) cytology or core biopsy for histology.

Examination of the surgical specimen should define the size, site and local extent of the primary lesion and the number and position of axillary nodes in the specimen. Histological review determines size, type of tumour, grade, assessment of excision margins, oestrogen-receptor status and lymph-node involvement. If the breast is preserved, the position of the tumour in relation to the surgical scar must be known and should be obtained from a surgical operative diagram.

Where inoperable primary tumours remain palpable after systemic therapy, they can be assessed by palpation and ultrasound, marked on the skin and a photograph taken.

PATIENT POSITION

The patient is treated supine, and her position should remain the same during planning, simulation and treatment. The slope of the chest wall can be corrected by insertion of a triangular wedge or inclined plane under the head and shoulders for a simulator or simulator-CT localization (Fig. 20.2). However, this technique is not CT compatible, and if three-dimensional CT planning is to be used, a supine position with both arms elevated and secured above the head is optimal for entering the CT scanner aperture. An immobilization device such as a unilateral or bilateral arm pole with a scale and a footboard to ensure reproducible positioning can be used for simulation, or a vacubag for CT planning. All patients should be aligned using a system of medial and lateral tattoos and laser lights. When tangential and lymph-node fields are used, careful consideration must be given to matching field edges to avoid inhomogeneity of dose distribution. Any junction between adjacent treatment fields is affected by normal respiration causing some patient movement, and verification should be carried out in each radiotherapy department when multiple diverging beams are used.

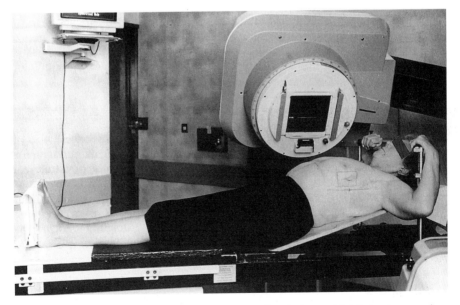

Fig. 20.2   Immobilization of a patient on an inclined plane with bilateral arm poles and a footboard for simulation of an isocentric breast technique.

DEFINITION OF TARGET VOLUME

For this complex treatment several target volumes must be defined.

Breast

The entire breast is included in the target volume, with a 1-cm margin around palpable breast tissue. The aim is to treat down to the deep fascia, but not the underlying muscle, rib-cage, overlying skin or excision scar. The superior border covers as much breast tissue as possible and lies at about the level of the suprasternal notch medially, and just below the level of the abducted arm laterally. The inferior border lies 1 cm below the breast. The medial and lateral borders are determined by the site of the primary lesion and the size of the breast. The medial border is usually in the mid-line, and the lateral border is in the mid-axillary line unless proximity of the primary site to this border means that the volume must be extended laterally. In selected patients these margins can be reduced, provided that the cover of the tumour bed is not compromised, in order to minimize the treatment volume and/or amount of lung in the high-dose zone. Irradiation of the rib-cage inferior to the inframammary fold is unnecessary unless the tumour bed encroaches on this margin or the breast is pendulous. The deep margin extends down to the deep fascia.

Chest wall

The target volume includes the skin flaps. Posteriorly, the deep margin extends to the deep fascia, inevitably including underlying muscle and rib-cage. Part of the surgical scar may have to be excluded medially or laterally in order to reduce the dose to the underlying heart and lung to acceptable tolerance limits. This is achieved by allowing a maximum central lung distance of 2 cm on the simulator film.

Tumour bed

This volume must be chosen by taking into account the initial site and size of the tumour determined clinically, by photographic record and by mammography, the position of the surgical scar in relation to the tumour from a surgical diagram, the depth of the tumour in relation to skin and chest wall, and histopathological reports. Surgical clips may help to locate the tumour bed if their exact relationship to the tumour is known. A 2-cm margin is allowed around this estimated clinical target volume, with a deep margin extending to the underlying muscle fascia, giving a PTV of 7–9 cm in diameter at the skin surface (i.e. electron applicator 8–10 cm in diameter).

Lymph nodes

The lymphatic drainage to the axillary and supraclavicular nodes forms an irregular volume lying anteriorly at its upper border in the supraclavicular fossa, and extending more posteriorly at the lower border to include all groups of axillary nodes. After positive axillary-node sampling, the entire target volume may be treated in continuity. However, after a positive complete axillary clearance, the supraclavicular lymph nodes alone may be treated using the technique described below, in order to avoid unnecessary morbidity.

The internal mammary nodes lie 2–3 cm lateral and deep to the mid-line. Since they cannot be treated satisfactorily with the breast target volume, and the incidence of clinical involvement is low, they are only treated in high-risk patients with large central or medial quadrant tumours with involved axillary lymph nodes.

Field arrangements

All fields should be treated with the patient in the same supine position as described above.

Breast technique

The patient lies supine with appropriate immobilization, and her position is aligned using laser lights. The borders of the target volume are marked on the skin with the centre points of the medial and lateral fields defined. Two reference tattoos are made at medial and lateral field centres, and a third one is made on the opposite side of the body, corresponding to the lateral field centre, to prevent rotation. Using the simulator, an isocentric technique is planned. The maximum depth of lung included in the tangential field is 2–3 cm (the central lung distance is usually less than 2 cm) as defined by simulation, simulator-CT or CT scanning (Fig. 20.3). The anterior border of the field in free air should be at least 1 cm

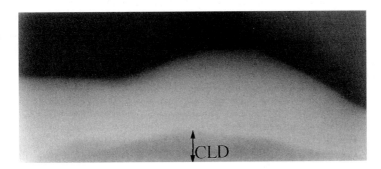

Fig. 20.3 Beam film of isocentric breast technique showing central lung distance (CLD) of 2 cm.

from the skin surface (to ensure a satisfactory dose distribution). A transverse cross-section of the patient is taken through the centre of the planning target volume using an external contour or computerized tomography. Beam divergence into the lung at the posterior border of the field can be reduced by using either independent collimators to block the posterior half of the beam, or a 5° gantry tilt to align the opposing posterior field borders.

A dose distribution is prepared across the target volume using a wedge as compensator to ensure dose inhomogeneity of no more than ±5 per cent (Fig. 20.4). Lung correction employing a correction factor within the range 0.2–0.3 may be used when calculating the dose distribution. Where the breast is large, outlines are taken through the centre of the volume and 5–8 cm above and below the centre; the simulator-CT facility is ideally suited to collecting these data. Dose distributions are produced at these three levels in order to check homogeneity and prepare tissue compensators if necessary.

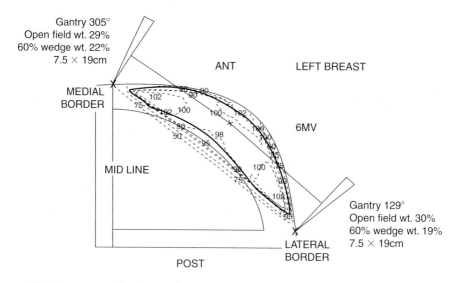

Fig. 20.4   Dose distribution for treatment of breast by tangential fields using an isocentric technique.

Chest-wall technique

Two tangential fields arranged as for the breast can be used. Bolus is usually only needed when treating recurrent disease, in order to maximize the dose to the skin. An alternative technique is to use a single anterior electron field of appropriate energy for the thickness of the chest wall determined by ultrasound or CT (usually 8–15 MeV).

Breast or chest wall and lymph nodes

ANTERIOR FIELD

The irregular three-dimensional target volume of the breast and regional lymph nodes makes it technically difficult to deliver an equal and adequate dose to all areas and to spare the lungs, heart and brachial plexus.

The tangential fields used to treat the breast or chest wall are planned as described above. For irradiation to the supraclavicular nodes only, a single anterior field is used with the patient in exactly the same position. The superior border extends at least 3 cm above the medial end of the clavicle, but leaving a margin of skin clear superiorly in order to reduce reaction. Medially the border is placed 1 cm lateral to the mid-line to avoid the larynx and spinal cord. The lateral border lies at the junction of the medial two-thirds and the lateral one-third of the clavicle. The inferior border is at the lower border of the clavicle.

If the axillary lymph nodes and supraclavicular fossa are to be included in the target volume, then the inferior border of the anterior field is extended caudally to match with the tangential field, with shielding of the apex of the lung where appropriate. The lateral border extends to the outer border of the head of the humerus, with lead shielding of the acromio-clavicular joint and the head of the humerus (Fig. 20.5a). Various techniques have been developed for matching the inferior border of the supraclavicular field with the superior border of the tangential fields. A gap of 5–10 mm may be left between the

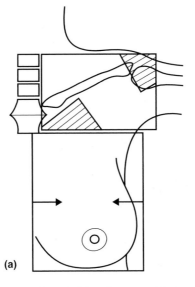

(a)

Fig. 20.5a Diagram showing three-field technique with tangential fields to the breast and anterior field to the supraclavicular and axillary nodes.

fields at the skin. The superior divergence of the tangential beams can be eliminated by rotating the couch through an angle of approximately 5° so that the superior edge of the fields lies horizontal and matches the straight upper border of the target volume. This manoeuvre increases the divergence inferiorly, but this is not usually clinically important. Divergence may then be removed from the inferior border of the anterior nodal field by moving the gantry a few degrees following a 90° couch rotation. Despite these two manoeuvres to remove divergence, matching at a skin junction is not perfect at depth, and movement of the patient due to respiration leads to inhomogeneity at the match line. Independent collimators can be used to produce half-beam blocking at the inferior border of the supraclavicular field and the superior border of the tangential field (Fig. 20.5b).

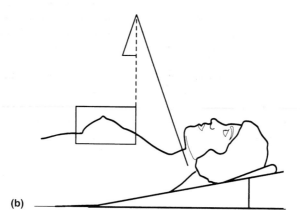

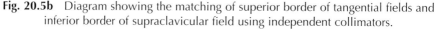

(b)

Fig. 20.5b   Diagram showing the matching of superior border of tangential fields and inferior border of supraclavicular field using independent collimators.

ADDITIONAL AXILLARY FIELD

A single anterior field encompassing the planning target volume is recommended for adjuvant radiotherapy to supraclavicular and axillary lymph nodes. For advanced, palpable axillary disease, an additional posterior axillary field may be needed to ensure an adequate dose to the axillary nodes. When the axillary separation exceeds 15 cm, the mid-plane dose to the axilla for a single anterior field falls below 80 per cent for 6-MV photons. An adequate mid-plane dose to the axilla can be achieved using a posterior axillary field treated every day, and weighted according to the separation in the axilla (e.g. for 16–18 cm, 1:10 weighting of posterior axilla: anterior SCF field applied doses). However, the hot spot at D_{max} (*c.* 2 cm below the anterior skin surface) increases for larger separations to 110 per cent. Care must be taken to stay within the tolerance range of the brachial plexus, and a dose distribution should be produced for each patient when this technique is used. The posterior axillary field is defined by palpating the apex of the axilla and aligning the infra-medial margin along the upper border of the rib-cage (Fig. 20.6).

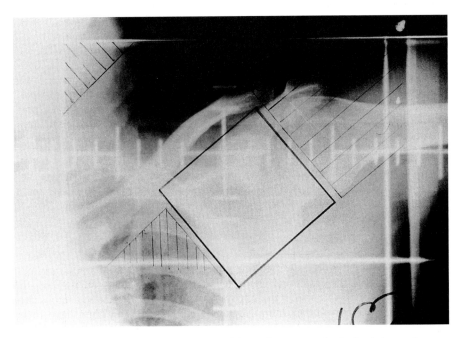

Fig. 20.6 Posterior axillary field with shielding of acromio-clavicular joint and upper humerus, apex of lung and chin to anterior field.

SINGLE ISOCENTRE, BREAST AND NODAL TECHNIQUE

A technique can be used where a single isocentre is set up at depth on the match-line of the anterior nodal and tangential fields (Fig. 20.7). The gantry is set up to treat the tangential fields by blocking the beam superior to the central axis and thereby shielding the nodal field. When the supraclavicular/axillary field is treated, the inferior part of the beam is blocked. This technique requires asymmetric collimators and good immobilization of the patient so that the isocentre does not move during the entire treatment. It is assumed that the effects of respiration are random. The technique requires large field sizes (a 40 × 40 cm field produces a maximum tangential field length of 20 cm). Special wedges may be needed for the maximum field length or the tangential half of the beam only. This technique can be time-consuming to simulate, and its accuracy depends on precise abutment of the jaws, as an under- or overlap of 1 mm can lead to significant inhomogeneity of dose.

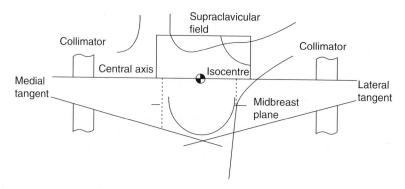

Fig. 20.7 Alignment of tangential breast and supraclavicular fields using a single isocentre and asymmetric collimators. Reprinted from *Radiotherapy and Oncology*, 28, Marshall, M.G., Three-field isocentric breast irradiation using asymmetric jaws and a tilt board, Page No's. 228–32, Copyright 1993, with permission from Elsevier Science.

INTERNAL MAMMARY NODE FIELD

Megavoltage anterior fields are no longer used to treat internal mammary lymph nodes because of the exit dose to the heart. For medial-quadrant disease, the tumour bed may lie so close to the internal mammary nodes that it is impossible to treat both target volumes homogeneously. Treatment may then have to be given to the primary tumour alone by moving the tangential field further across the mid-line on to the contralateral side. Alternatively, an electron field of electron energy 9–12 MeV can be used to treat the internal mammary nodes with a match to adjacent tangential fields. Care must be taken to ensure homogeneity of dose to the primary tumour bed, and attempts must be made to calculate the dose distribution at the electron–photon interface.

BILATERAL BREAST IRRADIATION

Where bilateral breast irradiation is indicated a combination of two- and three-field techniques is used, with particular care to prevent overlap of the tangential fields in the mid-line by leaving an appropriate gap. When a second primary tumour is diagnosed in a contralateral breast and radiotherapy is required, it is important to reconstruct any previous radiotherapy treatment to the original side in order to ensure that there is no risk of overlap, particularly in the mid-line and supraclavicular region. Doses to underlying spinal cord should be estimated.

IRRADIATION OF TUMOUR BED OR RESIDUAL DISEASE

Further irradiation is given to the tumour bed using a planning target area of around 7–9 cm in diameter at the skin surface. This requires an electron applicator 8–10 cm in diameter using 8–15 MeV electrons chosen to encompass the depth of the target volume by the 90 per cent isodose. Alternatively, small opposing tangential fields or an interstitial implant can be used.

INTERSTITIAL IMPLANTATION

For interstitial implantation, the distribution of sources to cover the target volume is chosen and a suitable perspex template used. Under general anaesthesia, rigid needles are passed through the breast and fixed at each end with a template (Fig. 20.8a). Undue pressure on the templates should be avoided as this can cause severe scarring.

The length of iridium wire loaded into a needle should position the end of the active wire 5–10 mm from the skin entry point. The superficial plane of wires should be approximately 1 cm below the skin surface (Fig. 20.8b). These measures ensure that the high dose rates around the wire do not cause telangiectasia or skin necrosis. For peripheral tumours or chest-wall recurrence where there is only sufficient tissue for a single-plane implant, a straight plastic tube technique can be used. Breast implants can be performed with remote afterloading; if this is done at a high dose rate, the treatment may need to be fractionated.

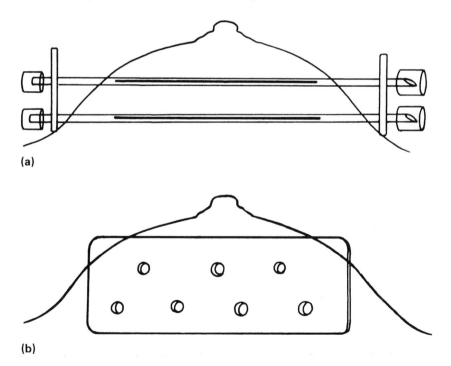

(a)

(b)

Fig. 20.8   (a) Interstitial implant with rigid needles inserted through template. (b) Geometry of source arrangement for two-plane implant.

Implementation of plan

Patient alignment is checked using sagittal and coronal laser lights to medial and lateral tattoos. Tangential fields are treated isocentrically, and anterior and posterior nodal and electron fields are treated at the machine FSD. Appropriate shielding is applied to the anterior field. Beam films are taken on the treatment unit in order to check the borders of the tangential fields and to ensure that the central lung distance included does not exceed 2 cm.

Dose prescription

BREAST AND CHEST WALL

50 Gy in 25 fractions given in 5 weeks.

Using tangential fields, skin doses are adequate for the intact breast, but bolus may sometimes be required for chest-wall irradiation for recurrent disease.

TUMOUR BED

10–15 Gy in 5 to 7 fractions to the 100 per cent isodose given in 7 to 9 days

or 20–25 Gy at the 85 per cent isodose given in 2 to 2.5 days by implant.

RESIDUAL TUMOUR

18–20 Gy given in 6 to 8 fractions

or 30–40 Gy at the 85 per cent isodose given in 3 to 4 days by implant.

NODAL IRRADIATION

50 Gy in 25 fractions given in 5 weeks.

The dose from the anterior supraclavicular field is prescribed to the 100 per cent point (build-up depth) on the central axis. The dose received at the mid-axillary plane from the anterior supraclavicular field is calculated using the axillary separation, and recorded.

If an additional contribution from a posterior axillary field is considered to be necessary to bring this dose up to 50 Gy, a dose distribution is essential. This additional dose should be given as small daily fractions, and the summated dose at the anterior bronchial plexus should be kept within the tolerance range according to guidance given.

Patient care

Patients are instructed to limit washing of the irradiated skin and to use aqueous cream to keep the skin moisturized. One per cent hydrocortisone cream may be used to relieve the discomfort of dry desquamation. If moist desquamation occurs, treatment is temporarily stopped and paraffin gauze or hydrogel applied until healing occurs.

Tight-fitting clothes should be avoided as much as possible in order to reduce friction and abrasion of the skin. Loose cotton garments are recommended.

Further reading

NHS Executive 1997: *Improving outcomes in breast cancer. The research evidence.* Leeds: NHS Executive.

Swedish Council of Technology Assessment in Health Care 1996: Radiotherapy for Cancer. Breast cancer. *Acta Oncologica* **35**(Suppl. 7), 54–63. Oslo: Scandinavian University Press.

Yarnold, J. 1995: Breast cancer. In Price, P. and Sikora, K. (eds), *Treatment of cancer*, 3rd edn. London: Chapman and Hall, 413–36.

CHAPTER 21

Central nervous system

Role of radiotherapy

The central nervous system (CNS) may be affected by many different tumours whose treatment is determined by histology, site and pattern of spread, as well as by the age and general condition of the patient.

LOW-GRADE ASTROCYTOMA AND OLIGODENDROGLIOMA

Excison is the mainstay of treatment. In patients with focal neurological signs or evidence of mass effect, the maximum safe resection should be performed. A less than total or radical subtotal excision is followed in adults by radiotherapy, which is also given for inoperable symptomatic lesions or for recurrence after previous excision. For patients with low-density lesions without mass effect, presenting with fits alone which are well controlled with anticonvulsants, observation until there are signs of progressive disease may be appropriate. Radiotherapy is not needed after complete or radical subtotal resection of cystic cerebellar or juvenile pilocytic astrocytomas. Radiotherapy is deferred as long as possible in young children with inoperable optic gliomas or with incompletely resected low-grade lesions because of the potentially serious sequelae of radiotherapy. With these approaches, the median survival overall is 7–10 years, and the 10-year survival varies between 58 and 95 per cent depending on a variety of prognostic factors.

HIGH-GRADE ASTROCYTOMAS

Radiotherapy prolongs the median survival and increases 3-year survival rates. For grade III lesions, 5-year survival rates of approximately 15 per cent can be obtained by radiotherapy after partial resection, but for grade IV tumours treatment remains essentially palliative, although radiotherapy increases the median survival from 3 to 9 months. Patients under 60 years of age with good performance status receive high-dose radiotherapy. For those with poor performance status, shorter palliative courses are preferable.

PITUITARY ADENOMAS AND CRANIOPHARYNGIOMAS

Initial management is by decompressive surgery. Patients with hyperprolacti-naemia or acromegaly may be treated with initial bromocriptine followed by radiotherapy without surgery. In patients who are unfit for surgery, radiotherapy can be used as the sole treatment. Radiotherapy may be withheld if resection is thought to be complete.

MENINGIOMA

Primary management is by complete surgical excision if possible. Postoperative radiation may be offered after incomplete excision in those cases where further surgery is likely to be difficult, or where histology suggests locally aggressive disease or malignancy. It may be used for recurrent tumours which would be difficult to excise.

Treatment dose

54–60 Gy in 1.8 to 2Gy fractions given in 5.5 to 6 weeks.

MEDULLOBLASTOMA AND EPENDYMOMA

Medulloblastoma is a chemosensitive disease. The role of chemotherapy has not been clearly defined except for patients who present with metastatic disease or who relapse following radiotherapy. Because of the infiltrative nature of the tumour, complete excision is rarely possible. Surgery must be followed by radio-therapy, which improves local tumour control and survival. High doses are needed to the primary tumour bed, which remains the commonest site of relapse, and to the brain and spine, to control seeding. Attempts to reduce doses to the spine have resulted in loss of efficacy.

High-grade infratentorial ependymoma is treated with similar craniospinal irradiation. Low-grade infratentorial lesions are commonly treated with pos-terior fossa radiation alone.

High-grade supratentorial ependymomas are treated as glioblastomas, and low-grade lesions are treated as low-grade astrocytomas.

LYMPHOMA

Biopsy is followed by postoperative radiotherapy using whole-brain radio-therapy followed by a boost to the primary site. The optimum use of chemo-therapy in this chemosensitive tumour has yet to be defined. Patients with poor performance status (especially those with HIV-associated disease) may be offered palliative radiotherapy alone.

LEUKAEMIA

CNS prophylaxis is usually accomplished with systemic chemotherapy. Trials comparing chemotherapy and radiotherapy for patients with high-risk disease are continuing. Craniospinal irradiation may be needed for patients with initial CNS involvement if total body irradiation and bone-marrow transplantion or peripheral stem-cell reinfusion are not planned. Any of the currently used approaches to treatment will reduce the incidence of CNS disease to a few per cent. Radiotherapy is ineffective unless the disease can first be controlled with chemotherapy.

GERM-CELL TUMOURS

These often arise deep in the mid-line where radical surgery is difficult. Biopsy or partial excision is undertaken. Localized germinomas are usually treated by craniospinal radiotherapy. Other types of germ-cell tumours and pinealoblastoma and patients with intra-axial spread (any histology at presentation) are treated with combination chemotherapy followed by craniospinal or local radiotherapy according to current trial protocols.

OTHER TUMOURS

In small-cell carcinoma of the lung, prophylactic whole-brain irradiation reduces the rate of CNS involvement. Radiotherapy may also be used for palliation of intracranial metastases from a variety of tumours.

Regional anatomy

Gliomas may occur throughout the central nervous system, including the spinal cord, but are most commonly found in the cerebral cortex. Extensive microscopic spread may occur, particularly across the corpus callosum.

The relationships of the pituitary gland are shown in Fig. 21.1. Tumour extension commonly occurs upwards into the suprasellar region, in proximity to the optic chiasma and hypothalamus, and inferiorly to erode the floor of the pituitary fossa.

When treating the meninges, their extensions into the retro-orbital space along the optic nerve and through the foramen magnum must be included.

ASSESSMENT OF DISEASE

A full neurological assessment is important in all patients, with additional endocrinological and neuro-ophthalmological evaluation for those patients whose

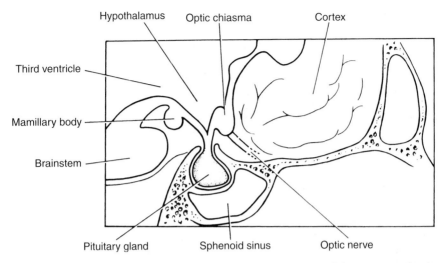

Fig. 21.1 Sagittal section of the brain to show relationships of the pituitary gland.

tumours involve the hypothalamic and pituitary regions. CT and MRI scanning (with or without contrast) have replaced other more invasive methods for defining tumour volume and identifying sensitive structures such as the eye, optic chiasma, hypothalamus, brainstem and spinal cord. Further information may be obtained at surgery. MRI of the spinal cord should be performed pre-operatively in patients with medulloblastoma, high-grade ependymoma or germ-cell tumours, and in patients with cytological evidence of CNS leukaemia in order to exclude macroscopic metastatic spread. Lumbar CSF should also be examined for cytological evidence of meningeal spread. AFP and β-HCG levels in lumbar CSF and blood should be obtained routinely in patients with suspected germ-cell tumours. In patients with leukaemia, bone marrow and CNS remission should be confirmed before prophylactic irradiation is started.

Gliomas

DEFINITION OF TARGET VOLUMES

Low-grade gliomas

The target volume encompasses the tumour as demonstrated on the most sensitive pre-operative imaging (which is usually the T2 image on MRI with a margin of 1–2 cm).

Fit patients with anaplastic astrocytoma or glioblastoma

Two phases of treatment are used. Phase 1 encompasses the primary lesion and associated oedema with a margin of 2–4 cm as demonstrated on pre-operative CT or MRI scanning. In phase 2 the target volume encompasses the primary lesion with a 2-cm margin.

For palliative treatments in unfit patients, the tumour volume with a margin of 2–3 cm is treated in a single phase.

LOCALIZATION

Patients are treated in a perspex shell. Tumours in the frontal lobes may be satisfactorily treated with the patient supine, but a prone or lateral shell may be needed for more posterior tumours and those in the temporo-parietal region.

CT localization

The shell is marked with a reference contour line in the scan plane and passing through the estimated centre of the target volume. Two radio-opaque markers are placed at lateral positions on this line. The mid-line is marked on the shell with a continuous radio-opaque marker. The patient is set up in the scanner as for treatment, and the reference contour is set to the zero couch position on the scanner. A lateral scout view is obtained. Intravenous contrast (typically 50 mL Niopam) is injected and scans are taken at intervals through the region of interest. Using the CT planning system, the shell contour, target volume and any relevant structures (e.g. eyes) are localized on multiple slices.

Conventional localization

If CT planning is unavailable or inappropriate, the shell is prepared with a localization grid and magnification markers. Orthogonal plain films are taken and the tumour drawn on to them using the clinical and imaging information. The target volume is then transferred to a transverse outline taken through the volume centre.

FIELD ARRANGEMENTS

For phase 1 treatments, opposing lateral fields may be appropriate. Smaller volumes usually require a three-field technique (Fig. 21.2). Care should be taken to position the baseline such that the eye is not included in either the incident beam or the exit beam.

IMPLEMENTATION OF THE PLAN

The laser alignment marks and field-entry portals are marked on to the shell. Treatment is given with a linear accelerator, treating isocentrically. In the lateral

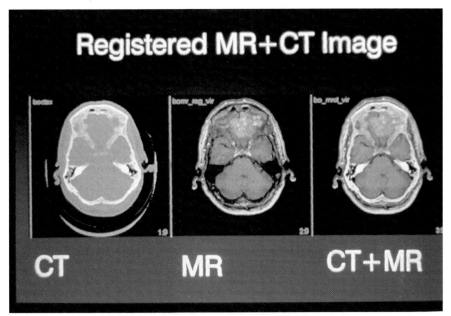

Plate 2.1 Image registration of CT and MRI for planning treatment of brain tumours. (Courtesy of Prof. D. Hawkes.)

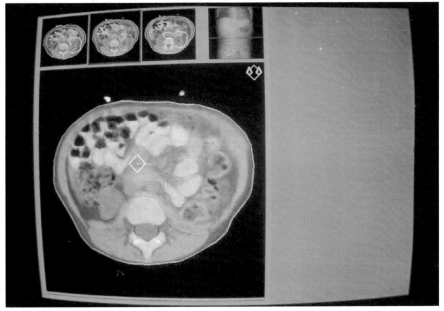

Plate 2.2 Transverse CT scan of patient with residual microscopic neuroblastoma outlining PTV (primary tumour bed and regional nodes, body contour, right kidney and spinal cord).

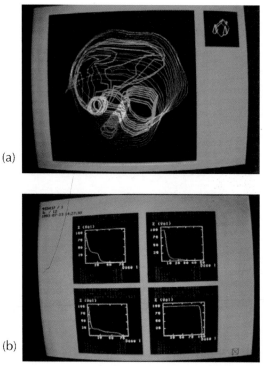

(a)

(b)

Plate 2.3 (a) Three-dimensional visualization of target volume (blue), liver (green), right kidney (yellow) and spinal cord (orange) and body contour for same patient as shown in Plate 2.2 (b) Dose–volume histograms for dose distribution to treat PTV shown in Plate 2.2. Top left = spinal cord; top right = right kidney; bottom left = liver; bottom right = target.

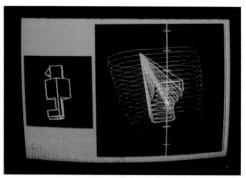

Plate 2.4 Beam's eye view showing field shaping for same patient as shown in Plate 2.2.

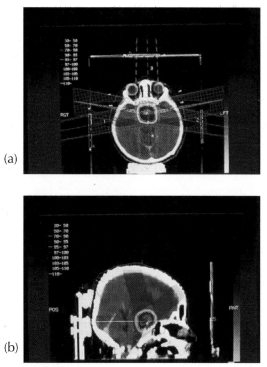

(a)

(b)

Plate 2.5 CT scans showing four fixed non-coplanar beams for treatment of craniopharyngioma with stereotactic radiotherapy. (a) Transverse section. (b) Sagittal reconstruction. (Courtesy of Dr M. Brada.)

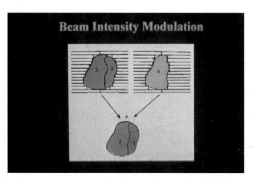

Plate 2.6 Diagram to demonstrate use of multileaf collimator to achieve beam intensity modulation. During a single treatment the collimator leaves are moved across the target to produce a non-uniform dose distribution. (Reproduced with permission from Webb, S. 1993: *The physics of 3D radiotherapy: conformal radiotherapy, radiosurgery and treatment planning.* Bristol: Institute of Physics.)

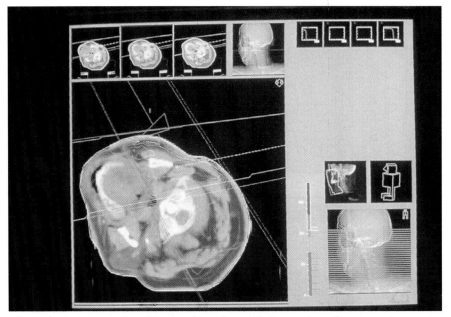

Plate 2.7(a) Transverse CT scan to show dose distribution from anterior and posterior wedged oblique fields to treat left parotid tumour.

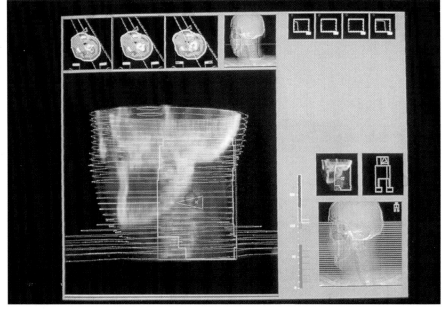

Plate 2.7 (b) Digitally reconstructed radiograph (DRR) of anterior oblique field obtained from planning system by projection of CT data along the direction of the beam.

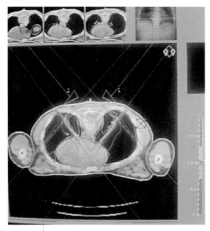

(a)

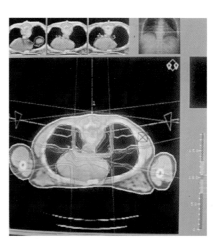

(b)

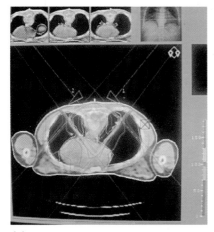

(c)

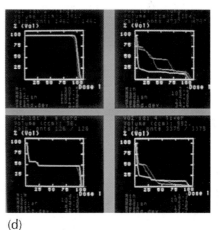

(d)

Plate 2.8   Three different plans produced to treat thoracic chordoma in a teenager. (a) Posterior oblique wedged fields. (b) Single posterior and two lateral fields. (c) Anterior and posterior opposing fields. (d) Dose–volume histograms show that all three dose distributions give satisfactory target volume doses (top left), but lower doses are produced in specified normal organs in Plate 2.8 (c).

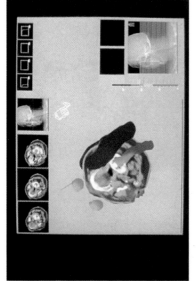

(a)

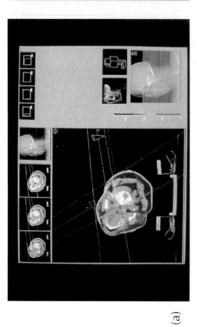

(b)

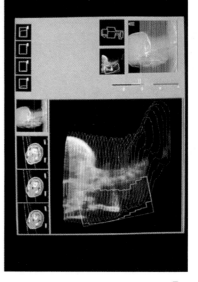

(c)

Plate 13.1 (a) CT scan of parotid tumour with patient in treatment position in a fixation shell. (b) Three-dimensional visualization of parotid tumour and adjacent nodes (red), spinal cord (yellow) and eyes (green). (c) Beam's-eye view of posterior oblique field on DRR.

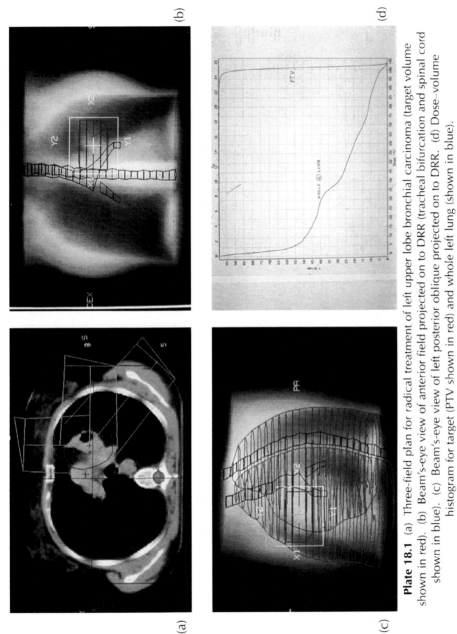

Plate 18.1 (a) Three-field plan for radical treatment of left upper lobe bronchial carcinoma (target volume shown in red). (b) Beam's-eye view of anterior field projected on to DRR (tracheal bifurcation and spinal cord shown in blue). (c) Beam's-eye view of left posterior oblique projected on to DRR. (d) Dose–volume histogram for target (PTV shown in red) and whole left lung (shown in blue).

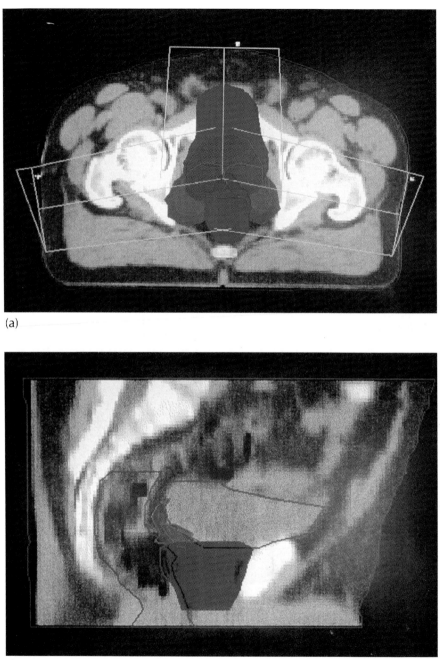

(a)

(b)

Plate 26.1 CT localization of the target volume (prostate shown in red and seminal vesicles shown in pink), rectum (posterior shown in blue) and bladder (anterior shown in blue). (a) Transverse section. (b) Sagittal section.

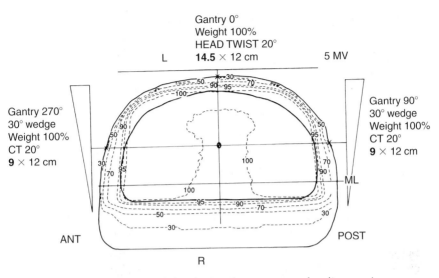

Fig. 21.2 Three-field distribution for treatment of a glioma using a left lateral cast. CT = couch twist.

position, the lateral field has a head twist (collimator angle) to avoid the eye. The anterior and posterior fields are aligned with laser lights and have a couch twist (rotation) to correspond to the head twist on the lateral field. For treatment in the supine position, the fields are set up isocentrically. Machine check films are taken to ensure correct positioning. Lead shielding may be used to protect the cornea and lens, and the scattered dose to the eyes may be measured using lithium fluoride thermoluminescent dosimetry.

DOSE PRESCRIPTION

Anaplastic glioma (in fit young patients)

Initial volume

40 Gy in 20 fractions given in 4 weeks.

Reduced volume

20 Gy in 10 fractions given in 2 weeks.

Glioblastoma (grade IV)

Two-phase treatment

As for anaplastic glioma (see above)

Single-phase treatment (patient under 60 years with good performance status):

45 Gy in 20 fractions treating twice daily over 2 weeks.

Palliative (unfit patients)

30 Gy in 6 fractions treating 3 times per week over 2 weeks.

Low-grade glioma

54 Gy in 28 fractions given in 6 weeks (1.8 Gy/fraction).

Volumes greater than 1000 mL:

45 Gy in 25 fractions given in 5 weeks.

PATIENT CARE

Hair loss is anticipated and may be permanent. Skin reactions are usually mild, and depend on the incident and exit doses. The shell should be cut away at the field entry portals, where possible, in order to preserve skin sparing. Most patients require dexamethasone during irradiation. If the intracranial pressure rises further, it can be controlled using mannitol. Otitis externa and otitis media may occur if the auditory canal is included in the field. Tiredness, lethargy and somnolence are common during treatment.

Pituitary tumours

DEFINITION OF TARGET VOLUME

Using surgical and CT-scan data, the tumour is reconstructed in the treatment plane (Fig. 21.3) and a 1 to 2 cm margin of clearance is allowed. The length and height of the volume are usually between 4 and 6 cm, and the width is determined from transverse CT sections. Care must be taken to include any extension into the sphenoid sinus.

LOCALIZATION

A supine cast is made with the chin flexed so that Reid's baseline (a line joining the external auditory meatus to the outer canthus) is as near perpendicular to the couch top as possible. The tumour and target volumes are localized on to a lateral simulator film taken in the treatment position. The baseline lies above the orbital margin in order to avoid irradiation of the eye. The target volume is transferred from the simulator films to a transverse outline taken around the cast

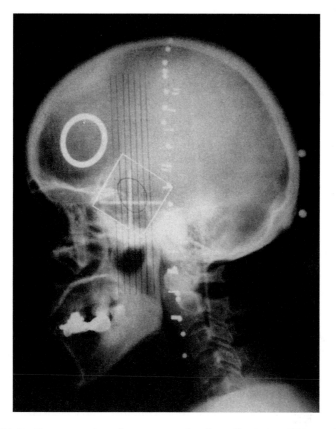

Fig. 21.3 Reconstruction of tumour on simulator film using CT scan data.

through the central plane. Where possible, therapy CT scans are taken postoperatively with the patient immobilized in the perspex shell. Ideally, a gantry angle is chosen so that scans are obtained parallel to the skull baseline in the treatment plane, for direct CT planning.

FIELD ARRANGEMENTS

A three-field technique is used as illustrated in Fig. 21.4, with an anterior and two lateral wedged fields. This technique is chosen in order to minimize the dose to the temporal lobes. The anterior field is positioned to lie above the plane of the eyes and exit through the occiput. An alternative three-field technique uses a superior and two lateral wedged fields, with the superior field exiting through the pharynx. It is possible to use opposing lateral fields, but this arrangement results in a higher dose to the temporal lobes and is not recommended. Rotational therapy of the pituitary gland is also satisfactory, but has no particular advantage. Stereotactic radiotherapy may be useful.

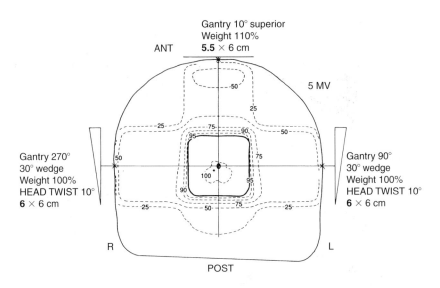

Gantry 10° superior
Weight 110%
5.5 × 6 cm

ANT

5 MV

Gantry 270°
30° wedge
Weight 100%
HEAD TWIST 10°
6 × 6 cm

Gantry 90°
30° wedge
Weight 100%
HEAD TWIST 10°
6 × 6 cm

R

L

POST

Fig. 21.4 Three-field distribution for treatment of pituitary tumour. x = laser reference point.

IMPLEMENTATION OF THE PLAN

Treatment is given isocentrically using a linear accelerator with the patient lying supine. The field entry points are aligned using laser lights (so defining the treatment plane). An appropriate collimator angle is applied to the lateral fields to match the skull baseline, and a corresponding gantry angle is applied to the anterior field with the couch rotated through 90°. Machine films are obtained in order to ensure correct positioning, and lithium fluoride is used to measure eye doses. All fields are treated daily.

DOSE PRESCRIPTION

Micro-adenoma and postoperative macro-adenoma

45 Gy in 25 fractions given in 5 weeks.

Large pituitary tumours

50.4 Gy in 28 fractions given in 5.5 weeks.

Craniopharyngioma

50.4 Gy in 28 fractions given in 5.5 weeks.

(Dose reduction may be required in children to give 40–45 Gy in 6 to 7 weeks with daily fractionation.)

PATIENT CARE

Temporary localized epilation and skin erythema occur. Attention should be paid to endocrine status, and full endocrinological assessment should be performed both before and at regular intervals after treatment. Visual fields should be assessed in all patients, especially those with suprasellar extension. Dexamethasone may be required if there is evidence of raised intracranial pressure.

Whole neuraxis

Neuraxis irradiation is used for medulloblastoma, high-grade infratentorial ependymoma, germ-cell tumours and some pineal tumours.

DEFINITION OF TARGET VOLUME

The whole brain and neuraxis are treated in the initial phase. The site of the primary tumour is treated in the second phase (Fig. 21.5).

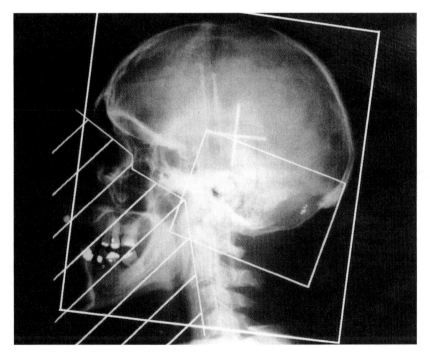

Fig. 21.5   Lateral simulator film showing two phases of cranial treatment for the whole neuraxis irradiation with shielding of extracranial structures.

Whole brain

The initial volume includes the whole brain and extends to the inferior border of the third or fourth cervical vertebra to allow an adequate margin below the primary tumour in the posterior fossa, and to facilitate matching of the spinal field.

Spine

The spine is treated from the fourth or fifth cervical vertebra to the second to fourth sacral foramina to include the theca and sacral nerve roots.

Primary tumour

The volume is reduced to cover the primary tumour. For medulloblastoma, the anterior border of the field passes behind the posterior clinoid process avoiding the pituitary gland. The inferior border lies at the bottom of the first cervical vertebra, and the superior and posterior borders are set to cover the contents of the posterior fossa. For other tumours, the phase 2 treatment encompasses the primary tumour as shown by CT or MRI scans with a small margin (1–2 cm).

IMMOBILIZATION

The patient is treated prone. An individual facial support is made. The shell is cast to immobilize the head, and extends over the shoulders to restrict movement there as well.

FIELD ARRANGEMENTS

Whole brain

In the simulator, opposing lateral fields are applied to the whole brain with a collimator rotation of 7–10° to match the divergence of the direct posterior spinal field. The lower border is at the C3/4 junction. A template is made to facilitate shielding of the extracranial structures (eyes, teeth, etc.; see Fig. 21.5). Particular care is required with the upper template border to ensure adequate cover of the frontal and temporal lobes, which have deceptive bony landmarks. After checking the template, the shell is marked and corresponding alloy blocks are cast.

Treatment is given isocentrically using a linear accelerator. The position of the lower cranial border is shifted by 1 cm every 7 treatments to change the level of the junction with the spinal field. The fields and shielding are verified with machine films, and eye doses are checked with lithium fluoride thermoluminescent dosimetry.

Spinal field

The lower border of the cranial field is tattooed. Lateral and PA simulator films of the vertebral column are then taken with the patient in the prone cast. The position of the spinal cord is marked on the lateral film, and the dose at its central axis is calculated over its entire length, which extends from the junction with the cranial field to the fourth sacral foramina (Fig. 21.6). If this dose varies by more than ±5 per cent, a wax compensator is used to improve the uniformity. The field width ranges from 4 cm in small children to 6 cm in adults (to cover the lateral spinal roots).

Despite the use of an FSD extended up to 140 cm, two adjacent fields are commonly required to cover the spinal cord in adults and older children. The technique for calculating the gap at field junctions is described in Chapter 1. Both this and the craniospinal field junction are moved caudally every 7 treatments.

×   Sites of maximum cord dose

•   Sites of minimum cord dose

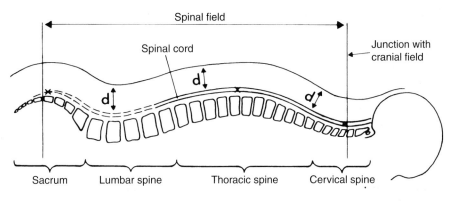

Fig 21.6   Diagram of simulator film showing patient in the prone position for CNS axis irradiation. d = depth for gap calculation.

DOSE PRESCRIPTION

The doses in both phases of the treatment are prescribed to the mid-plane of the reduced volume. Doses received at the mid-plane of the whole brain volume are also documented. If there is variation of more than ±5 per cent between the two central doses, compensators must be used. The spinal dose is prescribed to the central spinal axis (the middle of the spinal cord).

Medulloblastoma and high-grade infratentorial ependymoma

Phase 1 (whole brain)

30–35 Gy in 18–21 fractions given in 4 weeks (normally 35 Gy).

Spinal field (prescribed to mid-point of cord)

30–35 Gy in 18–21 fractions given in 4 weeks (normally 35 Gy).

The maximum dose to the skin must also be recorded. In some adults the cord dose may have to be reduced to 31.5 Gy in 18 fractions if the skin dose is too high because of cord depth and loss of skin sparing from the use of a compensator. Macroscopic disease identified on myelogram or MRI may be boosted to 45 Gy.

Phase 2 (primary tumour)

20 Gy in 11 fractions given in just over 2 weeks.

Infratentorial low-grade ependymoma

54 Gy in 30 fractions given in 6 weeks.

Supratentorial high-grade ependymoma

Phase 1 (whole brain)

40 Gy in 20 fractions given in 4 weeks.

Phase 2 (primary tumour)

20 Gy in 10 fractions given in 2 weeks.

Supratentorial low-grade ependymoma

54 Gy in 28 fractions given in 6 weeks.

Germinoma

Phase 1 (whole brain and spine)

30 Gy in 18 fractions given in 4 weeks.

Phase 2 (primary tumour)

15 Gy in 8 fractions given in 1.5 weeks.

Other germ-cell tumours (teratoma, pineoblastoma, etc.)

Phase 1 (whole brain and spine)

35 Gy in 20 fractions given in 4 weeks.

Phase 2 (primary tumour)

20 Gy in 10 fractions given in 2 weeks.

Doses must be amended according to trial protocols when primary chemotherapy is given.

Primary spinal cord tumours

Treatment must be individualized.

Lymphoma

Phase 1 (whole brain)

40 Gy in 20 fractions given in 4 weeks.

Phase 2 (primary lesion + 2 cm margin)

14 Gy in 7 fractions given in 1.5 weeks.

Palliative:

20 Gy in 5 fractions given in 1 week.

PATIENT CARE

Anaesthesia may be required for young children, but sedation is preferred because of the hazards of treatment in a prone cast. Care must be taken to ensure adequate nutrition, since meals may be missed because of sedation. Hair loss occurs, and may be permanent in the high-dose area. Acute skin reactions are common, and may be reduced by cutting out the cast over the ears where possible. Twice-weekly blood counts are required to monitor bone-marrow suppression when the whole spine is irradiated. Nausea is common, particularly early in treatment, and prophylactic anti-emetics may be of value. Dexamethasone may also be required.

CNS irradiation for acute leukaemia

Patients with high-risk disease who are assigned to receive prophylactic cranial irradiation by trial protocol receive treatment to the cranial meninges with their extensions retro-orbitally, and into the foramen magnum. For therapeutic irradiation, given to patients with initial CNS disease after remission has been obtained with intrathecal and systemic chemotherapy, the whole brain and spinal cord to the level of S4 are irradiated using a similar technique to that described for medulloblastoma.

Palliative treatment may be given for localized disease, such as facial nerve involvement or compression of the spinal cord, when the volume is determined by the extent of disease.

LOCALIZATION

For cranial irradiation, a supine cast is made and the outer bony canthi of the orbit marked with wire or lead pellets before simulation. Two opposing lateral fields are used to cover the whole of the cranium extending to the inferior border of the second cervical vertebra. The posterior half of the orbit is included in the field because of the meningeal reflection along the optic nerve. The anterior orbit and nasopharynx are protected by lead shielding as shown in Fig. 21.7. The exit dose to the contralateral eye may be reduced by angling fields posteriorly by 5° or, preferably, by placing the central axis of the beam at the anterior orbital margin with appropriate shielding.

A prone cast is made for therapeutic irradiation of the neuraxis using a technique similar to that described for posterior fossa tumours.

IMPLEMENTATION OF PLAN

The lateral cranial fields are treated isocentrically daily using a linear accelerator. Lasers are used to check alignment, and films are taken during the first treat-

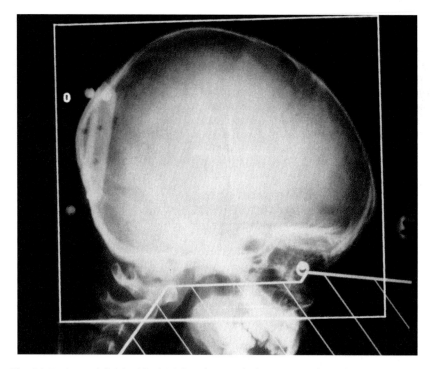

Fig. 21.7   Lateral field with shielding for prophylactic cranial irradiation in acute lymphoblastic leukaemia.

ment to ensure correct positioning of the fields and lead shielding. Lithium fluoride thermoluminescent dosimetry is used to measure the dose to the eyes, which should not exceed 10 per cent of the mid-plane dose.

DOSE PRESCRIPTION

Prophylactic irradiation

18 Gy in 10 fractions given in 2 weeks (whole brain).

Therapeutic irradiation

24 Gy in 12 fractions given in 2.5 weeks (whole brain).

10 Gy in 5 fractions given in 1 week (spinal cord).

Palliative irradiation

24 Gy in 6 fractions given in 8 days.

PATIENT CARE

Many patients have already lost their hair following chemotherapy, but radiotherapy will cause further temporary epilation. Acute skin reactions are mild. Weekly instillations of intrathecal methotrexate are continued during radiotherapy, and patients may develop headaches or nausea. Most experience somnolence at about 6 weeks after treatment, and should be warned that lethargy, nausea and anorexia are self-limiting and do not require special treatment.

Cranial metastases

Whole-brain irradiation is given using opposing lateral fields.

20 Gy in 5 fractions given in 1 week.

An additional boost may be given in selected patients with a solitary metastasis, who may also be treated with more protracted fractionation.

For small-cell carcinoma of the bronchus, where irradiation is given to prevent development of brain metastases:

20 Gy in 5 fractions given in 1 week

or 30 Gy in 10 fractions given in 2 weeks.

Base line - orbital ridge → EAM.
coll TWIST.

PATIENT CARE

Dexamethasone is needed because raised intracranial pressure may be exacerbated during irradiation.

Further reading

Brada, M. and Laing, R. 1994: Radiosurgery/stereotactic external beam radiotherapy for malignant brain tumours: the Royal Marsden Hospital experience. *Cancer Research,* **123**, 91–104.

Davies, E. and Hopkins, A. (eds) 1997: *Improving care for patients with malignant glioma.* London: Royal College of Physicians.

Thomas, D.G.T. (ed.) 1990: *Neuro-oncology. Primary malignant brain tumours.* London: Edward Arnold.

CHAPTER 22

Lymphomas

Role of radiotherapy

HODGKIN'S DISEASE

Approaches to the treatment of Hodgkin's disease vary considerably, and clinical studies are continuing to test the best way of combining chemotherapy and radiotherapy. Relapse after radiotherapy alone for early-stage disease usually responds favourably to chemotherapy, and similar results may be expected from *either* initial chemotherapy *or* radiotherapy, with chemotherapy if necessary for relapse. Patients with stage IA and small-volume stage IIA disease with good prognostic features may therefore be treated with radiotherapy alone, with survival rates of 90 to 95 per cent. Because the initial pattern of spread of disease is by contiguous node involvement, the mantle technique of extended field irradiation is usually used for supradiaphragmatic disease, and an 'inverted Y' technique for infradiaphragmatic disease. Patients with early-stage disease but poor prognostic features such as bulky nodes, more than three sites of involvement, systemic symptoms, high erythrocyte sedimentation rate (ESR) and mixed cellularity or lymphocyte-depleted histology should be treated with chemotherapy followed by radiotherapy to the initial sites of disease. Where there is bulky mediastinal involvement and associated lung infiltration with poor response to chemotherapy, subsequent radiotherapy may include low-dose lung irradiation.

Treatment of patients with more advanced disease is by chemotherapy alone. It may be followed by high-dose chemotherapy and/or local radiotherapy to improve outcome in poor responders.

NON-HODGKIN'S LYMPHOMAS

About 15 per cent of patients with nodular lymphomas present with stage I or II disease, and approximately 50 to 60 per cent of these may be cured by local field irradiation alone. The outcome is not improved in this group by the addition of chemotherapy. Patients with stage III and IV low-grade nodular disease who are symptomatic or show evidence of disease progression are treated with chemotherapy. Chemotherapy is recommended as the initial treatment for all stages of diffuse lymphoma (intermediate or high grade, B- or T-cell tumours). Radiotherapy may then be given to sites of initially bulky disease, or where residual node masses persist. Localized treatment fields are usually appropriate. Patients with non-bulky (<5 cm) stage IA disease who are unfit for chemotherapy may be treated with radiotherapy alone. Local radiotherapy may also be used for palliation of symptoms in patients either with disease that is uncontrolled by or who are unfit for chemotherapy.

TOTAL BODY IRRADIATION

Patients with a high risk of disease relapse may be considered for elective intensive therapy and bone-marrow transplantation. This is often preceded by conditioning with chemotherapy alone. If total body irradiation is to be included, areas of bulky disease may be boosted immediately before TBI. Special care is needed if mediastinal irradiation is also required (see Chapter 37 for a discussion of TBI). Similarly, for some high-grade non-Hodgkin's lymphomas with CNS involvement that are treated without bone-marrow transplantation, craniospinal irradiation may be needed (see Chapter 21). If intensive therapy is planned, a boost to the CNS can be given as described in Chapter 37.

Regional anatomy

Lymphomas may affect any of the lymph nodes in the body, as well as extra-nodal sites such as Waldeyer's ring, the thyroid, gastrointestinal tract, central nervous system, testes and skin. Spread occurs via the lymphatic pathways and also by the bloodstream to the spleen, liver, lungs and bone marrow.

Planning technique

ASSESSMENT OF DISEASE

Clinical examination should include measurement of peripheral lymph nodes and examination of the upper airways. Chest X-ray is used to detect mediastinal lymphadenopathy. CT scanning of the chest gives additional information about small-volume mediastinal disease, as well as detecting lung infiltration and enlarged nodes at the root of the neck.

CT scanning of the abdomen and pelvis is more useful than ultrasound for detecting enlarged para-aortic, pelvic, coeliac, mesenteric and splenic hilar nodes, and for demonstrating ureteric obstruction leading to hydronephrosis. It is not useful for detecting involvement of normal-sized lymph nodes or diffuse involvement of the liver or spleen. Histological assessment of the whole spleen and a liver biopsy are the only accurate means of determining such involvement. However, in most cases this information would not affect treatment decisions, and laparotomy is no longer performed routinely.

Gallium scanning may be helpful for assessing mediastinal and lung disease, and PET scanning performed pre- and post-chemotherapy can help to differentiate between fibrosis and functioning residual tumour when persistent lymph-node enlargement is detected on CT.

LOCAL FIELD IRRADIATION

Where radiotherapy is used alone to treat localized nodal disease, adjacent anatomical lymph-node areas may be included in the field. Examples of common situations are shown in Fig. 22.1. Where local field irradiation is given following chemotherapy, fields may be confined to the site of residual or original bulky disease alone.

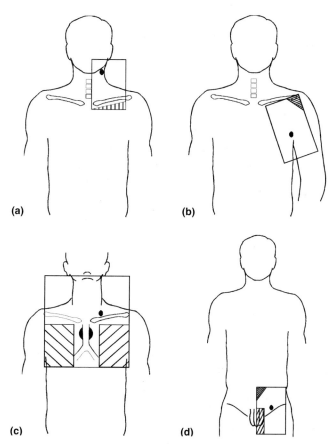

Fig. 22.1 Diagrams of opposing fields for local nodal irradiation. (a) Unilateral cervical field for stage IA high cervical node (with shielding to lung apex). (b) Axillary field (with shielding of humeral head). (c) Neck and mediastinum (with lung shielding). (d) Groin (with shielding of testes and small bowel).

'Mantle' technique

DEFINITION OF TARGET VOLUME

The target volume for a 'mantle' field includes the occipital, submental, submandibular, anterior and posterior cervical and supraclavicular nodes. In addition, it covers the infraclavicular, axillary, medial-pectoral, paratracheal, mediastinal and hilar lymph nodes. The volume is encompassed by a large field to the upper half of the body, with lead shielding of the oral cavity, larynx, lungs, humeral heads and cervical and thoracic spine, as appropriate.

The field extends from the tip of the mastoid process to the junction of the tenth and eleventh thoracic vertebrae, and it includes the axillae laterally.

LOCALIZATION

Patients must be seen by the radiotherapist before chemotherapy so that the sizes and sites of initial disease are documented with a view to designing fields for subsequent treatment. The target volume is localized using a simulator or CT-simulator when CT scanning images taken in the treatment position can be used for depth dose calculations and heterogeneity corrections.

It is desirable for anterior and posterior fields to be treated with the patient remaining in the same supine position, and with most modern linear accelerators this can usually be achieved by treating at 100 cm FSD either to the skin or isocentrically. A field size of about 40 × 40 cm is needed. With some machines with small maximum field sizes this can only be achieved with an extended FSD. If it is not possible to oppose the anterior field at an extended FSD with the patient lying supine, a change to the prone position is necessary for treatment of the posterior field.

The patient lies with their arms slightly abducted (to allow axillary skin sparing) and the neck extended in order to displace the oral cavity from the irradiation field. This position is difficult to maintain and reproduce accurately, and immobilization with vacuum bags or other devices is advisable. Lymph-node masses are outlined on the patient with lead wire so that they can be seen on simulator films.

A tattoo is placed on the skin in the mid-line over the mediastinum at the approximate field centre and the separation measured (in supine and prone positions if appropriate). Two lateral tattoos are placed at a set height above the table top in line with the central tattoo in order to minimize lateral rotation. A fourth tattoo is marked at a defined point inferior to the central tattoo in the mid-line. All of these tattoos are labelled with lead markers before simulator films are taken of the proposed treatment area. The lymph-node areas are mapped and appropriate shielding designed (Fig. 22.2).

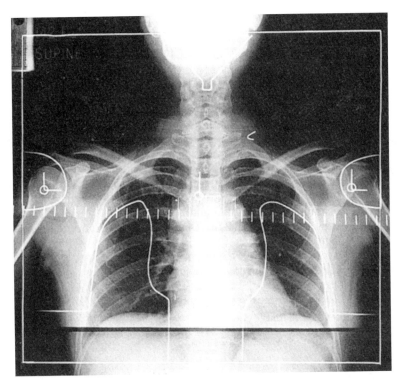

Fig 22.2   Simulator film of a template for 'mantle' field irradiation.

BEAM SHAPING

The lateral border of the lung shield lies just within the rib-cage to treat the lymphatic drainage of the medial pectoral nodes. The upper border curves centrally to spare the lung and to ensure inclusion of the infraclavicular nodes. The medial borders of the lung blocks are shaped so as to treat the hilar nodes with maximum sparing of the lungs and heart. A gap of 8–10 cm is left in the mid-line between the lung blocks to treat the mediastinal lymph nodes. Infero-laterally, lung blocks are extended to shield soft tissues, especially the breast, unless there is involvement of the axillary node. The head of the humerus is shielded unless there is axillary lymphadenopathy, when apical nodes might also be inadvertently shielded.

Individualized oral cavity and laryngeal shields are used in the anterior field, and the brainstem and cervical spinal cord are shielded in the posterior field, unless there is mid-line or upper cervical lymphadenopathy. The thoracic spinal cord is shielded from the posterior field after a mid-plane dose of 20 Gy has been reached, provided that there is no detectable mediastinal involvement. In some centres the heart is also shielded at 25–30 Gy if appropriate.

CONSTRUCTION OF LUNG BLOCKS

Expanded polystyrene is used to construct moulds for individual lung blocks which allow for beam divergence following a geometrical set-up corresponding to that used on the treatment unit. The divergent edges of the lung blocks reduce the penumbra that they create in the beam, and their position on the carrier tray prevents secondary electron contamination and enables small-sized blocks to be used (Fig. 22.3a). When a distance of 100 cm to the isocentre is adopted, blocks may be too heavy for routine use (depending on the area being shielded). At an FSD of 100 cm to the skin, blocks will be lighter and field sizes may be large enough for the patient to be treated in the supine position throughout. At 142 cm FSD, the blocks will be lightest, but the patient's position will be changed between fields and positioning errors of the blocks will be magnified.

The simulator film, with alloy shielding marked on it, is transferred by digitizer to the treatment-planning system. It is then demagnified and a template of appropriate magnification formed at a distance d (Fig. 22.3a). This template printout is used to construct a perspex template for the carrier tray and the lung blocks. The field centre is aligned with a mark on a polystyrene block which represents the centre of the beam. The outlines of the blocks are traced on to the polystyrene. Using a geometric set-up identical to that on the treatment unit, but inverted, the polystyrene is placed at a distance d from a target bar attached to a

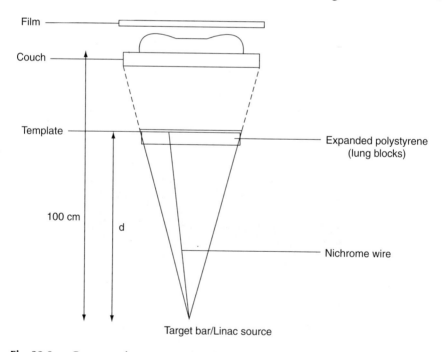

Fig. 22.3a Geometry for construction of divergent lung blocks showing relationship of blocks, template and treatment couch. d = distance from focus to template.

heated nichrome wire (Fig. 22.3b). The heated diverging wire is guided around the outline of lung shielding on the polystyrene in order to delineate the lung blocks (Fig. 22.3b). Alternatively, using a similar hot-wire system and appropriate geometry, a template and lung blocks are cut out of polystyrene by tracing directly from the simulator film. After checking the moulds against the templates for accuracy, they are positioned on the heat exchanger and clamped into position (Fig. 22.3c). The lung blocks are cast in an alloy with a low melting point of 70°C, which does not melt polystyrene. Lung blocks of 75 mm thick alloy reduce transmission of radiation to less than 10 to 15 per cent of the primary beam. The thickness of the lung blocks may be reduced in patients with hilar lymphadenopathy or lung infiltration in order to irradiate the lung in continuity with the mediastium, but to a lower dose.

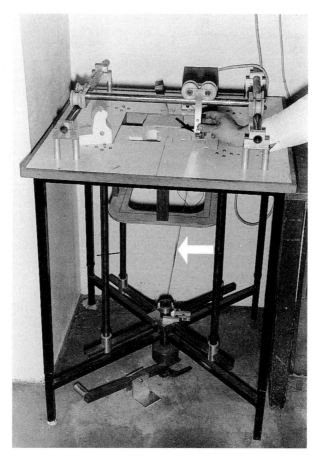

Fig. 22.3b   Technique using heated wire (white arrow) attached to stylus (black arrow) for cutting polystyrene mould for lung blocks.

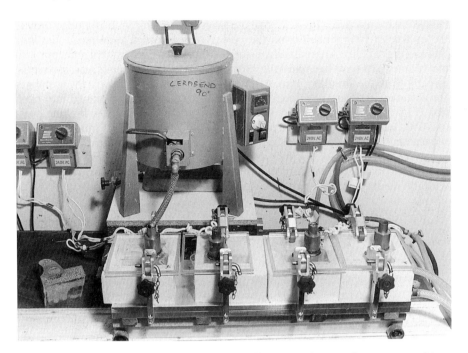

Fig. 22.3c Casting of lung blocks showing alloy poured into polystyrene moulds.

Simulator films are taken of the patient, aligned using tattoos and laser lights to check the position of lung blocks and template, and these films are compared with the original localization films before the patient receives treatment (Fig. 22.4).

FIELD ARRANGEMENTS

A linear accelerator is used for treatment which is given with anterior and posterior fields. The dose received at the mid-point of the fields is reduced by the lead shielding and is calculated as shown below.

Calculation of depth dose for 'mantle' field

When calculating the mid-plane dose (MPD) at the centre of the 'mantle' field, adjustment has to be made for the amount of scatter removed by the lead shielding. This amount is deducted from the central-axis depth dose for the open field obtained using tables of equivalent squares for rectangular fields. Figure 22.5 illustrates a 'mantle' field of 32×37 cm with an IPD of 18.5 cm at the centre of the field, point P. A rectangle wxyz (32×10 cm) is drawn around the central point P such that it contains minimal lead shielding.

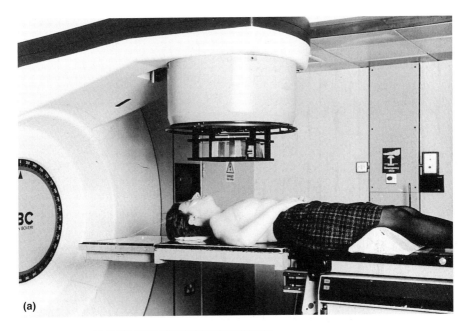

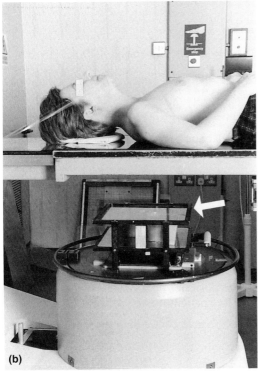

Fig. 22.4 Patient in position for 'mantle' irradiation with template and lung blocks in a double tray attached to treatment machine head. (a) anterior field. (b) Posterior field (arrow to template).

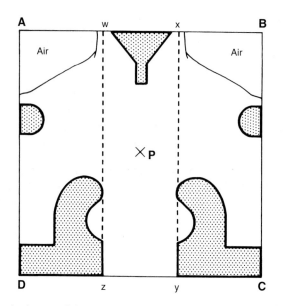

Fig. 22.5 Calculation of the mid-plane dose at the centre point **P** of a 'mantle'.

Equivalent square of wxyz = 13.9

Percentage depth dose at 9.25 cm = 70 per cent (where IPD is 18.5 cm)

For an open field ABCD without lead shielding centred on point P

Equivalent square of ABCD = 30

Percentage depth dose at 9.25 cm = 74 per cent.

However, lead shielding and air occupy approximately two-thirds of the remaining area (ABCD−wxyz), and do not contribute any scattered dose to point P.

Therefore the additional effective area contributing scatter is one-third (ABCD−wxyz) = one-third (30−13.9).

Thus the total dose to point P at a depth of 9.25 cm

$= 70 + \frac{1}{3} (74-70)$ per cent

$= 71.33$ per cent.

The percentage depth dose for the posterior field is calculated in a similar way using the new IPD, and for this patient it is 70 per cent.

Therefore, the mid-plane dose to the field centre in the mediastinum in this patient

$= 71.33 + 70 = 141.3$ per cent.

Supraclavicular fossa and axillary dose

The dose to these sites is calculated using a similar method, with rectangles drawn round the point of calculation. The separations at the axilla and supraclavicular fossa are measured on the treatment unit using callipers. The IPD is measured from the couch top to the anterior skin surface at each site.

Figure 22.6 shows that the FSD is greater than 100 cm at the supraclavicular fossa, and that the separation is much less than that at the mediastinum. The increase in FSD is given by the differences in measurement of the IPD at the two sites (in this example $20-12 = 8$ cm). The FSD at the supraclavicular fossa is therefore $100 + 8 = 108$ cm.

For a separation of 10 cm, the mid-plane dose at 5 cm with an FSD of 100 cm is read from percentage depth dose charts. To obtain a percentage depth dose at the increased FSD, an inverse square correction must be made as follows.

Percentage depth dose at 5 cm with FSD of 108 cm

$$= \text{percentage depth dose at 5 cm with FSD of 100 cm} \times \frac{(100 + 5)^2}{(108 + 5)^2}$$

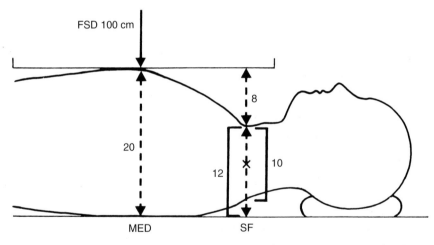

Fig. 22.6 Calculation of a dose at supraclavicular fossa (SF). MED = mediastinum.

IMPLEMENTATION OF PLAN

Treatment is given with a linear accelerator, and for mantle treatments this may be at an FSD of 100 cm to the skin or with an appropriately extended FSD. The mid-line tattoos on patient and template are used to ensure correct alignment each day, with the position of the lateral tattoos checked in order to prevent rotation. Shielding blocks are placed to correspond with marks on the template which lies on the carrier fitted to the head of the machine. On the first day of treatment, check films are taken of anterior and posterior fields. Both fields are treated every day. *In-vivo* dosimetry with lithium fluoride may be used to verify calculations of the dose at sites of lymph-node involvement.

Dose prescription

HODGKIN'S DISEASE

Radiotherapy as the sole treatment

Mediastinal dose:	35 Gy in 20 fractions given in 4 weeks.
Other sites of involvement:	40 Gy in 20 fractions in 4 weeks.
After chemotherapy:	30 Gy in 17 fractions given in 3.5 weeks.

Similar doses are given when the mantle technique is used. Because of the variation in the FSD and patient separation, the dose to the supraclavicular and axillary nodes is increased by 10 to 20 per cent relative to the dose to the mediastinum. This is satisfactory for involved sites where a total dose of 40 Gy is planned. However, shielding may need to be added to the neck and axillae if a uniform dose to all node sites is required.

If whole-lung irradiation is needed, 15–20 Gy in 20 fractions are given in 4 weeks using lung blocks of reduced thickness as appropriate to deliver this dose to the lung, with a full dose to the mediastinum given in the same overall time.

NON-HODGKIN'S LYMPHOMA

Stage IA or active disease

40–45 Gy in 22–25 fractions given in 4 to 5 weeks.

5–10 Gy additional dose to residual disease if needed in 3–5 fractions.

After chemotherapy

30 Gy in 17 fractions given in 3.5 weeks.

PATIENT CARE

Skin reaction occurs mainly in the axillae, supraclavicular region and neck. These areas are kept dry and one per cent hydrocortisone cream is applied sparingly if necessary. Dry shaving is recommended if appropriate. Patients who are being treated with the mantle technique or a high field to neck nodes should be warned to expect temporary hair loss over the occipital region. Hoarseness may occur if the larynx is not shielded. Nausea occasionally occurs during wide-field irradiation, often during the first few days, but it rarely persists. Anti-emetics should be given before treatment if necessary. Dysphagia may occur towards the end of a course of mantle treatment due to mild radiation oesophagitis, and this may be treated with mucaine or soluble paracetamol. Cough due to mild pneumonitis may occur. Lhermitte's syndrome may be seen when cervical or thoracic spinal shielding has to be omitted.

'Inverted Y' technique

DEFINITION OF TARGET VOLUME

The volume includes the pelvic, para-aortic and inguinal nodes bilaterally.

The margins of the target volume extend from the junction of the tenth and eleventh thoracic vertebrae or below the calculated gap from the previous 'mantle' field, to the bottom of the obturator foramina. In its upper part, the field is 8–10 cm wide to cover lymph nodes demonstrated by CT scanning. Splenectomy is rarely performed, and irradiation of the splenic axis does not usually have to be considered. However, if there is evidence of gross splenic disease that is unresponsive to chemotherapy, and for which radiotherapy is needed, the position of the spleen may be marked on the skin by CT or ultrasound scanning. The left kidney lies immediately adjacent to the spleen, and shielding must be considered if appropriate.

LOCALIZATION

Localizing films are taken in the same treatment positions as for the 'mantle' technique with 1-cm lead cups placed around the testes. Lead wire is used to outline palpable node masses. The lower border of the previous 'mantle' field is reconstructed using the tattoos and marked with wire to aid in calculation of the gap between fields.

A central tattoo is placed over the junction of the fourth and fifth lumbar vertebrae in the mid-line, with two further tattoos placed at fixed points above and below. Lateral tattoos are placed over the iliac crests at the level of the inferior tattoo, and the height of these above the couch top is recorded. The IPD at the central tattoo is measured with the patient in the treatment position.

BEAM SHAPING

The 'inverted Y' field shown in Fig. 22.7 is obtained by applying lead to the lateral borders of a rectangular field, thereby shielding the kidneys, whose positions are taken from abdominal CT scans. A central lead block is used in the pelvis to shield the bladder, small bowel and ovaries if transposed.

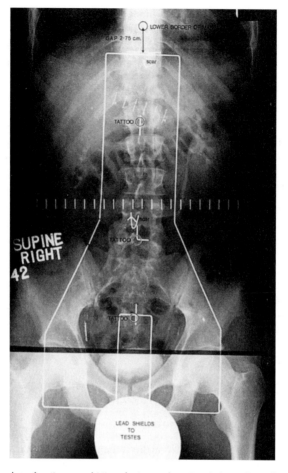

Fig. 22.7 Template for 'inverted Y' technique showing bilateral nephrograms and lead shields to testes. The gap below lower border of previous 'mantle' field is shown.

TEMPLATES

Perspex templates are made to define the shielding for the anterior and posterior fields. Wire can be used to outline the field margins and the templates checked following administration of intravenous contrast to demonstrate the kidneys. To ensure simulation under treatment conditions, 1 cm thick lead cups are placed around the testes. With this shielding used during irradiation, the testicular dose is reduced to about 0.6–1 Gy for a prescribed nodal dose of 40 Gy.

FIELD ARRANGEMENTS

Anterior and posterior fields are used. Calculation of the mid-plane dose is made using the 'equivalent squares method' described for the 'mantle' technique.

IMPLEMENTATION OF PLAN

The patient is treated using a linear accelerator with lead shields placed around the testes. The template is aligned using the three mid-line tattoos and laser lights. The height of the lateral tattoos above the couch is also checked with lasers to ensure that there is no rotation. Shielding blocks are placed on the template on the carrier tray and treatment is then given. Both fields are treated each day.

Dose prescription

Hodgkin's disease

35 Gy in 20 fractions given in 4 weeks.
40 Gy given to involved sites.

Non-Hodgkin's lymphoma

40–45 Gy in 20–25 fractions given in 4 to 5 weeks.
5–10 Gy additional dose to residual disease in 3 to 5 fractions.

PATIENT CARE

Nausea and vomiting may occur in the first few treatment days, but often settle spontaneously or in response to the use of anti-emetics. Diarrhoea is not usually troublesome but may require treatment (see Chapter 30). Skin reaction is usually mild, but temporary epilation occurs over the treatment area. The groins should be kept dry and 1 per cent hydrocortisone cream applied if the skin reaction is marked.

COMBINED MANTLE AND INVERTED Y TECHNIQUES

This approach is now rarely used as patients with extensive disease are initially treated with chemotherapy. If combined supra- and infradiaphragmatic irradiation is needed, overlap at depth is inevitable because of beam divergence, and a suitable gap at the skin must be calculated so that this overlap does not occur in the region of the spinal cord (see Chapter 1). Lateral films centred at the level of the junction of the tenth and eleventh thoracic vertebrae are taken on a simulator with the patient supine (and also prone if appropriate). The positions of the

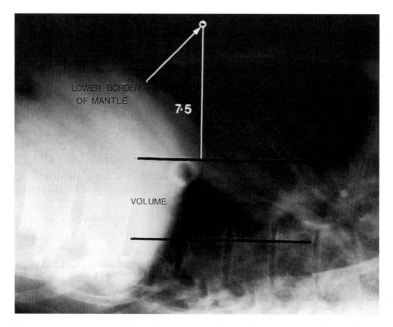

Fig. 22.8   Lateral simulator film to show matching of anterior mantle and inverted Y fields at anterior border of target volume.

skin tattoos at the inferior border of the previous mantle field (Fig. 22.8) or the superior border of the previous abdominal field are marked with lead on the patient. The position of the spinal cord, the volume of the lymph nodes and the depth at which the beams should match are marked. This match point is chosen at the anterior border of the target volume for matching anterior fields, and at the posterior border of the target volume for matching posterior fields. This results in a higher dose area lying within the target volume, with sparing of the lungs anteriorly and the spinal cord posteriorly.

Further reading

Cosset, M., Henry-Amar, M., Meerwaldt, J. *et al.* 1992: The EORTC trials for limited stage Hodgkin's disease. *European Journal of Cancer* **28A**, 1847–50.

Gospodarowicz, M.K., Sutcliffe, S.B., Bergsagel, D.E. and Chua, T. 1992: Radiation therapy in clinical stage I and II Hodgkin's disease. *European Journal of Cancer* **28A**, 1841–6.

Rosenberg, S. and Kaplan, H. 1985: The evolution and summary results of the Stanford randomised clinical trials of the management of Hodgkin's disease 1962–1984. *International Journal of Radiation Oncology, Biology and Physics* **11**, 5–22.

CHAPTER 23

Pancreas

Role of radiotherapy

Patients with pancreatic adenocarcinoma have a 1 to 4 per cent 5-year survival rate because of difficulty in diagnosis, early spread of tumours to lymph nodes and liver, and a lack of effective systemic therapy. Highly selected patients with localized tumours of the head of the pancreas may show up to 20 per cent 5-year survival rates following radical surgery. Combined chemoradiotherapy given either pre- or postoperatively extends the median survival to 20 months, compared with around 12 months after surgery alone.

The role of radiotherapy in the palliation of locally advanced disease is unclear, as pain is often better controlled with medication or a coeliac axis nerve block. Intra-operative radiotherapy with electron beam irradiation is under investigation.

Regional anatomy

The pancreas is closely related to other upper abdominal structures as shown in Fig. 23.1. The radiation dose is limited by tolerance of the adjacent duodenum and kidneys. Small bowel lying anteriorly may be damaged if its normal mobility is impaired following laparotomy.

Tumour extension is predominantly local, with invasion of the peripancreatic lymph nodes. Metastatic spread also occurs along perineural lymphatics.

Planning technique

ASSESSMENT OF PRIMARY DISEASE

If chemoradiation is given postoperatively, the findings of laparotomy are important for defining the extent of any residual disease, and for recording the tumour size and margins, histological features and any involvement of regional lymph nodes. Where treatment is given pre-operatively, the diagnosis may be made by fine-needle aspiration cytology under CT control, and contrast-enhanced CT scans are used to define the extent of primary disease (Fig. 23.2)

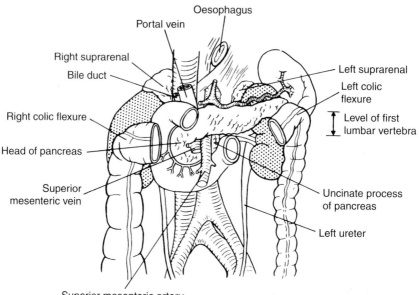

Oesophagus

Portal vein

Right suprarenal

Bile duct

Right colic flexure

Head of pancreas

Superior
mesenteric vein

Left suprarenal

Left colic
flexure

Level of first
lumbar vertebra

Uncinate process
of pancreas

Left ureter

Superior mesenteric artery

Fig. 23.1 Relationships of the pancreas.

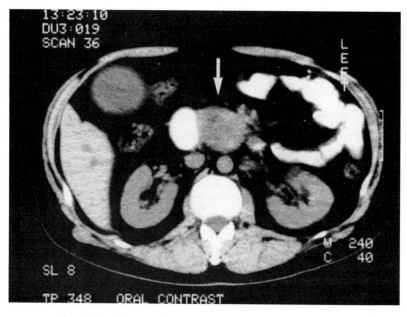

Fig. 23.2 CT scan showing pancreatic tumour (arrowed).

and to exclude liver metastases. CT is particularly useful for showing posterior extension of the tumour to the pre-vertebral fascia and around the aorta, and may detect involved lymph nodes.

DEFINITION OF TARGET VOLUME

The target volume includes the primary tumour with adjacent margin of normal lymph nodes, allowing a margin of 1–2 cm.

The dose-limiting organs are the kidneys, duodenum, spinal cord and liver. Irradiation of the entire gland is limited by the tolerance of the left kidney, which is closely applied to the tail of the pancreas.

CT LOCALIZATION

CT scanning should be used when radical radiotherapy is to be given. The patient is scanned with their arms securely immobilized above their head. Records are made of the patient and arm positions. A skin tattoo at the level of the first lumbar vertebra is marked on the anterior abdominal wall with barium paste, oral contrast medium is given to outline the small bowel, and a topogram is taken for localization. Two lateral tattoos are also made to prevent lateral rotation, and their height from the couch top is recorded. CT scans are then taken through the upper abdomen to determine the target volume and position of normal organs such as the adjacent duodenum, kidneys, small bowel and spinal cord. For two-dimensional treatment planning, the CT section at the centre of the target volume is used for calculation of isodose distributions, ensuring that this encompasses the tumour throughout the length of the target volume. For three-dimensional treatment planning, the target volume and normal organs are outlined on each CT slice. CT scans should be taken using 5-mm slice thickness at 5-mm intervals so that three-dimensional localization and subsequent calculations can be performed.

CONVENTIONAL LOCALIZATION

If palliative treatment is indicated, the target volume can be localized on to an anterior simulator film after administration of oral barium as shown in Fig. 23.3, and should not exceed 12 × 12 cm. The centre of the target volume is tattooed and field borders are marked on the patient.

Field arrangements

An anterior and two lateral wedged fields are used (Fig. 23.4a), with the angle of the lateral field chosen to minimize the renal dose, which should not exceed

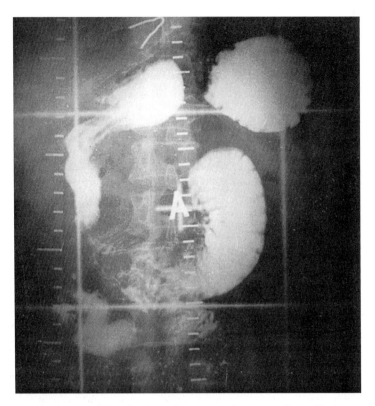

Fig. 23.3 Conventional localization of a pancreatic tumour for palliative treatment with opposing anterior and posterior fields. A = skin tattoo.

15–20 Gy except to very small areas (Fig. 23.4b). The lateral fields may be weighted to reduce the exit dose to the spinal cord from the anterior field. The spinal cord dose should be limited to 45 Gy with fractions of 2 Gy per day. If the volume lies to the right of the mid-line, anterior and right lateral wedged fields may be used to spare the small bowel and left kidney.

Alternatively, opposing anterior and posterior fields may be used for lower-dose palliative treatments.

Implementation of plan

The patient is treated supine with their arms immobilized above their head and skin tattoos aligned using laser lights to ensure accurate reproducibility of patient position. An isocentric technique is used on a linear accelerator and the interplanar distance is checked regularly so that the correct pin depth is main-

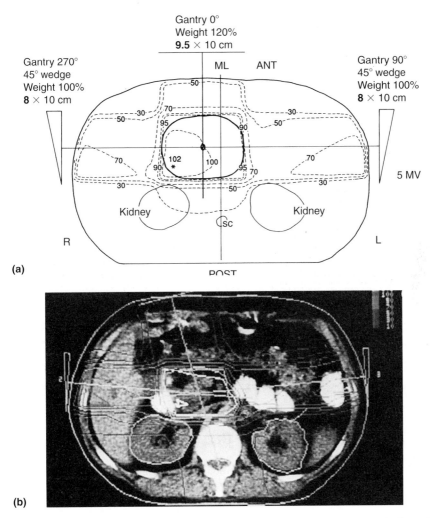

Gantry 0°
Weight 120%
9.5 × 10 cm

ML   ANT

Gantry 270°
45° wedge
Weight 100%
8 × 10 cm

Gantry 90°
45° wedge
Weight 100%
8 × 10 cm

5 MV

Kidney

Kidney

sc

R

L

POST

(a)

(b)

Fig. 23.4   (a) Field arrangement used to treat pancreatic tumour. sc = spinal cord.
(b) CT plan showing three-field arrangement with angled lateral fields to
reduce renal dose.

tained. The pin setting is adjusted according to the plan and all three fields are
treated each day. Where three-dimensional conformal therapy is used, the
instructions are followed for shielding with alloy block or the multileaf
collimator and careful verification is performed.

Dose prescription

Radical treatment

45–60 Gy in 20–30 fractions given in 5 to 6 weeks with daily fractionation.

The final dose depends on the treatment volume, the patient's general condition, any concomitant chemotherapy administration, and whether radiotherapy is given alone or with surgery.

Palliative treatment

40–50 Gy in 20–25 fractions given in 4 to 5 weeks.

Patient care

Nausea, vomiting and diarrhoea are common, particularly in patients who have had surgery. Oral medication is given as required. An adequate fluid intake must be maintained. If gastrointestinal side-effects are severe, treatment should be suspended.

Further reading

Hoffman, J.P., Weese, J.L., Solin, L.J. *et al.* 1995: Pilot study of pre-operative chemo-radiation for patients with localised adenocarcinoma of the pancreas. *American Journal of Surgery* **169**, 77–8.
Warshaw, A.L. and Fernandez-Del Castillo, C. 1993: Pancreatic carcinoma. *New England Journal of Medicine* **326**, 455–65.

CHAPTER 24

Rectum

Role of radiotherapy

Surgery is the mainstay of treatment for carcinoma of the rectum, and gives overall 5-year survival rates of 73 to 94 per cent, 60 to 82 per cent and 17 to 33 per cent for Dukes' A, B and C disease, respectively. For tumours of the lower rectum, surgery results in a permanent colostomy, although for tumours higher in the rectum, an anastomosis of the bowel with sphincter preservation is usually possible with a temporary colostomy. Surgical technique is crucial in determining outcome, particularly with regard to local recurrence. Total mesorectal excision with its low rates of local recurrence is increasingly practised. However, despite advances in surgical practice the local recurrence rates in most reported series are still of the order of 20 per cent or more. Radiotherapy can reduce this figure by 25 to 50 per cent, and recent evidence suggests a survival benefit when radiotherapy is added to surgical resection.

Pre-operative radiotherapy reduces small bowel toxicity, but results in over-treatment of early tumours. Pre-operative radiotherapy in a short 5-day course for mobile, operable tumours gives excellent results (Swedish Rectal Cancer Trial). For operable, mobile tumours a trial is in progress comparing pre- and postoperative radiotherapy. If an operative specimen shows involvement of the radial resection margin, local recurrence is likely and radiotherapy is indicated.

Fixed or tethered tumours should be treated with pre-operative radiotherapy over 4–5 weeks, often with concomitant chemotherapy. A delay of 6–8 weeks before surgery allows time for tumour shrinkage.

Early operable tumours of the lower rectum can be treated by local radiotherapy in selected cases. Superficial exophytic tumours are amenable to endocavitary radiotherapy, and more infiltrative tumours can be treated by a combination of endocavitary treatment and interstitial iridium-192 brachytherapy.

Inoperable disease/local recurrence can be palliated by local radiotherapy (often with concomitant chemotherapy) which may offer durable relief of symptoms and disease control for long periods.

Regional anatomy

The rectum extends from the external sphincter to the recto-sigmoid junction at approximately 20 cm from the anal margin. Carcinomas arise in the mucosa, and may be exophytic, ulcerated or annular, when they may produce obstruction of the lumen. Tumours extend through the wall of the serosa to invade surrounding organs such as the bladder, prostate and vagina, with direct extension to the pre-sacral region in advanced cases. The lymphatic drainage of the rectum is to the pararectal lymph nodes which lie along the course of the superior haemorrhoidal blood vessels. These drain into nodes at the level of the bifurcation of the inferior mesenteric artery. There is also drainage to hypogastric and presacral lymph nodes as shown in Fig. 24.1. Spread towards the anal margin may be associated with inguinal lymphadenopathy. The surgical specimen is used to assess the histological staging of the tumour according to Dukes' classification.

Planning technique

ASSESSMENT OF PRIMARY DISEASE

Digital rectal examination, sigmoidoscopy, colonoscopy and double-contrast barium enema are used to assess the extent of the primary tumour and to exclude other lesions in the colon. Biopsy of the tumour is taken for histology. If treatment is given pre-operatively, pathological staging is not available, and CT scanning of the pelvis may then be useful for determining the extent of disease (Fig. 24.2) and for planning radiotherapy treatment. Estimation of carcino-embryonic antigen levels may be used to monitor response to treatment.

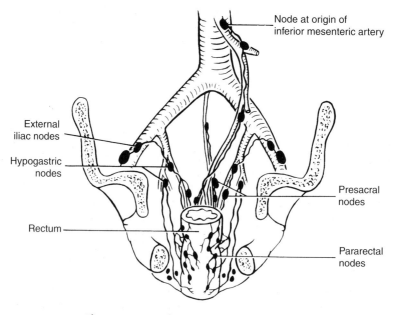

Fig. 24.1 Lymphatic drainage of the rectum.

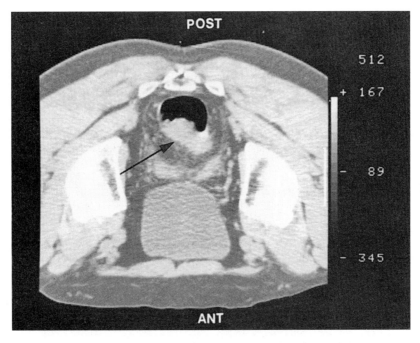

POST

512

+ 167

- 89

- 345

ANT

Fig. 24.2   CT scan of primary rectal carcinoma (arrowed).

At laparotomy, the primary tumour and lymph nodes up to the inferior mesenteric artery are removed and examined histologically. Liver metastases may be detected by inspection and palpation at laparotomy, or subsequently by ultrasound or CT scanning.

DEFINITION OF TARGET VOLUME

The target volume includes the primary tumour or tumour bed, adjacent lymph nodes, and the presacral region. The inferior mesenteric nodes are not irradiated, either because they are removed at surgery, or because their inclusion in a palliative treatment volume would increase morbidity.

The target volume extends from the top of the sacrum to 5 cm below the primary tumour or tumour bed, and laterally it includes the pelvic side-walls and internal iliac nodes. Posteriorly, the presacral lymph nodes and sacral hollow are covered, and anteriorly an adequate margin is left in front of the surgical anastomosis or the tumour (including the posterior vaginal wall in females). If there is a high risk of tumour recurrence in the perineum, the inferior border should cover the perineal scar.

For inoperable or recurrent tumours, small bowel toxicity is minimized by using a small volume which covers the sacrum and the soft-tissue mass as defined by CT scanning.

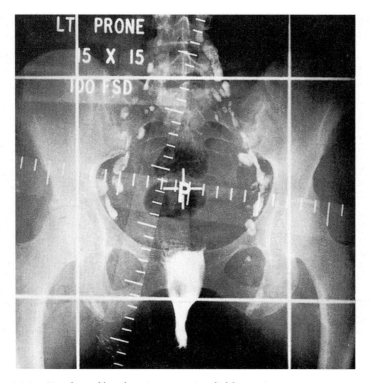

Fig. 24.3 Simulator film showing posterior field margins to encompass target volume.

LOCALIZATION

Using the simulator (Fig. 24.3) or CT scanner, the target volume is localized with the patient in the prone position with a full bladder (to displace the small bowel anteriorly and superiorly). In the simulator, barium for contrast is introduced into the rectum and vagina as appropriate, and a wire marker is placed on the anal margin or perineal scar. Postero-anterior and lateral simulator films are taken, and the target volume is marked on a transverse outline taken through the centre.

CT scanning delineates the tumour more clearly and, when the rectum has been removed in male patients, is the best way of determining the anterior margin (Fig. 24.4). Loops of small bowel may be visualized with oral contrast media so that their position can be taken into account when choosing the dose distribution.

When palliative treatment is given using anterior and posterior opposing fields, the field margins are determined by screening and marked on the patient's skin. This technique is not commonly used and small volumes should be treated.

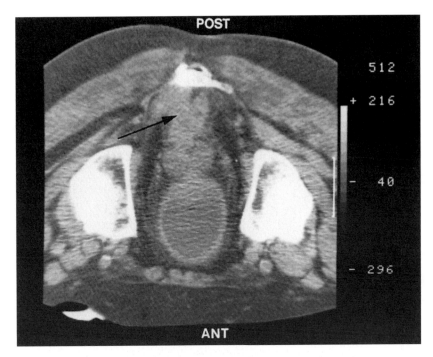

POST

512

+ 216

− 40

− 296

ANT

Fig. 24.4 CT scan showing recurrent carcinoma of the rectum in the presacral region (arrowed).

Field arrangements

A homogeneous dose to the target volume with minimum dose to small bowel and bladder is achieved using a direct posterior field with reduced weighting, and either two lateral or posterior oblique wedged fields depending on the shape of the patient. Posterior oblique fields at a gantry angle of 45–60° will produce a rounded volume with some anterior spread of dose, whereas lateral fields give a sharp cut-off anteriorly, reducing the small bowel dose (Fig. 24.5). Angles less than 45° are not used as this causes overlap of the fields posteriorly, increasing skin reaction in the natal cleft. In special circumstances other field arrangements may be needed. A four-field plan (see Fig. 30.5) or anterior and posterior fields, for example, may be used where there is bladder or anterior abdominal wall involvement, in order to increase the dose anteriorly. Perineal disease may be best treated by lying the patient prone over a barrel-shaped support, and using inferior and superior oblique fields. Alternatively, a direct perineal field may be used, with the patient in the lithotomy or lateral decubitus position.

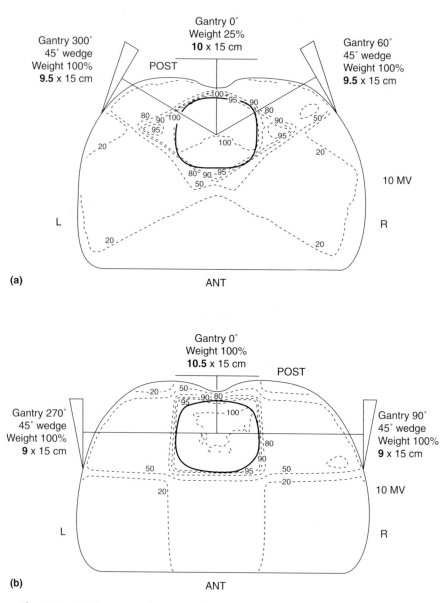

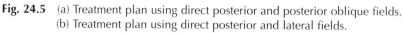

Fig. 24.5 (a) Treatment plan using direct posterior and posterior oblique fields.
(b) Treatment plan using direct posterior and lateral fields.

Implementation of plan

Patients are treated prone with a full bladder, using a linear accelerator. Lasers and skin tattoos are used to align the patient, and lateral rotation is prevented by means of lateral tattoos over the iliac crests. All three fields are treated isocentrically each day. For anterior and posterior opposing fields, the IPD is used to calculate the mid-plane dose.

Dose prescription

Chemotherapy with schedules containing 5-fluorouracil is often given concomitantly and will affect morbidity.

Pre-operative dose

Either

> 44 Gy in 22 fractions given in 4.5 weeks followed 6 to 8 weeks later by surgery (for fixed tumours).

Or

> 25 Gy in 5 fractions given in 1 week followed immediately by surgery (for mobile tumours).

This must be done using a 3 or 4 field plan.

Postoperative dose

> 45–50 Gy in 25 fractions given in 5 weeks. Where there is residual macroscopic disease, a further 10–15 Gy in 5–7 fractions may be given to a small volume to a total dose of 55–60 Gy in 6.5 to 7 weeks.

Local control is improved by increasing the total dose, but morbidity due to small bowel damage is often the dose-limiting factor, particularly if mobility is reduced by postoperative adhesions. It is desirable to image small bowel and shield it wherever feasible if high doses are given.

Inoperable or recurrent disease

> 45–50 Gy in 20–25 fractions given in 4 to 5 weeks.

For maximum local control where prolonged survival is expected, an additional 10–15 Gy in 5–7 fractions may be given to a small volume to a total dose of 55–60 Gy in 6.5 to 7 weeks.

Alternative fractionation regimen (for palliation when hospital visits need to be reduced)

36 Gy in 6 fractions given in 3 weeks.

Patient care

Skin reaction in the sacral and perineal region is common and difficult to treat. Exposure to air and keeping the skin as dry as possible are helpful. One per cent hydrocortisone cream is given where there is erythema or irritation. A low-residue diet is given, and diarrhoea is treated with drugs if necessary (see Chapter 30). If it is severe, treatment may be suspended or the dose per fraction reduced.

Further reading

Abulafi, A.M. and Williams, N.S. 1994: Local recurrence of colorectal cancer: the problem, mechanisms, management and adjuvant therapy. *British Journal of Surgery* **81**, 7–19.

Påhlman, L. and Glimelius, B. 1997: Improved survival with pre-operative radiotherapy in resectable rectal cancer. Swedish Rectal Cancer Trial. *New England Journal of Medicine* **336**, 980–7.

CHAPTER 25

Anus

Role of radiotherapy

The histology, natural history and management of tumours in this region are determined by whether the tumour arises in the anal canal or, as is less common, at the anal margin. The prognosis is governed by tumour size and depth of invasion, with anal margin tumours having a better prognosis than those of the anal canal.

T_1N_0 tumours are treated with radiotherapy alone. The treatment of choice for other anal canal tumours is concurrent chemotherapy and radiotherapy which produces 5-year survival rates of 50 to 60 per cent, equal to those of abdomino-perineal resection, but with preservation of the rectum in the majority of patients. Ongoing studies are evaluating new chemotherapy regimens and their scheduling with radiotherapy in order to reduce treatment toxicity while maintaining local control rates. Radiotherapy is given using external beam therapy with interstitial implantation in selected cases.

Small well-differentiated tumours of the anal margin are commonly treated by wide local surgical excision, giving 5-year survival rates of 70 to 83 per cent. External beam radiotherapy or electron therapy may be used, with preservation of the external sphincter, giving equally good local control rates. For more extensive lesions, and those with high-grade histology, where the risk of lymphatic spread is increased, external beam therapy is given to the primary tumour and adjacent inguinal lymph nodes. This gives overall survival rates of 30 to 50 per cent, with the advantage of retaining the anal sphincter in 70 to 80 per cent of patients.

Lymphatic spread to the inguino-femoral regions occurs with tumours at the anal margin and in the distal anal canal. Although 40 per cent of patients have palpable inguinal nodes at presentation, only about 50 per cent of these are found to be involved with tumour on biopsy. When combined chemotherapy and radiotherapy is given, the target volume includes irradiation of the inguinal region. If there is no palpable inguinal lymphadenopathy at presentation, the risk of involvement is low, and prophylactic radiotherapy is not generally given because of the risk of increased toxicity. Survival rates of 60 per cent can be obtained by deferred block dissection for the 10 to 20 per cent of patients who will subsequently develop disease in this site.

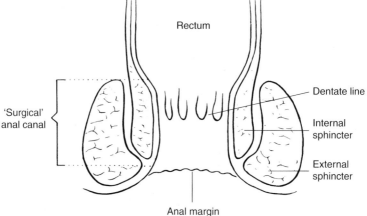

Fig. 25.1 Anatomy of the anus.

Regional anatomy

Definition of the anal canal varies widely, making classification of tumours and comparison of results difficult. The 'surgical' anal canal extends from the ano-rectal ring composed of upper fibres of the internal sphincter to the anal margin as shown in Fig. 25.1. The anal margin consists of the area of skin around the anal orifice. Tumours of the anal margin are slow growing and tend to infiltrate locally within the perineum, with late spread to lymph nodes. Tumours of the anal canal most commonly arise in the transitional zone just above the dentate line, and tend to spread proximally in the submucosa to the distal rectum. Tumours invade anteriorly into the vagina and uncommonly to the prostate, laterally to the ischio-rectal fossae, and posteriorly along the ano-coccygeal ligament to the coccyx. Anterior spread to the prostate may be limited by Denonvilliers' fascia, and inferior spread may be limited by the suspensory ligaments.

Lymphatic drainage from the anal margin and peri-anal skin is to the super-ficial inguinal and femoral lymph nodes, and thence to the external iliac nodes. The lymphatic drainage of the anal canal, proximal to the dentate line, is to the superior rectal, superior haemorrhoidal, hypogastric, obturator and presacral lymph nodes (Fig. 25.2). Tumours distal to the dentate line drain to superficial inguinal nodes as well as to pararectal nodes.

Planning technique

ASSESSMENT OF PRIMARY DISEASE

Inspection of the perineal skin and digital rectal examination are used to assess the site and extent of anal tumours. Vaginal examination is performed to detect

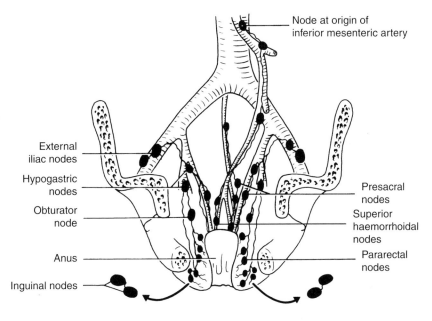

Fig. 25.2 Lymphatic drainage of the anus.

any involvement of the posterior vaginal wall. Trans-ano-rectal ultrasound may help to define the depth of tumour invasion. Endoscopic examination should be perfomed under general anaesthetic if pain or spasm are a problem. Proctoscopy and sigmoidoscopy are essential to define the upper limit of the tumour and to biopsy the primary lesion. The size of any palpable lymph nodes in the inguinal region must be documented, and fine-needle aspiration cytology or excision biopsy should be performed for diagnosis.

Double-contrast barium enema studies may be used to exclude synchronous lesions in the colon. CT scanning of the abdomen may be useful for excluding involvement of lymph nodes and for identifying liver metastases, which occur in less than 5 per cent of patients.

DEFINITION OF TARGET VOLUME

The target volume will depend on the site and size of the primary tumour, local extension of disease, histological involvement of lymph nodes, and whether concomitant chemotherapy is being given.

Anal margin – T_1 tumours

The target volume encompasses the primary tumour with a 2-cm margin.

Anal margin – T_2–T_4 tumours (and small tumours of the distal anal canal)

Initial treatment covers the primary tumour, anal canal, pararectal and presacral nodes. The inguinal nodes are not included for prophylactic treatment as the risk of involvement is relatively low. The volume must include superficial tissues and perineal skin because of the risk of local infiltration.

The target volume for a second phase of treatment encompasses the primary tumour alone.

All other tumours

Initial treatment includes the primary tumour, anal canal, lower rectum and the pararectal, obturator and hypogastric lymph nodes, as shown in Fig. 25.3. The volume extends from the anal verge, with a margin of perineal skin as appropriate, to the bottom of the sacro-iliac joints. The lateral margins encompass the internal iliac nodes within the true pelvis. The volume extends from the sacrum posteriorly to encompass all disease anteriorly.

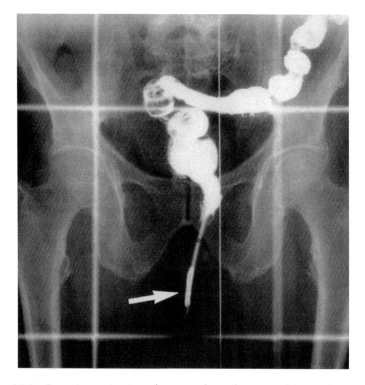

Fig. 25.3 Posterior projection of target volume for external beam therapy of carcinoma of the anal canal, with ring marking anal margin (arrowed).

The target volume for a second phase of treatment encompasses the primary tumour alone.

Inguinal lymph nodes

The target volume for inguinal node irradiation is localized by palpation and estimation of the depth of lymphadenopathy.

LOCALIZATION

For external beam treatments, CT scanning is used to localize a posterior pelvic volume. Patients are scanned while prone in the treatment position with the bladder full in order to displace the small bowel out of the pelvis. The buttocks may be taped apart to reduce skin reaction, and barium paste is used to mark a skin reference tattoo on the coccyx, to localize the anal margin and to mark two lateral tattoos to prevent rotation. Since the depth of the target volume varies from the presacral region superiorly to the anal canal inferiorly, multiple scans are used to ensure adequate cover of tumour and nodes at all levels. A scan through the centre of the volume is used for initial two-dimensional treatment planning, with three-dimensional localization and planning where available.

Alternatively, barium may be placed via a catheter in the rectum, with a tampon in the vagina and a wire ring marking the anal margin. Postero-anterior and lateral films are taken in the prone position on the simulator and used to localize the target volume on a transverse outline taken through the centre.

Field arrangements

ANAL MARGIN – T_1 TUMOURS

These tumours are best treated with the patient lying prone over a barrel-shaped support. A direct electron field of appropriate energy is used to encompass the target volume in the 90 per cent isodose. It is difficult to obtain accurate geometry for these lesions with interstitial implantation, and this technique is rarely used for these small superficial anal margin tumours.

ANAL MARGIN – T_2–T_4 TUMOURS (AND SMALL TUMOURS OF THE DISTAL ANAL CANAL)

Initial treatment may be given by a direct perineal field with the patient in the lithotomy position or lying prone over a barrel-shaped support. The field margins are marked on the skin and treatment is given at the standard FSD. Bolus may be needed to increase the dose superficially, especially where there is infiltration of the perineal skin. 8 MV photons are used to give an adequate depth dose (e.g. 75 per cent at 9 cm for a 10 × 10 cm field). A more uniform dose to the presacral region may be obtained by using superior and inferior wedged fields with the patient in the same position, employing a sagittal body outline.

Residual primary tumour in the anal canal may be treated by interstitial implantation as described below.

ALL OTHER TUMOURS

Initial treatment can be given with a three-field technique using a direct posterior field with reduced weighting and two posterior oblique fields, at a gantry angle of 45–65° depending on the shape of the volume and its proximity to the skin surface (Fig. 25.4). Angles of less than 45° are not used because they cause over-lap with fields posteriorly, increasing skin reaction in the natal cleft. Bolus may be needed inferiorly at the site of the primary tumour. This technique reduces the dose to the small bowel lying anteriorly compared with opposing anterior and posterior fields.

If at the initial assessment the tumour is considered to be small enough for interstitial implantation, this is performed 6 weeks after external beam therapy has been completed to allow for tumour regression and healing of the skin. Sometimes continuation of external beam treatment with reduced fields is more appropriate.

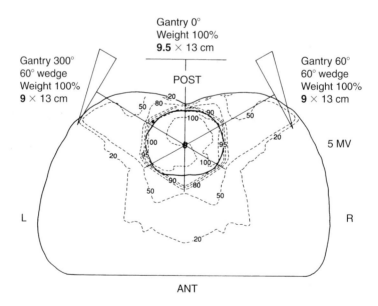

Fig. 25.4   Dose distribution using three-field technique for irradiation of anal tumour.

Interstitial implantation

This technique is used as a boost to the site of the primary tumour after external beam therapy for anal canal lesions. Patients are prepared by two daily enemas prior to implantation and are established on oral codeine phosphate and a low-residue diet. The conical shape of the peri-anal region and the anal canal creates a high risk of convergence or divergence of implanted sources, so a template technique is needed to achieve parallelism of sources. Implantation is performed under general anaesthesia with the patient in the lithotomy position and with a urinary catheter in place.

It is essential to have a full description of the primary tumour at presentation before chemotherapy or external beam radiotherapy, so that the target volume can be defined using this information. Following initial treatment there may be considerable tumour regression, which makes the volume for implantation difficult to delineate.

Most implants are performed in a semicircular plane about 3 cm in diameter with a separation of 1 cm between the needles encompassing not more than two-thirds of the anal circumference, in order to reduce the risk of stenosis. The stainless steel guide needles are passed through the template parallel to the anal canal, with a finger in the rectum so that they are positioned approximately 5 mm below the mucosa. It is usual to use five to seven needles, each being 5–8 cm in length depending on the depth of the target volume and limited by the sacral prominence. The template is sutured to the perineal skin and a hollow tube is inserted into the rectum and sutured to displace the uninvolved mucosa away from the implant and to maintain parallelism (Figs 25.5a and b).

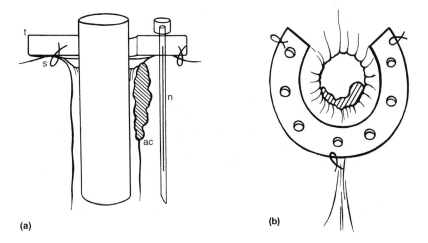

(a)
(b)

Fig. 25.5   (a) Technique for implantation of anal carcinoma with iridium wires, showing template sutured to anal margin and guide needle inserted through template. s = suture; ac = anal carcinoma; t = template; n = needle. (b) Circular arrangement of sources for iridium wire implant of anal canal tumour.

The length of the active wire is chosen to allow for lack of crossing of the deep ends of the implant, using a greater length than the target volume if possible and clinically appropriate. Active wire often has to pass through the anal margin to cover the target volume, but if this can be avoided, the risk of painful necrosis will be reduced. Removal of the implant with adequate analgesia but without general anaesthesia is usually well tolerated.

INGUINAL LYMPH-NODE IRRADIATION

Where there is inguinal node involvement, the three-field technique can be combined with anterior electron fields to both groins with the patient lying supine. However, overlap of these anterior fields with the posterior direct field may occur within the pelvis, and summated doses should be calculated at depth.

Because this technique requires a change of treatment position from prone to supine, with consequent inaccuracies of summated dosimetry, it is preferable to treat the patient in the supine position only. Inguinal nodes can then be treated in continuity with the primary tumour by large anterior and posterior fields as shown in Fig. 25.6. Additional treatment is given to the primary tumour using a three-field technique as described above, and to the inguinal region using electrons to spare the underlying femoral heads. Inguinal and perineal skin reactions may be severe when this opposed-field technique is used.

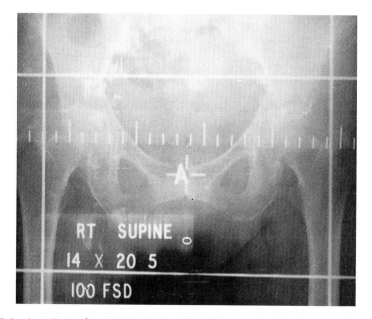

Fig. 25.6 Anterior and posterior opposing fields to treat primary anal margin tumour and inguinal lymph nodes in continuity.

Implementation of plan

For the prone three-field technique, patients are treated with a full bladder, and lasers are used to align the skin reference tattoo and lateral tattoos over the iliac crests to prevent rotation. All fields are treated isocentrically each day with a linear accelerator. The IPD is checked and the pin depth measured from the treatment plan. The gantry angle is set appropriately, with care taken to calculate the reduced weighting of the posterior field. It is important that the set-up is seen on the first day by the radiotherapist to ensure that there is adequate cover of the primary tumour by the inferior borders of the fields.

For treatment of the pelvis and inguinal region in the supine position, the IPD is measured at the centre of the field and the mid-plane dose is calculated. Anterior and posterior fields are treated isocentrically using a central tattoo as a reference point, and lateral tattoos to prevent rotation.

Small anterior inguinal fields are matched to skin marks using an applicator to define the machine SSD for electron or orthovoltage therapy.

Dose prescription

INITIAL TARGET VOLUME

40–45 Gy in 20–25 fractions given in 4 to 5 weeks.

For a direct perineal field, doses are prescribed to the centre of the target volume on the central axis, with calculation of skin doses and minimum and maximum target volume doses.

PRIMARY TUMOUR ALONE

Interstitial implantation

20–25 Gy to the 85 per cent reference isodose.

External beam therapy

20–25 Gy in 10–13 fractions in 2 to 2.5 weeks to give a total dose to the primary tumour of 60–65 Gy in 6.5 to 7 weeks.

INGUINAL NODE IRRADIATION

Initial target volume (including primary tumour and inguinal nodes)

40–44 Gy in 20–22 fractions given in 4 to 4.5 weeks.

Additional electron therapy to include palpable lymphadenopathy using a direct anterior field to a target volume encompassed within the 90 per cent isodose curve.

10–20 Gy in 5–10 fractions given in 1 to 2 weeks.

Direct anterior field (to inguinal nodes alone)

The electron energy should be chosen to include the target volume within the 90 per cent isodose curve.

55–60 Gy applied dose in 27–30 fractions in 6 weeks, treating daily.

Patient care

The perineal and inguinal tissues are particularly sensitive to irradiation and skin reactions may be brisk and painful. The skin should be kept as dry as possible, and if moist desquamation occurs treatment may have to be suspended. A low-residue diet is advised, and diarrhoea is treated with appropriate medication.

Further reading

Cummings, B.J. 1995: Anal cancer: radiation, with and without chemotherapy. In Cohen, A.M. and Winawer, S.J. (eds), *Cancer of the colon, rectum and anus*. New York: McGraw-Hill.

United Kingdom Co-ordinating Committee for Cancer Research (UKCCCR) 1996: Anal Canal Cancer Trial Working Party. Epidermoid anal cancer: results from the UKCCCR randomised trial of radiotherapy alone versus radiotherapy, 5-fluorouracil and Mitomycin C. *Lancet* **348**, 1049.

CHAPTER 26

Prostate

Role of radiotherapy

The screening and management of patients with prostate cancer are controversial. For patients with T_1 and T_2N_0 tumours, the options for therapy are radical surgery, radical radiotherapy (brachytherapy or external beam) or a watch policy. In early disease, surgery and radiotherapy are probably equally effective, but the morbidity differs. The patient's life expectancy and attitude to the benefits or risks of interventions should be considered in choosing treatment. The prognosis is worse with an increase in either local extent of tumour at presentation, prostate-specific antigen (PSA) level or histological Gleason grading score.

After radiotherapy, 70 to 90 per cent of patients with T_1/T_2 tumours and 50 to 70 per cent of those with T_3/T_4 lesions are alive at 5 years. By 10 years, the survival rates have fallen to 30 to 70 per cent depending on the stage – results similar to those obtained by radical prostatectomy. Local control is difficult to assess, but a nadir PSA level after treatment of $< 2\,ng/mL$ within 2 years appears to predict long-term control. The significance of this in terms of improved survival has yet to be determined. Short-term neo-adjuvant androgen deprivation before and during radiotherapy has proved beneficial. Reports of a 25 to 50 per cent reduction in prostate target volume may allow improvements in therapeutic ratio with subsequent conformal therapy.

There is conflicting evidence with regard to the value of elective radiotherapy to the pelvic lymph nodes. The relatively small potential benefit from such treatment should be balanced against the increased toxicity which may occur with whole pelvic radiotherapy (see Chapter 30). Patients found to have enlarged pelvic nodes on staging CT scan are treated with primary hormone therapy.

Patients with disease confined within the prostate capsule (i.e. T_1 and T_2) tumours can be treated by brachytherapy. For tumours with a risk of capsular involvement, brachytherapy can be used as a boost after external beam therapy. Brachytherapy techniques are described at the end of this chapter.

The value of postoperative radiotherapy when margins after prostatectomy are positive is not yet clear.

Palliative radiotherapy is useful in patients with metastatic disease, to relieve symptoms from local prostatic disease, bone metastases or soft-tissue masses.

Gynaecomastia from oestrogen therapy may be prevented by breast irradiation.

Regional anatomy

The prostate gland lies between the pubic symphysis and the anterior rectal wall, and is closely applied to the bladder neck and seminal vesicles (Fig. 26.1). Local extension occurs through the prostatic capsule, especially posteriorly, at the apex, and at the junctions between the base and bladder neck and seminal vesicles, and may correlate with perineural invasion. Denonvilliers' fascia reduces spread towards the rectum.

Lymphatics drain from the prostate gland to the obturator, presacral, internal and external iliac nodes, and thence to the common iliac and para-aortic nodes (Fig. 26.2). Lymph-node involvement increases with increasing tumour stage and histological grade.

Planning technique

ASSESSMENT OF DISEASE

The local extent of the primary tumour is defined by digital rectal examination, cystocopy and transrectal ultrasound (TRUS). For patients with T_1/T_2 tumours who have PSA levels of less than 20 ng/mL, no bony symptoms and well-differentiated histology, isotope bone scanning is unnecessary. It is performed to exclude bone metastases in all other groups of patients, in addition to a chest X-ray. Where PSA levels are greater than 20 ng/mL and histology shows Gleason grade 7 or more, CT or MRI of the abdomen and pelvis is performed in order to detect involvement of the obturator, internal, external and common iliac or para-aortic nodes. MRI may be particularly useful for distinguishing capsular invasion, seminal vesicle involvement and peri-apical extension. CT scanning

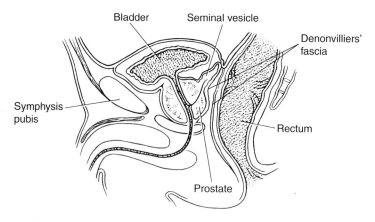

Fig. 26.1   Sagittal section through pelvis to show the relationships of the prostate gland.

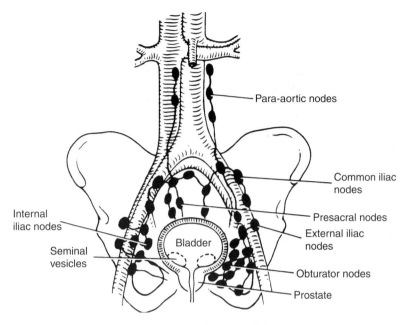

Fig. 26.2 Lymphatic drainage of the prostate.

for treatment planning is performed in all patients to define the extent of primary tumour and spread to the extra-prostatic tissues, seminal vesicles or bladder (Fig. 26.3).

DEFINITION OF TARGET VOLUME

The margins of the target volume are determined by the tumour extent as palpated rectally and visualized on CT scanning. Nomograms for predicting the percentage probability of seminal vesicle involvement are based on clinical T-stage from rectal examination, Gleason score and PSA level. The gross tumour volume consists of the total prostate gland as defined by clinical and radiological staging, with inclusion of the base of the seminal vesicles. If there is either high risk of or known seminal vesicle involvement, the volume must be extended posteriorly and superiorly to include all of the seminal vesicles. To allow for microscopic spread and positional variation, a PTV is created which allows a margin of 1–1.5 cm inferiorly around the prostatic apex, superiorly above the tip of the seminal vesicles and anteriorly towards the pubic symphysis. The posterior border includes a 1 cm margin of anterior rectal wall which may be reduced for a high-dose prostatic boost. The volume is usually $7 \times 7 \times 7$ cm, but is extended to around $9 \times 9 \times 9$ cm where there is seminal vesicle involvement. Shaping of the target volume by shielding blocks or multileaf collimators can reduce irradiation to normal tissues by around 30 per cent.

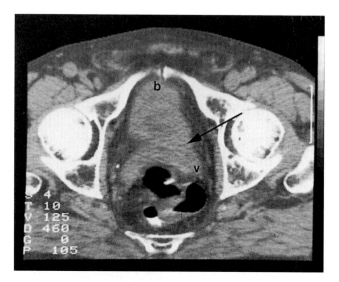

Fig. 26.3   CT scan showing involvement of the left seminal vesicle by carcinoma of the prostate (arrowed). b = bladder; v = seminal vesicle.

PATIENT POSITIONING

Verification studies show that patient position can be maintained and reproduced either by the use of alpha cradles or shells, or by careful positioning of the patient in a supine position with leg restraints and a co-ordinated system of midline and lateral skin tattoos and laser lights for accurate alignment (Fig. 26.4). It is essential that each department has a good procedure for positioning the patient which has been verified with portal imaging, particularly if conformal therapy is to be used.

LOCALIZATION

The patient is immobilized supine as for treatment, with skin tattoos placed anteriorly over the pubic symphysis and laterally over the iliac crests to prevent lateral rotation. These are labelled with barium paste and radio-opaque catheters. Although a full bladder can be used to displace the small bowel, studies have shown that the prostate is displaced by overfilling of the bladder or rectum, leading to variations in its position. A comfortably full bladder is therefore required for scanning and treatment, and CT planning scans are taken of the pelvis after normal fluid intake and voiding of the rectum. If the rectum is found to be overfilled by gas or faecal contents, a repeat scan may be necessary to provide an acceptable baseline for planning. CT scans are usually taken at 5-mm intervals

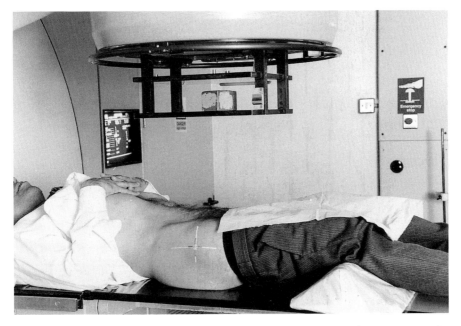

Fig. 26.4 Position of patient supine with knee pads to prevent pelvic rotation and mid-line and lateral skin tattoos aligned using laser lights.

contiguously using a slice thickness of 4–5 mm throughout the pelvis (Fig. 26.5). No oral, rectal or intravenous contrast should be used.

Two-dimensional localization

The superior and inferior borders of the gross tumour volume are obtained from serial images and a margin of 1–1.5 cm is added. The CT section at the centre of the volume is used as the main planning slice to outline patient contour, target volume, rectum and bladder on the CT planning system (Plates 26.1a and b). For two-dimensional planning, the PTV is outlined on multiple sections to ensure that the entire tumour is also encompassed at all levels by the target volume defined on the central section. The rectum curves anteriorly to lie adjacent to the base of the prostate within the high-dose zone in the superior part of the target volume, so the rectal outline must also be transposed on to the central section in order that the dose can be adequately estimated.

CT scanning is the standard method of localization, but where this facility is not available, a cystogram is performed with the patient supine. Contrast medium (20 mL) and air (10 mL) are introduced into the bladder via a urinary catheter, with 20 mL of contrast medium in the catheter balloon which is pulled down onto the bladder base. An AP film is taken on the simulator (Fig. 26.6), barium is inserted into the rectum and a lateral film is taken. The target volume is marked on to a transverse outline taken through the centre of the volume.

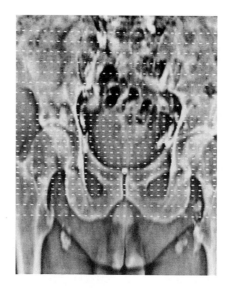

Fig. 26.5 CT topogram of the pelvis with radio-opaque catheter in the plane of the skin tattoo marked by barium paste.

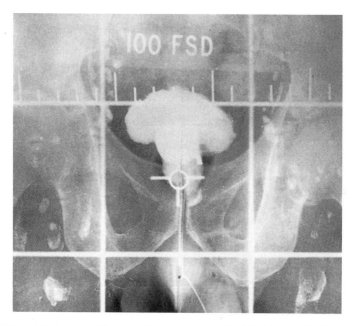

Fig. 26.6 AP simulator film showing contrast in the bladder and balloon of the urinary catheter.

Three-dimensional localization

Where three-dimensional planning and dose calculations are available, the GTV and PTV should be constructed on each CT slice. In addition, all normal organs, i.e. rectum, bladder, small bowel and femoral heads, should also be outlined. The rectum should be outlined from the anus to the recto-sigmoid junction – a length of approximately 12 cm in most patients.

Field arrangements

TWO-DIMENSIONAL PLANNING

The technique chosen depends on the size and shape of the target volume. Three-field techniques using an anterior and two posterior oblique or two opposing lateral fields give a high dose to the prostate with the lowest dose to the posterior rectal wall. The posterior fields may be wedged to compensate for patient contour, and are usually angled at 110–120° (Fig. 26.7). An anterior rotation of the gantry decreases the dose to the rectum but increases the dose to the femoral heads, which may be of concern in the case of patients who have had a total hip replacement. A four-field box technique increases the dose posteriorly and may produce a better dose distribution when the seminal vesicles are included in the target volume.

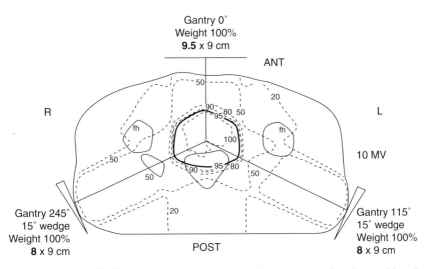

Fig. 26.7 Three-field technique for irradiation of the prostate. fh = femoral head.

THREE-DIMENSIONAL PLANNING

The three- or four-field techniques used for two-dimensional planning or six coplanar fields may be used, namely two lateral opposing fields and two pairs of lateral oblique fields. The angle of the oblique fields will usually be at 35–40° from the lateral beams. Shaping of the fields to conform to the PTV can be achieved with the use of either alloy blocks or multileaf collimators, and recorded on simulator or digitally reconstructed radiographs. Provided that contrast media has not been used for CT scanning and rectal gas is minimal, pixel-by-pixel dose inhomogeneity corrections can be made for pelvic bone. When shielding is applied, care must be taken to ensure accurate immobilization of the patient and precise target volume definition, as any day-to-day variations may lead to shielding of tumour or a marginal miss.

Implementation of plan

The patient is treated supine on a linear accelerator (preferably at a high energy) with a comfortably full bladder, after rectal voiding if necessary. The patient is immobilized using knee pads, and accurate alignment is ensured by using anterior and lateral laser lights to check the position of mid-line and two lateral skin tattoos in order to prevent lateral rotation. The field centre is marked with reference to the anterior tattoo of the pubic symphysis. The interplanar distance is checked and the pin depth measured from the treatment plan. All fields are treated isocentrically every day with shielding as instructed. Verification is performed using portal films or an on-line portal imaging system, and the results are compared with simulator images or digitally reconstructed radiographs.

Dose prescription

64 Gy in 32 fractions given in 6.5 weeks.

Dose escalation with conformal therapy is under study.

Patient care

Severe skin reactions may occur over the sacrum and the natal cleft. A low-residue diet is advised to prevent diarrhoea, which is treated with loperamide as necessary. If diarrhoea is severe, irradiation may be suspended or the dose per fraction reduced. Proctitis and tenesmus during treatment are common. If symptoms of cystitis or urinary frequency occur, a midstream urine specimen is taken for bacteriological examination. This is often negative, and a high fluid intake should be advised.

Male breast irradiation prior to hormone therapy for prostate cancer

9–12 MeV electron therapy using a circular field (7–9 cm diameter) to breast tissue.

15 Gy in 3 fractions given in 3 days.

Brachytherapy

Patients with disease confined within the prostate capsule (T_1 and T_2) can be treated by brachytherapy. The inclusion criteria for brachytherapy are as follows:

- life expectancy greater than 10 years;
- biopsy-confirmed adenocarcinoma of prostate;
- disease confined within the prostate capsule;
- bone scan negative;
- CT or MRI showing no pelvic or abdominal lymph-node enlargement;
- prostate volume less than 50 cm^3 (if larger and otherwise suitable, 3 months of neo-adjuvant hormone treatment will usually bring the volume down to 50 cm^3 or less);
- no prior transurethral resection of prostate (TURP);
- PSA less than 20 ng/mL.

The most commonly used technique is transrectal ultrasound and template-guided percutaneous implantation of iodine-125 seeds. The number and position of seeds required is obtained from a planning transrectal ultrasound scan performed in the lithotomy position. This defines the volume of the prostate and template co-ordinates which can be used for insertion of the needles that carry the radioactive seeds.

The implant is performed under spinal or general anaesthesia at a later date. The patient is first placed in the lithotomy position so that the prostate ultrasound slices are the same as those used for planning. The iodine-125 seeds are inserted into the prostate percutaneously via a thin needle, using the template and real-time ultrasound to guide it into the pre-planned position. Between 20 and 30 needles containing 60 to 120 seeds are implanted depending on the volume and seed activity. The needles are then removed, leaving the seeds permanently in place. The patient is usually able to return home the following day. Post-implant dosimetry cannot change the seed distribution, but is useful for quality control.

CT images of the prostate can be obtained using 5-mm slices and isodose contours calculated to evaluate the dose actually delivered to the prostate. This provides a permanent record of the dose delivered. Check films are also taken of the seeds in order to confirm the number of seeds implanted and their position. (Fig. 26.8).

For treatment by brachytherapy alone, the plan aims to deliver a dose of 160 Gy to a volume which includes the prostate capsule plus a margin of 2–3 mm.

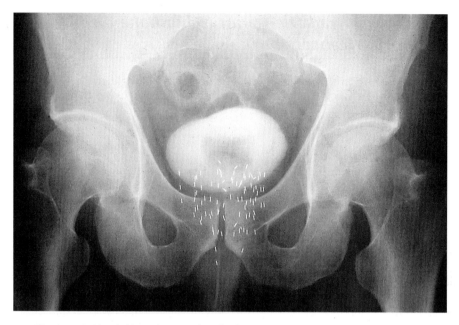

Fig. 26.8 Check films showing brachytherapy treatment of the prostate using iodine-125 seeds.

For patients at risk of capsular involvement, brachytherapy can be used as a boost after external beam therapy. Remote afterloading techniques can also be used with TRUS and template guidance. These usually employ high-dose-rate (HDR) radiation and have to be fractionated. They can only be used as a boost after prior external beam therapy.

Further reading

Blasko, J.C., Grimm, P.D. and Ragde, H. 1995: Prostate-specific antigen-based disease control following ultrasound guided ^{125}I implantation for stage T_1/T_2 prostate carcinoma. *Journal of Urology*, **154**, 1096–7.

Perez, C.A. 1997: Prostate. In Perez, C.A. and Brady, L.W. (eds), *Principles and practice of radiation oncology*, 3rd edn. Philadelphia, PA: Lippincott-Raven, 1583–694.

CHAPTER 27

Bladder

Role of radiotherapy

Radical cystectomy and radical radiotherapy as single modality treatments have never been compared in a prospective randomized controlled trial, and comparison of results from a series of single-modality treatments is difficult because of selection bias and the non-surgical staging of radiotherapy patients. Selection of treatment has therefore often depended on available experience as well as patients' wishes and motivation. Centres in the UK, Canada and Europe have more often used primary radiotherapy with salvage cystectomy, whereas in the USA initial cystectomy with or without chemotherapy has been used more widely. Brachytherapy has had a particular role in some European countries.

For well-differentiated T_1/T_2 tumours where lymph-node involvement is uncommon, cure rates of up to 80 per cent can be obtained with surgery. Recurrent or multiple T_1 tumours and multifocal T_{1S} tumours are treated with intravesical chemotherapy or immunotherapy (BCG), giving control rates of around 80 per cent, with salvage cystectomy for fit patients who fail treatment. The role of radiotherapy in grade 3 stage T_1 transitional cell carcinoma is still under investigation. Series reporting local radiotherapy to the bladder and perivesical tissues give 5-year survival rates of 40 to 60 per cent, while results for T_1T_2 tumours treated by primary cystectomy are of the order of 60 to 80 per cent. Radiotherapy may not be suitable for patients with a small contracted bladder, or following extensive intravesical treatment.

Radical radiotherapy for T_3 tumours produces 5-year survival rates of less than 35 per cent, which may be increased to 45 to 60 per cent in selected patients after salvage cystectomy. Radical primary cystectomy with urinary reconstruction has a low operative mortality in specialist centres, and produces survival rates of 40 to 50 per cent. This approach may be preferred in young patients.

So far no overall advantage has been shown for chemotherapy added to radiotherapy in the management of advanced T_2–T_4 tumours. Neo-adjuvant chemotherapy with or without radiotherapy before cystectomy is under investigation for locally advanced tumours. The role of adjuvant pre- or postoperative radiotherapy has yet to be defined.

Palliative radiotherapy treatment is useful for the relief of symptoms such as haematuria and pain for patients with T_4 bladder tumours. Nodal involvement is usually considered as an indication for palliative treatment in the UK, although 5-year survival rates of 10 to 35 per cent have been reported from a series of American patients treated radically.

Regional anatomy

Tumours originate in the bladder epithelium and infiltrate deeply into the muscle layers, penetrating through the bladder wall into perivesical fat and adjacent pelvic organs (Fig. 27.1 and see Fig. 26.1).

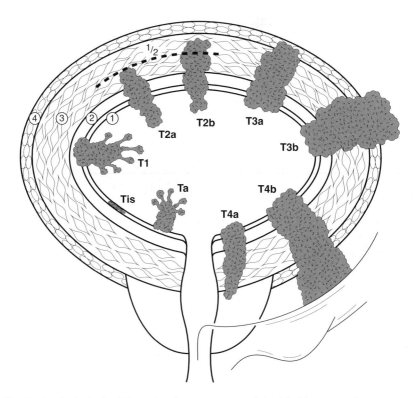

Fig. 27.1 Pathological T staging for carcinoma of the bladder, according to UICC Classification (1997). T_a = non-invasive papillary carcinoma; T_{is} = carcinoma *in situ*; T_1 = tumour invading subepithelial connective tissue; T_2 = tumour invading muscle; T_{2a} = tumour invading superficial muscle (inner half); T_{2b} = tumour invading deep muscle (outer half); T_3 = tumour invading perivesical tissue; T_{3a} = microscopically; T_{3b} = macroscopically (extravesical mass); T_4 = tumour invading any of the following: prostate, uterus, vagina, pelvic wall, abdominal wall; T_{4a} = tumour invading prostate or uterus or vagina; T_{4b} = tumour invading pelvic wall or abdominal wall. 1 = epithelium; 2 = subepithelial connective tissue; 3 = muscle; 4 = perivesical fat. (Reproduced with permission from Hermanek, P., Hutter, R. V. P. and Sobin, L. H. (eds) 1997: *International Union Against Cancer TNM atlas. Illustrated guide to the TNM classification of malignant tumours*, 4th edn. Berlin: Springer-Verlag.)

Lymphatic spread is first to the hypogastric, obturator, internal, external and common iliac lymph nodes (Fig. 27.2), and thence to the para-aortic and inguinal nodes. The risk of lymph-node metastases is proportional to the depth of tumour invasion, namely 20 per cent for invasion of lamina propria, 30 per cent with superficial muscle invasion and 60 per cent with full-thickness muscle invasion.

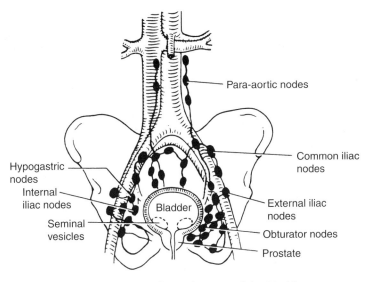

Fig. 27.2 Lymphatic drainage of the bladder.

Planning technique

ASSESSMENT OF DISEASE

The extent of the primary tumour is assessed by cystoscopy and bimanual pelvic examination under anaesthesia. Biopsy of the tumour defines the histological type and grade; biopsy of the base of the resected tumour shows the degree of invasion. Random mucosal biopsies of the bladder identify the presence of carcinoma *in situ*. An intravenous urogram may demonstrate a filling defect in the bladder at the site of the primary tumour, hydroureter secondary to tumour obstruction of the ureteric orifices, or other urothelial tumours.

CT scanning shows the tumour as a soft-tissue mass, and may reveal previously undetected extravesical extension, including spread into the seminal vesicles. It also demonstrates enlarged internal, external, common iliac and para-aortic nodes.

DEFINITION OF TARGET VOLUME

Lymphatic involvement occurs in about 30 per cent of patients with T_2 tumours and 60 per cent of patients with T_3 tumours, and radiation may be given to the whole pelvis in selected patients. Radiotherapy is given to the bladder alone for the majority of patients and when synchronous chemotherapy is given.

Large volume

The initial target volume includes the primary tumour and its local extensions, the whole bladder and the pelvic lymph nodes. The volume extends from the upper border of L_5 to include the common iliac nodes and inferiorly to cover the lower border of the obturator foramen. If the tumour involves the urethra, the volume must be extended inferiorly. The lateral margins lie 1 cm outside the bony pelvic walls. The anterior border lies 1–2 cm in front of the anterior bladder wall and the posterior border at the S2/3 junction encompasses the internal iliac nodes and the entire bladder.

Small volume

The planning target volume includes a margin of 1.5–2 cm around the bladder, with a minimum 2-cm margin at the tumour site to encompass any extension. CT scanning is used to define the target volume, which is usually 8–10 cm^3. The patient empties their bladder before the CT scan and before treatment each day in order to ensure that the tumour remains within the planned target volume.

LOCALIZATION

A skin tattoo is placed over the pubic symphysis and marked with barium paste, with two additional lateral tattoos placed over the iliac crests to prevent lateral rotation. With the patient in the treatment position, a CT scan is performed with the bladder full. This gives the most accurate information about the tumour extent (Fig. 27.3). These scans are used to plan treatment to the whole pelvis, which is given with the bladder full. A scan is repeated after the patient has emptied their bladder, and these scans are used to plan small-volume treatments. Using the CT planning system, the patient contour, target volume, rectum and femoral heads are localized on the CT section at the centre of the volume for two-dimensional planning. Multiple scans are used to check that the tumour is encompassed within the volume throughout its length. Three-dimensional treatment planning is performed when available.

When CT scanning is not available, a cystogram is performed on the simulator after the patient has emptied their bladder. A urinary catheter is inserted, 20 mL of contrast and 10 mL of air are introduced into the bladder, without draining residual urine, and an AP film is taken (Fig. 27.4). Following insertion of barium into the rectum, a lateral film is obtained. The target volume and rectum are localized on to a transverse outline taken through the centre of the volume.

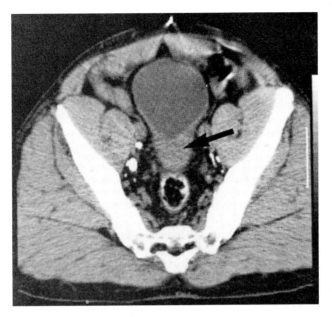

Fig. 27.3 CT scan of T_{3b} bladder tumour with posterior extension (arrowed).

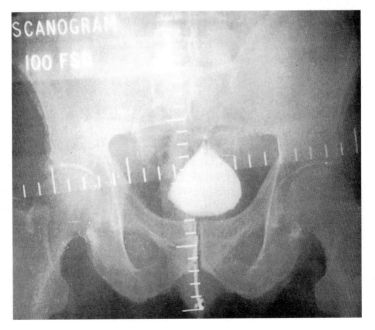

Fig. 27.4 AP simulator film with contrast and air in the bladder.

Field arrangements

LARGE VOLUME

An anterior and opposing lateral wedged fields are chosen, since this arrangement gives a homogeneous distribution shaped to the target volume with a sharp cut-off posteriorly to spare the rectum as shown in Fig. 27.5. This technique is discussed in Chapter 30, and the dose distribution is shown in Fig. 30.8.

SMALL VOLUME

Treatment may be given with the three-field technique described above, or with an anterior and two posterior oblique wedged fields, depending on the bladder contour. The angle between the posterior oblique fields is usually 110°, to spare the rectum (Fig. 27.6). For palliative treatment of some T_4 tumours, opposing anterior and posterior fields are chosen, following a simulator film to outline the soft-tissue bladder shadow or localizing cystogram if necessary. This arrangement is satisfactory for lower doses of palliative irradiation, to control haematuria in frail patients.

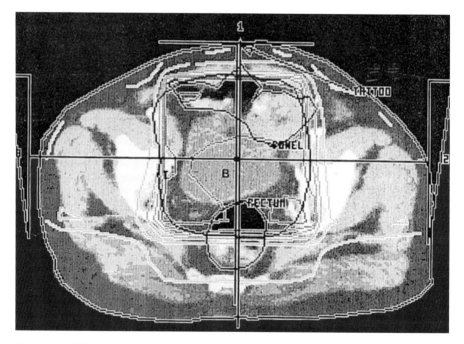

Fig. 27.5   CT scan with isodose distribution for whole pelvic irradiation. B = bladder.

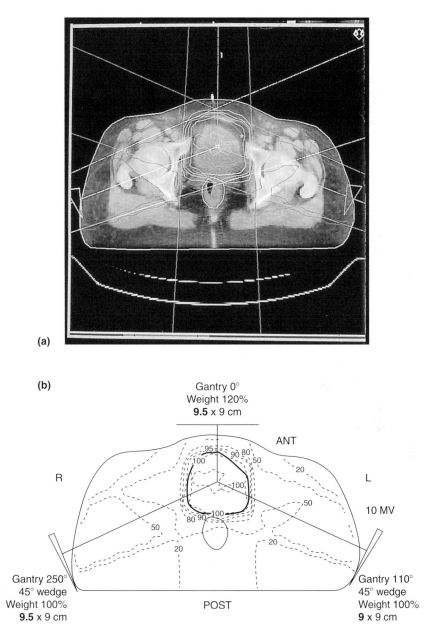

(a)

(b)

Gantry 0°
Weight 120%
9.5 x 9 cm

ANT

R

L

10 MV

Gantry 250°
45° wedge
Weight 100%
9.5 x 9 cm

POST

Gantry 110°
45° wedge
Weight 100%
9 x 9 cm

Fig. 27.6   Three-field technique for small-volume irradiation to the bladder. (a) CT scan with isodose distribution. (b) Diagram to show 95 per cent isodose encompassing target volume.

Implementation of plan

For whole pelvic irradiation, treatment is given with the patient supine and the bladder full in order to displace the small bowel out of the pelvis. For small-volume treatments, the bladder is empty to minimize the target volume and to ensure that all of the tumour is included. The bladder volume will inevitably vary from day to day because of residual urine, but this variation may be reduced by asking the patient to empty their bladder immediately before treatment each day. The patient is aligned using an anterior laser beam to check the mid-line and two lateral lasers to align lateral skin tattoos and prevent rotation. The field centre is marked with reference to the tattoo over the pubic symphysis. The interplanar distance (IPD) is checked and the pin depth measured from the treatment plan.

Most plans are treated isocentrically, but in an obese patient the IPD may vary widely from day to day. For whole pelvic treatment it may then be more accurate to measure the entry point of the lateral fields from the couch top in order to avoid any discrepancy in the pin depth, and to treat at 100 cm FSD.

Dose prescription

RADICAL TREATMENT

Initial target volume (whole pelvis)

44 Gy in 22 fractions given in 4.5 weeks.

Boost to bladder alone (after whole pelvic irradiation)

20 Gy in 10 fractions given in 2 weeks.

Small volume (bladder alone)

64 Gy in 32 fractions given in 6.5 weeks.

PALLIATIVE TREATMENT

35 Gy in 10 fractions given in 2 weeks

or 21 Gy in 3 fractions given in 1 week.

Patient care

A low-residue diet should be advised. Diarrhoea should be controlled with oral medication or suspension of treatment. If symptoms of cystitis or urinary frequency develop, a midstream urine specimen is taken for bacteriological examination. This is often negative, and a high fluid intake should be advised. Urinary catheterization is avoided where possible, since this may predispose to chronic infections or inflammation.

Further reading

Ozen, H. 1997: Bladder cancer. *Current Opinion in Oncology* **9**, 295–300.

CHAPTER 28

Testis

Role of radiotherapy

SEMINOMA

More than 70 per cent of patients with testicular seminoma present with stage I disease. Following orchidectomy, they are treated with radiotherapy to the para-aortic lymph nodes, and 5-year survival rates of 95 to 100 per cent are obtained. Studies are in progress to determine whether lower doses of irradiation produce the same control with a reduction in toxicity. Surveillance of patients with stage I seminoma reveals in a 15 to 20 per cent relapse rate at 5 years, with most patients curable by subsequent chemotherapy. However, since there are no reliable tumour markers, this policy requires intensive and prolonged restaging investigations over up to 8 years, and is only used in selected patients where prophylactic radiotherapy is contraindicated. Adjuvant single-agent carboplatin chemotherapy is currently being investigated as an alternative to radiotherapy for stage I disease. Patients with small-volume IIA disease also have a high cure rate (85 to 90 per cent) with radiotherapy alone.

Patients with bulky stage II, stage III and stage IV disease are treated with chemotherapy.

Relapse after chemotherapy alone is most common in sites of initial bulky disease, but the overall incidence is low (around 12 per cent) and the role of radiotherapy is therefore still controversial.

TERATOMA

A surveillance policy is followed for patients with stage I teratoma. Between 70 and 80 per cent will be cured by orchidectomy alone, and patients who relapse may also be cured with chemotherapy (90 per cent). Adjuvant chemotherapy is currently under trial for patients with stage I disease who have one or more high risk factors for relapse, such as embryonal carcinoma, or lymphatic and/or vascular invasion which predicts a relapse rate of 40 per cent. For symptomatic relief, radiotherapy may be used to control inoperable bulky disease after chemotherapy, or in patients with cerebral, lymph-node or bony metastases.

TESTICULAR INTRA-EPITHELIAL NEOPLASIA (TIN)

Five per cent of patients have TIN on random biopsy of the contralateral testis at the time of orchidectomy. The highest rates are associated with young patients and those with testicular atrophy. Low-dose radiotherapy is the preferred treatment for TIN, as it preserves the testes and Leydig cell function, and eradicates TIN effectively. The role of routine biopsy of the contralateral testis and the optimal dose of radiation therapy are still under investigation.

Regional anatomy

Regional spread is predominantly by the lymphatic pathways from the testis to the para-aortic, renal hilar and retrocrural lymph nodes, with involvement of the contralateral nodes occurring in 15 to 20 per cent of cases (Fig. 28.1). The pattern of lymphatic drainage may be distorted after hernia repair, orchidopexy or surgery to the scrotum. Tumour involvement of the tunica vaginalis or scrotum may lead to inguinal lymphadenopathy. Malignant teratomas also have a propensity for early spread via the bloodstream to the lungs and liver.

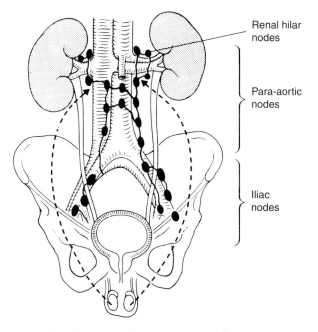

Renal hilar nodes

Para-aortic nodes

Iliac nodes

Fig. 28.1 Lymphatic drainage of the testis.

Planning technique

ASSESSMENT OF DISEASE

Clinical examination should include palpation of the contralateral testis, lymph-node areas (especially the supraclavicular fossa and abdomen) and breasts, to exclude gynaecomastia. Estimation of serum alpha-fetoprotein and beta human chorionic gonadotrophin levels, chest X-ray and CT scanning of the chest and abdomen are used to detect metastatic spread. PET scanning also defines disease extent with a high level of sensitivity and specificity.

DEFINITION OF TARGET VOLUME

The target volume includes lymph-node areas at high risk of microscopic involvement, i.e. para-aortic, renal hilar and retrocrural nodes bilaterally. If there has been previous orchidopexy, herniorrhaphy, surgery to the scrotum or tumour involvement of the tunica vaginalis, extended-field radiotherapy may include ipsilateral pelvic and inguinal lymph nodes and the ipsilateral scrotal sac. If there is involvement of the lower para-aortic nodes with a risk of retrograde spread to the pelvis, bilateral pelvic lymph nodes are also treated.

The margins of the target volume extend from the junction of the tenth and eleventh thoracic vertebrae to the junction of the fifth lumbar with the first sacral vertebrae. The field width is usually 8–10 cm and should include the renal hilar nodes (Fig. 28.2).

When designing the target volume it is essential to review the abdominal CT scans both to exclude a horseshoe kidney and to locate the position of both kidneys as critical normal organs to be avoided.

LOCALIZATION

The patient lies supine with his arms by his sides and his head comfortably positioned on a pad, and is aligned using laser lights in the mid-line. The superior and inferior margins of the target volume are localized as described above. The position of the kidneys is located using the abdominal CT scans, and the appropriate field width is chosen to include the para-aortic and renal hilar nodes while excluding the renal parenchyma. Tattoos are made at the centre of the target volume, the superior and inferior border, and laterally in the plane of the central tattoo to prevent rotation. Intravenous contrast may be given to define the position of the kidneys on simulator films of the target volume. The interplanar distance is measured at the central tattoo.

When extended-field radiotherapy is given to include the ipsilateral pelvic and inguinal nodes, a large rectangular field is drawn and shielding added to protect the kidneys, bladder and bowel, giving a 'dog-leg' configuration (Fig. 28.3). It is important to ensure adequate cover of lymph nodes lying at the mid-level of the fifth lumbar vertebra between the para-aortic and pelvic nodes. Lead shields

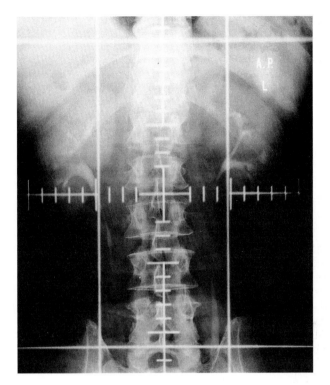

Fig. 28.2 Simulator film showing field margins for para-aortic lymph node irradiation.

1 cm thick are used to protect the remaining testis from scattered irradiation and to preserve fertility when the dog-leg configuration is treated. Measurements using thermoluminescent dosimetry have shown that the radiation dose to the testis is thus reduced by more than 50 per cent to 0.5–0.7 Gy. If scrotal irradiation is necessary, the inferior border of the dog-leg is tattooed after films taken on the treatment unit have been checked. The scrotal field using electron therapy of appropriate energy is then matched to this tattoo to include the lower inguinal nodes and scrotal sac on the involved side. A lead cut-out is made in the mould room to shield the penis and remaining testis. The dose to the contralateral testis is then about 1–1.5 Gy.

Field arrangements

Anterior and posterior fields are treated isocentrically on a linear accelerator, using perspex templates to shield critical structures when extended-field configurations are treated. Calculation of the dose distribution for the dog-leg field is made as for other irregular fields, such as the mantle (see Chapter 22).

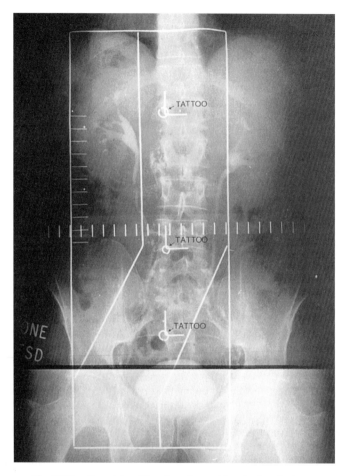

Fig. 28.3   Simulator film showing a 'dog-leg' technique.

Implementation of plan

The patient lies supine on the treatment couch, and laser lights are used to align his position with the anterior and lateral tattoos. The correct position of the lateral tattoos above the couch ensures that there is no rotation. When extended-field dog-leg irradiation is used, a template is needed to align lead shielding. When scrotal irradiation is given, electron therapy is used with a direct anterior field. The lead cut-out is positioned to match the lower border of the dog-leg field using the skin tattoo at this level.

Dose prescription

Seminoma stage I

30 Gy in 15 fractions given in 3 weeks.

(The results of lower dose trials of 20 Gy in 10 fractions given in 2 weeks are awaited.)

Seminoma stage IIA

35 Gy in 17 fractions given in 3.5 weeks.

Seminoma Stage IIB/IIC (for residual disease after chemotherapy)

35 Gy in 17 fractions given in 3.5 weeks.

Scrotal irradiation with electron therapy using a lead cut-out

30 Gy applied dose in 15 fractions given in 3 weeks.

Teratoma

Individualized, usually 35–45 Gy given in 3.5 to 4.5 weeks with daily fractionation.

TIN

18 Gy in 9 fractions daily given in 2 weeks.

Studies are currently in progress looking at lower doses of 10 Gy in 5 fractions given in 1 week.

Patient care

Nausea and vomiting may occur on the first few treatment days, but are usually self-limiting. If necessary, anti-emetics are prescribed. If the patient has a previous history of peptic ulceration, prophylactic treatment with an H_2-receptor antagonist and anti-emetics is recommended. Skin reaction is usually mild, but temporary epilation does occur over the treatment area. The scrotal skin should be kept dry and 1 per cent hydrocortisone cream prescribed, if necessary, for erythema.

Further reading

Horwich, A. 1995: Testicular tumours. In Horwich, A. (ed.), *Oncology. A multidisciplinary textbook*. London: Chapman & Hall, 485–98.

CHAPTER 29

Penis

Role of radiotherapy

Surgery is the standard treatment for elderly patients with carcinoma of the penis unless preservation of function is required, when radiotherapy is recommended. Small tumours limited to the prepuce can be treated by circumcision, and well-differentiated lesions can be excised by laser. Adequate surgical treatment of tumours involving the corpora cavernosa or urethra necessitates partial or complete amputation of the penis.

Radiotherapy with interstitial implantation or external beam therapy is recommended for young patients and those who do not wish to have an amputation. Tumours limited to the prepuce or glans penis (stage I) can be treated using electron beam therapy or an interstitial implant where the tumour measures less than 3 cm in every plane. Tumours with deep invasion of the shaft or corpora cavernosa (stage II) require irradiation of the entire penis using megavoltage therapy, and are not suitable for implantation.

Palpable mobile inguinal lymph nodes occur in 30 to 50 per cent of patients at presentation, but half of these will be related to infection rather than tumour. If tumour is confirmed by cytology or histology, then a radical block dissection of the affected groin is performed with postoperative radiotherapy if excision is incomplete. If the nodes are fixed, palliative radiotherapy may be given. In patients without proven lymphadenopathy there is no evidence that prophylactic node dissection is of greater benefit than delayed surgery.

Cure rates of 100 per cent can be obtained with T_1 tumours, falling to 40 to 70 per cent for T_2 and T_3 tumours, with the better results being obtained for small tumours at the distal end of the shaft.

Regional anatomy

The prepuce and skin of the penis drain to the superficial inguinal lymph nodes. The glans penis and corpora have a very rich lymphatic supply which drains to the deep inguinal and external iliac lymph nodes, as shown in Fig. 29.1.

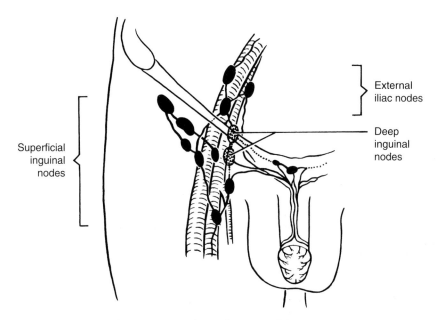

Fig. 29.1 Lymphatic drainage of the penis.

Planning technique

ASSESSMENT OF PRIMARY DISEASE

Careful inspection and palpation of the primary tumour are essential to determine the extent of infiltration before biopsy. Lymphadenopathy is assessed clinically by palpation of the femoral canals, groins and pelvis. Needle aspiration or
biopsy of enlarged nodes is performed to distinguish between infection and
tumour. If tumour involves the nodes, a CT scan of the abdomen is performed in
order to exclude involvement of other lymph nodes in the pelvis or abdomen
before inguinal node dissection.

INTERSTITIAL IMPLANTATION

It is essential that circumcision is performed before implantation. The implant is
performed under general anaesthesia following insertion of a urinary catheter.

The target volume is defined by allowing a margin of 1–2 cm around the palpable and visible tumour. For very small superficial tumours, a single-plane
implant may sometimes be considered, but for the majority of cases the entire
circumference of the penis is enclosed in a two-plane implant. It is usual to use
two or three sources in each plane and to maintain parallelism by the use of a

small template (Fig. 29.2a). The separation between the sources is usually 12–15 mm, but it may sometimes be up to 18 mm between the planes as determined by the thickness of the shaft of the penis.

The implant is usually performed with the axis of implantation at right angles to the axis of the penis. Only a small part of the track of the needle may be within the penis, and at the apex, where the glans has a conical shape, one or more needles may be entirely free in air but maintained in position with the template. The active length of iridium wire is usually 4–5 cm, which means that there is active wire extending through the skin on either side of the lesion (Fig. 29.2b).

Care must be taken not to pass iridium wire through the urethra. This can usually be avoided by making sure that the catheter moves freely.

In order to prevent the radioactive material from coming into contact with either the skin of the thigh or the testes, the shaft of the penis is supported erect in a foam block. For those patients for whom it is important to conserve fertility, a sheet of 2-mm-thick lead placed over the thighs will reduce the dose to the testes to a safe level.

EXTERNAL BEAM THERAPY

If implantation is not feasible, electron therapy is used for tumours limited to the prepuce or glans penis, with an energy chosen to give appropriate depth doses.

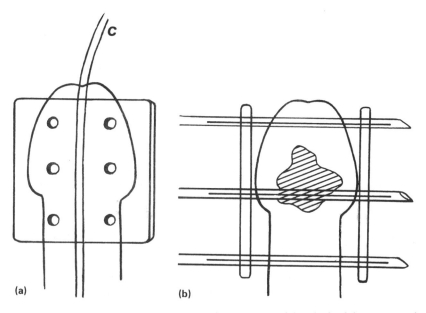

(a)   (b)

Fig. 29.2 Technique for implantation of carcinoma of the shaft of the penis with iridium wires. (a) Rigid needles inserted though template. (b) Iridium wires held in position by template. c = catheter.

A lead cut-out is made to treat the tumour with a 2-cm margin. A skin dose of 100 per cent is ensured by placing perspex on the cut-out directly over the lesion, or on the applicator which is used to define the SSD.

If there is evidence of tumour extension to the corpora cavernosa of the penis, the entire organ must be treated using a cobalt-60 unit or a 4-MV linear accelerator. The penis is covered with gauze tubigrip and placed between the two halves of a wax block within a central cavity. The box is closed, the gauze is then drawn up through a hole in the top and a wax plug is inserted to maintain the penis in position. The wax block allows even build-up, and a homogeneous dose is obtained using opposing lateral fields treating isocentrically. The testes and groins are shielded from scattered irradiation by a lead sheet, and on a cobalt-60 unit the lower edge of the beam is trimmed with a lead block (Fig. 29.3).

For inguinal or iliac node irradiation, a direct anterior field or opposing anterior and posterior fields are used with a central lead shield to cover the bladder. Electrons or photons from a cobalt-60 unit or a linear accelerator may be used according to the treatment depth required.

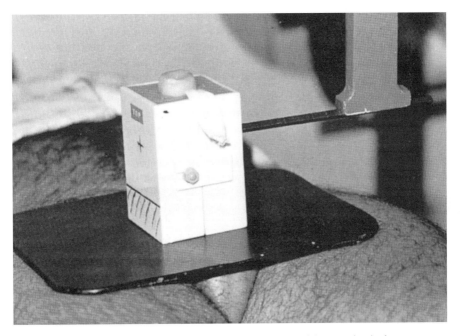

Fig. 29.3 Treatment technique for carcinoma of the penile shaft.

Dose prescription

External beam therapy

60 Gy in 30 fractions given in 6 weeks.

Interstitial implantation

65 Gy to the 85 per cent reference isodose given in 6 to 7 days using the Paris system.

Lymph-node irradiation

45–60 Gy in 4.5 to 6 weeks with daily fractionation.

Patient care

Systemic antibiotics and circumcision may be needed prior to irradiation in order to control infection and to prevent radiation-induced oedema leading to urethral obstruction. Treatment is poorly tolerated. Dysuria and difficulty with micturition are common symptoms, and a high fluid intake should be encouraged. A midstream urine specimen should be sent for bacteriological examination and antibiotics prescribed if appropriate. Skin reactions are often severe and are treated with exposure to air and 1 per cent hydrocortisone cream.

Meatal stenosis may occur following interstitial implantation or, to a lesser extent, after external beam therapy, and will require intermittent dilatation.

Further reading

Gerbaulet, A. and Lambin, P. 1992: Radiation therapy of cancer of the penis: indications, advantages and pitfalls. *Urologic Clinics of North America* **19**, 325–32.

CHAPTER 30

Pelvis

Role of radiotherapy

Irradiation of the whole pelvis may be used in the treatment of tumours of the bladder, prostate, cervix, uterus and rectum. The rationale for treatment of the pelvic lymph nodes is discussed under individual tumour sites. The decision as to whether regional lymph nodes are included in the target volume depends on the grade of histology, the T-stage of the tumour, and the pattern of local and distant spread. For example, in carcinoma of the cervix, pain and leg oedema from involvement of lymph nodes on the pelvic side-wall may be a major problem, whereas in carcinoma of the prostate, bone metastases are more common with advanced T-stage or high-grade histology.

For all of these tumour sites, there is conflicting evidence as to whether microscopic lymph-node metastases can be eradicated by radiotherapy, and any effect on survival is controversial.

The maximum dose given to the pelvic lymph nodes is determined by the tolerance of the surrounding normal organs. Factors affecting this include the following:

- the age of the patient;
- their general condition;
- diabetes;
- arteriosclerosis;
- previous bowel disease;
- the size of the target volume;
- previous surgery;
- previous or concurrent chemotherapy.

The treatment is less well tolerated with increasing age and poor general condition. Vascular changes associated with diabetes or hypertension, or previous surgery or chemotherapy may all reduce bowel tolerance. The upper pelvis is normally filled with small bowel which is freely mobile, and the dose to the whole pelvis is limited by small bowel tolerance to 45 Gy in 4.5 to 5 weeks.

Radical doses to the primary tumour will be tolerated if normal bowel mobility is maintained, but adhesions will prevent day-to-day changes in the segment of bowel being irradiated. CT scanning has clearly demonstrated that a full bladder does displace mobile small bowel out of the pelvis and hence out of the target volume. All patients who are receiving treatment to the pelvis should therefore be treated with the bladder full (Fig. 30.1).

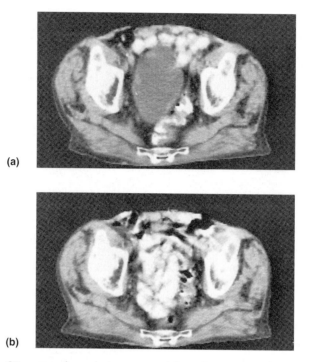

(a)

(b)

Fig. 30.1   CT section through the centre of the pelvic target volume with the bladder (a) full and (b) empty, showing small bowel replacing distended bladder.

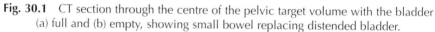

Other structures within the pelvic irradiation field include part of the recto-sigmoid colon and the femoral heads through which the lateral fields pass. Proctitis and tenesmus may result from doses needed to control nodal disease, and although avascular necrosis of bone is now rare with megavoltage irradiation, the risk must be considered, especially if radiation is combined with chemotherapy.

Regional anatomy

Lymphography will demonstrate nodal involvement with an accuracy of about 80 per cent, but is invasive, time-consuming and difficult to perform, and has therefore been largely superseded by CT scanning. This technique also has the advantage of delineating the first lymph-node stations (Fig. 30.2) for pelvic tumours, which are the obturator and hypogastric nodes, the internal iliac, pararectal and presacral lymph nodes, as well as the external iliac and common iliac nodes (Fig. 30.3). However, it does not detect involvement by tumour in nodes of normal size. MRI scanning is more sensitive than CT for primary tumour staging, but has no proven benefit over CT for nodal involvement. For

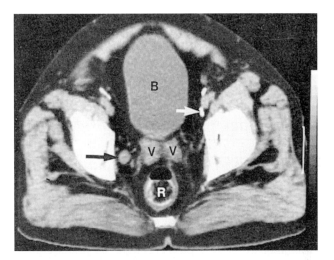

Fig. 30.2 CT scan illustrating the position of opacified external iliac nodes (white arrow) and obturator node (black arrow) in transverse section. B = bladder; V = seminal vesicles; R = rectum.

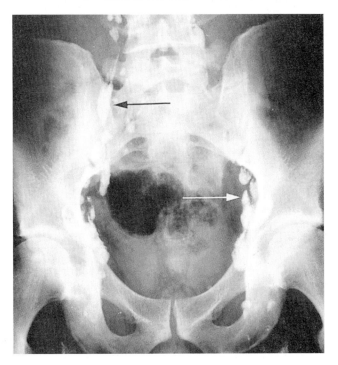

Fig. 30.3 Lymphogram illustrating position of the external iliac lymph nodes (white arrow) and common iliac nodes (black arrow) within the pelvis.

some gynaecological tumours treated with postoperative radiotherapy, surgical specimens may provide histological confirmation of involvement suspected radiologically. Fluorodeoxyglucose (FDG)-PET scanning shows promise.

Inguinal nodes are assessed by palpation, although involvement of enlarged nodes can only be proved by histological or cytological examination.

Planning technique

DEFINITION OF TARGET VOLUME

The target volume includes the primary tumour and the pelvic lymph nodes up to and including the common iliac nodes.

The superior field margin is therefore at the upper border of the fifth lumbar vertebra and the lower margin is at the inferior border of the obturator foramen which marks the floor of the true pelvis. For certain primary tumours, such as those of the anus or vagina, the lower margin must be extended inferiorly to encompass the primary tumour adequately, and the upper border is usually lower than the standard L4/5. The lateral borders include the pelvic nodes as demonstrated by CT and usually lie 1 cm outside the bony pelvic walls (Fig. 30.4). The anterior and posterior borders are more variable (according to the site

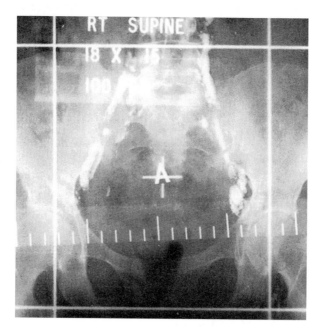

Fig. 30.4   AP simulator film showing anterior field margins to cover target volume for treatment of whole pelvis. A = central tattoo.

of the primary tumour), but usually extend from the mid-symphysis pubis anteriorly to the middle of S2 posteriorly.

LOCALIZATION

Palpation of the primary tumour by rectal or vaginal examination (including EUA) is vital in order to define the inferior border of the target volumes.

Radio-opaque markers are used as aids to localization where CT scanning is not available. For gynaecological lesions, barium is placed on an impregnated tampon in the vagina and by catheter in the rectum with a metal marker on the introitus and the patient lying supine. For urological tumours, a cystogram is performed and barium is placed in the rectum. For rectal tumours, the patient lies prone and barium is placed in the rectum and vagina where appropriate. Anteroposterior (AP) or PA and lateral simulator films are taken and the target volume as defined above is drawn on the films. A tattoo is placed at the centre of the volume and a transverse outline taken with plaster of Paris or wire. The target volume, rectum and femoral heads are marked on to this outline. For whole pelvic irradiation, CT may help to define AP borders of the target volume by showing the position of the bladder, rectum and internal iliac nodes in particular.

If a second phase of treatment is given to a reduced volume, another outline is needed through the new centre. For small-volume treatments, CT is used to localize the primary tumour, but clinical examination remains essential for definition of the lower border. Where localization is performed in one plane, the varying position of the rectum due to its posterior curvature must be taken into account.

Field arrangements

The two main considerations in whole pelvic irradiation are how to achieve homogeneity of dose in a large target volume and how to minimize dose to the rectum. The tolerance of the rectum is determined by length of bowel and proportion of circumference irradiated, as well as by total dose and fraction size. Since there is no single ideal technique, the choice of field arrangement will depend on the site of the primary tumour and associated lymph nodes within the pelvis. Higher energy photons 8–16 MV may be more appropriate than standard 5–6 MV beams.

In most situations, particularly for the treatment of gynaecological tumours or those with posterior tumour extension or potential involvement of internal iliac nodes, a four-field 'brick' arrangement is chosen. This employs anterior, posterior and lateral opposing fields with an appropriate wedge as tissue compensation (Fig. 30.5). This technique achieves good homogeneity but may give a high rectal dose depending on the position of the rectum. It is time-consuming because all fields must be treated daily.

Opposing anterior and posterior fields alone may be used where ease of setup is important e.g. palliative treatment (Fig. 30.6). Using photons of 5–8 MV,

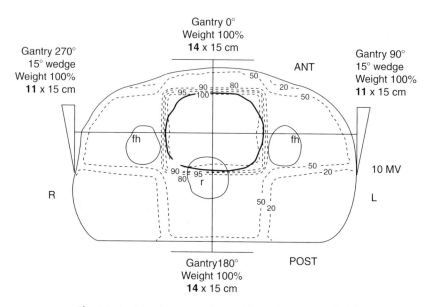

Gantry 0°
Weight 100%
14 x 15 cm

Gantry 270°
15° wedge
Weight 100%
11 x 15 cm

ANT

Gantry 90°
15° wedge
Weight 100%
11 x 15 cm

fh   fh

10 MV

R   L

Gantry180°
Weight 100%
14 x 15 cm

POST

Fig. 30.5 Anterior, posterior and lateral opposing fields giving a 'brick' configuration. r = rectum; fh = femoral heads.

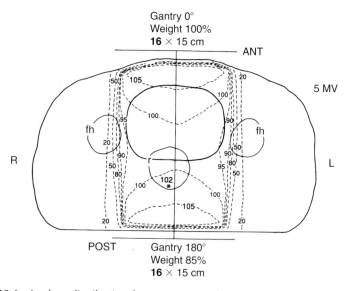

Gantry 0°
Weight 100%
16 × 15 cm

ANT

5 MV

fh   fh

R   L

POST

Gantry 180°
Weight 85%
16 × 15 cm

Fig. 30.6 Isodose distribution from anterior and posterior opposing fields using 5-MV photons (unequal weighting). r = rectum; fh = femoral heads.

the rectal dose is high and homogeneity poor, but with higher energies (16–20 MV) more satisfactory distributions may be obtained (Fig. 30.7).

When rectal doses must be kept as low as possible, an anterior field and lateral wedged opposing fields give a homogeneous distribution with a sharp fall-

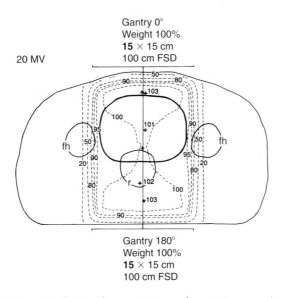

Fig. 30.7 Isodose distribution from anterior and posterior opposing fields using 20-MV photons. r = rectum; fh = femoral heads.

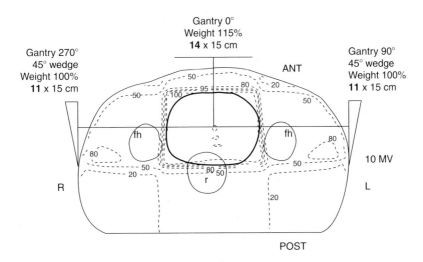

Fig. 30.8 Three-field technique using an anterior open and lateral opposing fields with a 45° wedge.

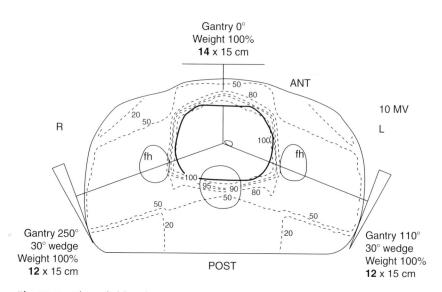

Fig. 30.9   Three-field technique using an anterior and two posterior oblique fields.

off in dose posteriorly (Fig. 30.8). Alternatively, an anterior field and two poste-rior oblique wedged fields may be used. The angle of the posterior fields lies between 110° and 120°. Increasing the angle between the wedged fields decreases the dose to the rectum but increases the dose to the femoral heads. This arrangement produces a homogeneous distribution where the target volume is rounded rather than rectangular (Fig. 30.9).

For rectal tumours, patients are treated prone with a three-field technique encompassing a posterior volume as described in Chapter 24. Where a high dose may be indicated (as for rectal cancer) efforts should be made to exclude as much small bowel as possible from the field. This may require opacification of small bowel so that it can be imaged and appropriate shielding blocks positioned to exclude it without shielding the target volume.

Implementation of plan

Except for some cases of rectal cancer, the patient lies supine with a full bladder in order to displace small bowel out of the pelvis, and is aligned using an ante-rior laser in the mid-line and lateral lasers to match lateral skin tattoos and pre-vent rotation. All techniques are treated isocentrically. It is important that the patient's IPD correlates with the measurement on the computer plan to ensure the correct pin depth. In obese patients the IPD may vary widely from day to day, giving a discrepancy in pin depth and leading to error when an isocentric tech-nique is used. For these patients it is more accurate to use an anterior field and two lateral fields with the entry point of the lateral fields measured up from the couch top and treated at 100 cm FSD. All fields must be treated every day.

Dose prescription

44 Gy in 22 fractions given in 4.5 weeks (bladder and prostate tumours).

40–50 Gy in 20–25 fractions given in 4 to 5 weeks (gynaecological tumours).

Patient care

Skin reaction occurs over the sacrum and natal cleft from combined anterior and posterior fields. If the patient develops diarrhoea, a low-residue diet is advised and loperamide hydrochloride, 4 mg initial dose followed by up to 2 mg 6-hourly, may be prescribed. If diarrhoea is severe, the treatment may be suspended or the dose per fraction reduced. Frequency or dysuria may occur. A midstream urine specimen should be taken for culture and antibiotics prescribed as appropriate if there is proven infection.

Further reading

Bentel, G.C. 1996: Treatment planning – pelvis. In *Radiation therapy planning*, 2nd edn. New York: McGraw-Hill.

CHAPTER 31

Cervix uteri

Role of radiotherapy

The choice of treatment for carcinoma of the cervix depends on the stage of the disease, the histology of the tumour, and the age and general condition of the patient. The UICC-FIGO staging system is used. In addition to defining the extent of the primary tumour, the important prognostic factors of tumour volume and lymph-node involvement must be considered.

Surgery alone is the treatment of choice for all patients with carcinoma *in situ* and micro-invasive disease. A Wertheim's hysterectomy is performed for FIGO stage IA disease (micro-invasive) unless the patient is unfit for surgery, when intracavitary treatment is given.

For small-volume stage IB and IIA carcinoma without lymph-node involvement, equivalent local control rates are achieved with Wertheim's hysterectomy or radical radiotherapy. Surgery may be favoured in younger patients, and the choice of modality will depend on clinical prediction of the relative morbidity of each treatment and patient preference. When surgery is inappropriate for these patients, external beam therapy may be given in combination with intracavitary treatment to control the primary tumour and its local infiltration, and microscopic involvement of pelvic nodes.

When pelvic nodes are found to be involved at surgery, the survival rate falls from 90 per cent at 5 years (for stage I patients) to less than 30 per cent. Postoperative pelvic irradiation may be given to reduce relapse at the pelvic sidewall. Although morbidity increases with the addition of radiotherapy to radical surgery, analysis of relapse patterns suggests that this approach reduces the unpleasant complications of local recurrence.

For all other stages of disease, initial external beam therapy is given to encompass bulky disease, and subsequent intracavitary therapy is used. Pelvic lymph nodes are included in external beam fields to eradicate micrometastatic disease. Where nodal involvement is demonstrated by CT scanning, a higher total nodal dose is given. Involvement of common iliac or para-aortic lymph nodes makes cure very unlikely, but palliative irradiation may be considered on an individual basis.

Regional anatomy

Local infiltration of tumour occurs from the cervix to the vaginal fornices and parametrial tissues, and may spread anteriorly to invade the bladder base or posteriorly to involve the uterosacral ligaments and the rectum. The ureters lie in the broad ligament below the uterine artery, 1 cm lateral to the supravaginal cervix. At this site they are at particular risk of compression by local tumour infiltration.

The lymphatic drainage from the cervix passes to paracervical nodes, through the broad and uterosacral ligaments and then to the obturator, presacral, internal and external iliac lymph nodes (Fig. 31.1a). The risk of involvement is increased in high-grade tumours and those with extensive local infiltration, and ranges from 15 to 20 per cent for stage IB to 60 per cent for stage IIIB lesions.

Planning technique

ASSESSMENT OF PRIMARY DISEASE

After general clinical assessment, a vaginal examination is performed to determine the extent of tumour in the vagina and cervix. Any vaginal spread is

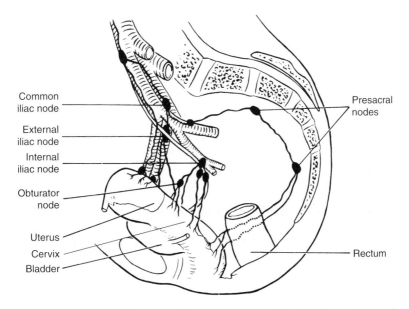

Fig. 31.1a Lymphatic drainage of the cervix. (Reproduced with permission from Johnston, T.B., Davies, D.V. and Davies, F. 1958: *Gray's anatomy*, 32nd edn. Edinburgh: Churchill Livingston.)

visualized using a speculum. Bimanual examination determines whether the uterus is enlarged or of impaired mobility. Rectal examination defines the involvement of parametria and uterosacral ligaments, and fixation to the pelvic side-wall. Examination under anaesthesia is carried out in all patients for biopsy and accurate assessment of the extent of the lesion according to the FIGO staging system. Cystoscopy is performed in order to look for invasion of the bladder base. The renal tract is assessed by CT scanning in order to detect ureteric obstruction or hydronephrosis, and to exclude a pelvic kidney. It will also demonstrate enlarged pelvic and para-aortic nodes, but will not exclude microscopic involvement of normal-sized nodes. MRI scanning is now the investigation of choice for assessing the local extent of disease in soft tissue (Fig. 31.1b).

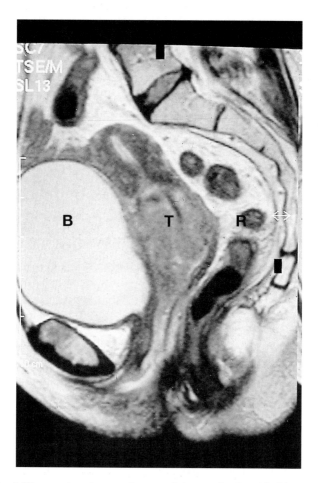

Fig. 31.1b   MRI scan showing carcinoma of the cervix (B = bladder, T = tumour, R = rectum). Courtesy of Dr. B. Carey.

DEFINITION OF TARGET VOLUME

When external beam radiation is given initially, the target volume is the whole pelvis (see Fig. 30.4) encompassing the extent of the primary tumour and pelvic lymph nodes. However, the superior margin is the lower border of the fifth lumbar vertebra, to reduce toxicity. The lateral borders usually lie 1 cm outside the bony pelvic side-walls. For early-stage low-volume disease the anterior border is 3 cm anterior to the anterior margin of the fifth lumbar vertebral body, and the posterior border is 2 cm anterior to the posterior aspect of the sacral hollow. For more advanced disease, clinical examination and CT or MRI may indicate a need for wider margins, and it is sometimes necessary to give much of the dose with parallel opposed fields so that the risk of geographical 'miss' is minimized. An introital marker must be used to define the lower border of the vagina in all patients.

Field arrangements and sequencing of external beam radiation with brachytherapy

With the exception of stage IA disease, which can be treated by brachytherapy alone, all patients are treated with a combination of external beam radiation, given to the primary tumour and the pelvic lymph nodes, and brachytherapy, given to raise the dose to the primary tumour and paracervical tissues. Because of the limited dose range of brachytherapy and the difficulty of shielding the inhomogeneous high-dose volume with subsequent external beam radiation, many centres deliver fractionated external beam radiation first and boost the tumour with brachytherapy afterwards. The shrinkage of tumour achieved by 4 to 5 weeks of external beam radiation brings the tumour closer to the intracavitary sources so that higher doses can be delivered. This sequence also obviates the need to attempt to shield the central high-dose volume from the external beam therapy.

The balance between external beam radiation and intracavitary radiation is modified according to the extent of disease and the risk, or known presence, of pelvic node involvement. For low-stage, low-volume disease, 40 to 45 Gy are given to the whole pelvis in 2-Gy fractions and 20 to 25 Gy are given to point A with continuous low-dose-rate brachytherapy. For more advanced disease, the dose to the pelvis is increased to 45 to 50 Gy and an extra 5 Gy may be given to boost known sites of disease on the pelvic side-wall. Brachytherapy applications also contribute a dose to point B, which is usually on the pelvic side-wall, and amounts to approximately one-third of the dose given to point A. Care must therefore be taken to summate the total doses given to critical pelvic structures.

In some centres, stage IA, IB and IIA small-volume node-negative disease is treated with a much greater contribution from brachytherapy, which is given before or during the external beam radiation. In these cases it is necessary to shield the high-dose central volume during external beam radiation in order to avoid toxicity to small bowel, bladder and rectum. It is difficult to match the inhomogeneous radiation from brachytherapy with external beam treatment and to position shielding accurately to avoid overlap. Individualized CT planning with the applicators in place may allow demonstration of dose distribution in three dimensions, and computerized planning can make it possible to construct an accurate shield. In practice, many centres use a standardized 4-cm-wide lead block (Fig. 31.2) or a shaped wedge inserted into anterior and posterior opposing fields. The positioning of the shielding may be assisted by insertion of a radio-opaque marker into the cervix at the time of brachytherapy. This central shielding can usually only be achieved from anterior and posterior fields and not from lateral fields when using a four-field plan.

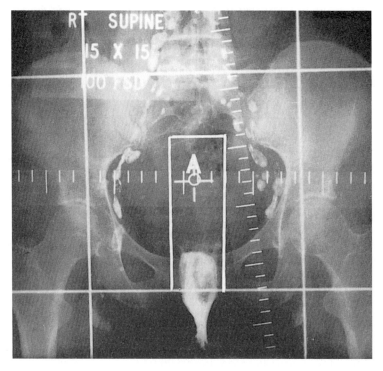

Fig. 31.2 Simulator film showing anterior field with 4 cm wide central lead shield.

When intracavitary treatment is not technically feasible, e.g. when the cervical os is obstructed, external beam radiation may be continued to a smaller volume.

The para-aortic region is treated with anterior and posterior opposing fields extending from the top of the first lumbar vertebra to the junction with the pelvic field (Fig. 31.3). The width of the volume is usually 8 cm and the dose is calculated to the mid-point of the volume. The calculation for the gap between the fields is performed using the technique discussed in Chapter 1.

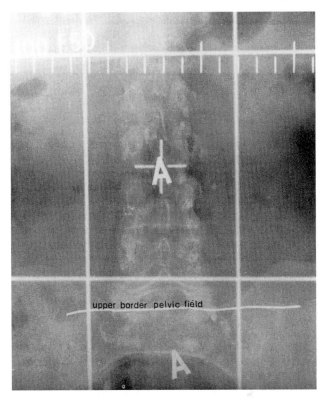

Fig. 31.3 Simulator film showing field margins to treat para-aortic lymph nodes.

Intracavitary irradiation

Intracavitary irradiation allows delivery of a very high dose to the central tumour volume to obtain maximal local control without exceeding the tolerance of the surrounding normal tissues. It is feasible because the normal uterus and vaginal vault are relatively radio-resistant, and there is a rapid fall-off of dose at a distance from the cervix, protecting the adjacent rectum, bladder and small bowel.

Dose specification

CLASSIC (MANCHESTER DERIVED)

Manchester point A is defined as a point 2 cm lateral to the central uterine canal and 2 cm superior to the lateral fornix in the plane of the uterus. It lies within the paracervical tissues near the uterine artery and ureter, and was chosen to take into account the tolerance of adjacent dose-limiting normal structures. This point is not necessarily the same anatomically in all patients, and it may vary considerably with individual intracavitary insertions. In general, current practice with rigid afterloading systems is to specify a prescribed dose of irradiation at a specific point which is 2 cm above and 2 cm lateral to the flange of the intra-uterine tube at the external os. This point is taken to be equivalent to Manchester point A. Point B is defined as being 3 cm lateral to point A, i.e. 5 cm from the mid-line on the lateral axis, and it is used to provide an indication of dose to the distal parametria. An additional point 1 cm lateral to the bony pelvic margin may be used to specify the nodal dose.

REPORTING DOSE FOR INTER-CENTRE COMPARISONS

The ICRU report No. 38 states that, as the dose gradient is steep in the vicinity of the sources, and the dose within the target volume is highly non-uniform, specification of the dose should not be at a single point. It is recommended that the dose be recorded in terms of a reference volume incorporating the target volume. The target volume, containing demonstrable tumour and subclinical disease, should be described independently of the dose distribution.

An absorbed dose level of 60 Gy is chosen as an appropriate reference level for classic low-dose-rate therapy. This represents the total dose of all intracavitary applications, or the combination of external beam and intracavitary treatments. For advanced-stage disease, for example, 45 Gy will be contributed by external beam therapy and hence $60 - 45 = 15$ Gy will be the reference isodose. Where medium- or high-dose-rate therapy is given, the clinician is expected to indicate a dose level equivalent to 60 Gy given at a low dose rate. The ICRU Report No. 38 also recommends recording the absorbed dose at reference points for the bladder, rectum, lymphatic trapezoid and pelvic wall.

The availability of imaging techniques that are able to demonstrate the position of the source carriers, the adjacent normal tissues and the tumour makes it possible to report doses and volumes much more accurately than was possible at the time of the ICRU Report No. 38. This new information may well form the basis of a revised report.

Intracavitary techniques

The three classic systems of intracavitary treatments (Stockholm, Paris and Manchester) were designed so that a quantity of radium was loaded into a specific spatial configuration for a defined period to enable clinically reproducible effects despite the rapid change of dose rate across the target volume.

Currently used afterloading techniques were developed both to reduce radiation exposure to staff and to allow sources of varying strengths to be used. Irradiation with low (0.4–2 Gy/hour), medium (2–12 Gy/hour) and high (> 12 Gy/hour) dose rate therapy is now possible (ICRU Report No. 38 definitions). High-dose-rate therapy using a Cathetron or Selectron loaded with cobalt-60 sources can be given on an out-patient basis, and is well tolerated and cost-effective. However, multiple insertions may be necessary to maximize the therapeutic ratio (as for a fractionated course of external beam therapy), because short treatment times do not allow for normal tissue recovery.

Theoretically, low-dose-rate therapy, as in the classic Paris system, may give the best therapeutic ratio, but such treatments – which require admission to hospital – may be inconvenient and uncomfortable. Clinical studies are continuing to develop optimal treatment schedules and delivery systems.

EXAMPLE OF AN AFTERLOADING TECHNIQUE

A variety of different applicators are available that are designed to reproduce the dose configuration of standard pre-loading techniques. Rigid applicators are used for medium- and low-dose-rate insertions in order to preserve the applicator position and configuration of sources during the treatment, which lasts approximately 24 hours. Flexible applicators are being developed for high-dose-rate sources to allow the possibility of short out-patient treatments without anaesthesia. The use of CT scanning and rapid computerized dosimetry means that source-loading and time patterns can be varied to give optimized intracavitary treatment.

After examination of the patient under anaesthesia, the cervix is dilated, the width of the vaginal vault is determined and the length of the uterus is measured with a uterine sound. Appropriate applicators are then positioned within the patient. Unless there is extensive invasion of the body of the uterus, it is not necessary to load the whole length of the intra-uterine tube. This will allow some reduction of dose to the small bowel, which may be lying over the fundus of the uterus. The empty source applicators are fixed or packed within the vagina and connected to hollow flexible plastic tubes which project from the introitus. A urinary catheter is inserted, and radiographs (Fig. 31.4) or CT scans with dummy sources are taken in order to delineate the position of the applicators within the uterus and vagina.

The relationship of these applicators to the tumour volume, defined by previous clinical, ultrasound and CT examination, determines whether a standard loading system is used or whether individual source arrangements are needed. A computerized dose distribution is obtained for each patient, and may be adapted to compensate for asymmetrical anatomy. The loading of the sources is achieved later, in the ward, by remote control using an automated device such as a Selectron machine (Fig. 31.5), and varying treatment times can be used for different sources in order to obtain the optimal dose distribution.

For low- or medium-dose-rate treatments, following insertion of the applicators containing dummy sources, AP and lateral or 'shift' films are taken to show the position of the sources and to obtain a magnification factor for calculation of the dose distribution. The dose to point A is calculated and the treatment time adjusted to deliver the prescribed dose. Computed dose distributions specify doses to points A and B (Fig. 31.6) and maximum doses to the rectal mucosa and bladder. These calculated doses can be checked by *in-vivo* dosimetry using micro-sources in the applicators and a rectal probe, which correlate well.

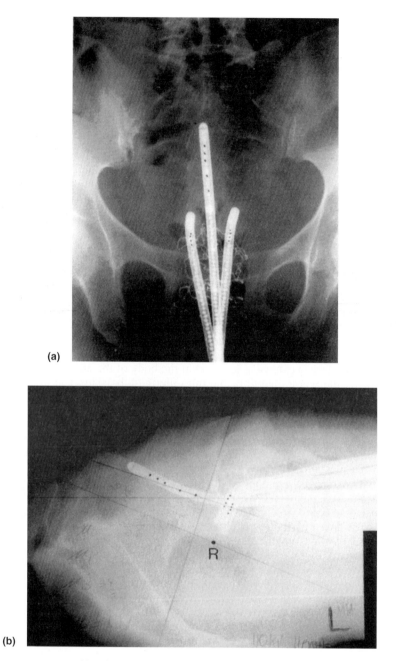

(a)

(b)

Fig. 31.4 (a) AP film showing source applicators for intracavitary therapy positioned in uterus and vagina. (b) Lateral film showing position of applicators and point for estimation of rectal dose (R).

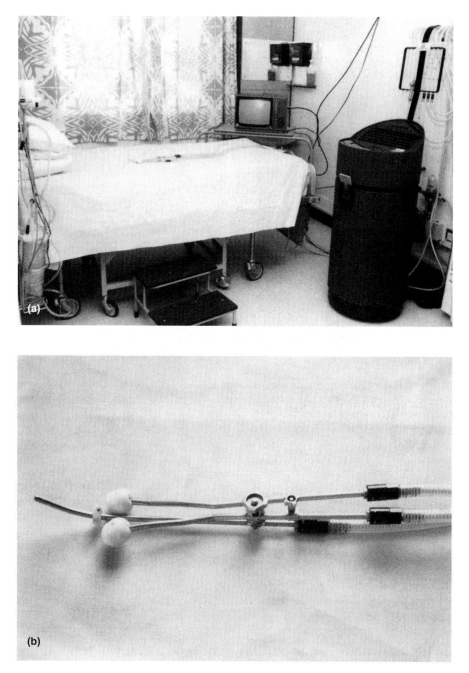

Fig. 31.5 (a) Selectron low/medium dose rate remote afterloading system. (b) Rigid applicators for afterloading uterine and vaginal sources. (Courtesy of Nucletron.)

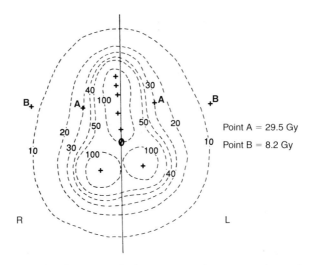

Point A = 29.5 Gy
Point B = 8.2 Gy

Fig. 31.6　Isodose distribution (with dose expressed in Gy) in plane of uterine canal from low-dose-rate (1.5 Gy/hour) Selectron Cs-137 insertion.

High-dose-rate (HDR) afterloading

The principles of applicator insertion are the same as those for low-dose-rate (LDR) and medium-dose-rate (MDR) application. Some systems use a shielded retractor instead of packing for the vagina. Because of the high dose rate, the brachytherapy must be fractionated. Where external beam radiation is given first, central disease is boosted with 2 to 3 fractions of HDR brachytherapy, which delivers 5 to 7 Gy per fraction to point A. For low-stage, low-volume disease, 5 to 7 fractions of HDR (5–7 Gy per fraction) brachytherapy are given first, followed by external beam radiation plus central shielding to treat the pelvic nodes.

As the treatment time is so short, it is necessary either to use a range of standard source arrangements to deliver a fixed dose to point A as defined from the catheter position, or to wait until radiographs are available to individualize the dose distribution before loading. Dosimetry can be modified if there is a significant change in source or normal tissue geometry during the course of fractionated treatment.

Dose prescription

STAGE IA (PATIENTS UNSUITABLE FOR SURGERY)

67.5 Gy to point A from two Selectron insertions at medium dose rate in 18–24 hours each.

STAGE IB/IIA SMALL-VOLUME (CT/MRI NEGATIVE NODES)

55 Gy to point A from two Selectron insertions

or 5 to 7 fractions of 5–7 Gy with HDR brachytherapy followed by:

external beam therapy to the pelvis with opposing fields and central lead shield.
36–40 Gy in 18 to 20 fractions given in 4 to 5 weeks.

ALL OTHER STAGES

External beam therapy

40–50 Gy in 20 to 25 fractions given in 4 to 5 weeks.

Intracavitary therapy

25–30 Gy to point A from a single Selectron insertion

or 21–25 Gy to point A in 3 to 5 fractions (5–7 Gy per fraction)
of HDR brachytherapy.

The increase in dose rate to around 1.5–1.7 Gy/hour has reduced the therapeutic index compared with classic low-dose-rate therapy of around 0.5 Gy/hour for radium. Morbidity from treatment must be carefully monitored, as small changes in dose may produce clinically detectable differences in side-effects. It may not always be possible to give additional pelvic side-wall doses of irradiation because of the difficulty in accurately shielding the high-dose zone centrally, and the subsequent risk of overlap over critical structures.

External beam boost

If intracavitary therapy is technically impossible, an additional 10–15 Gy are given to a central small volume to give a total dose of 55–60 Gy with daily fractionation. This dose cannot safely be given to the whole pelvis.

Para-aortic nodes

45 Gy in 25 fractions given in 5 weeks.

Patient care

Diarrhoea may occur during external beam irradiation of the whole pelvis, and is treated with loperamide hydrochloride and a low-residue diet. If necessary, treatment may have to be interrupted. If urinary frequency develops, a specimen should be sent for bacteriological examination and antibiotics prescribed if necessary. A good fluid intake should be encouraged. Severe vulval or natal cleft skin reactions are treated with 1 per cent hydrocortisone cream. Exposure to air and the use of a small fan may help, and regular bathing is allowed.

Further reading

International Commission on Radiological Units and Measurements. 1985: *Report No. 38. Dose and volume specification for intra-cavitary therapy in gynaecology.* Bethesda, MD: International Commission on Radiological Units and Measurements.
Khoury, G.G., Bulman, A.S. and Joslin, C.A. 1991: Long-term results of cathetron high dose rate intracavitary radiotherapy in the treatment of carcinoma of the cervix. *British Journal of Radiology* **64**, 1036–43.

CHAPTER 32

Corpus uteri

Role of radiotherapy

A total abdominal hysterectomy with bilateral salpingo-oophorectomy or extended hysterectomy is the mainstay of treatment for carcinoma of the corpus uteri. Radiotherapy is given postoperatively to reduce the incidence of vaginal vault recurrence, and to control disease in the pelvic lymph nodes.

Histological staging and prognostic factors are determined from the surgical specimen. Pre-operative brachytherapy may modify these, making it difficult to identify patients at high risk of recurrence who may benefit from further treatment. Patients are therefore commonly referred after surgery when histopathological information about the stage and grade of the tumour is available. Patients with well-differentiated tumours with minimal myometrial involvement are at low risk of vaginal vault recurrence, and any reduction in this incidence must be balanced against the risk of morbidity from intravaginal brachytherapy (vaginal stenosis and cystitis).

In selected patients for whom there is a high risk of loco-regional recurrence, postoperative pelvic radiotherapy is given. Poor prognostic features are high-grade histology or papillary or clear cell type, lymphovascular space invasion, invasion of the myometrial wall to more than one-half of its thickness (stage IC), and involvement of the cervix, ovaries or lymph nodes. With high-grade histology, lymph-node disease is found in 15 per cent of patients with minimal myometrial invasion, and in up to 35 per cent where this is more extensive. Postoperatively, external beam radiotherapy is given to the whole pelvis and may be followed by a single caesium insertion or high-dose-rate (HDR) iridium application to the vagina.

For more advanced disease, radiation is the primary treatment using combined external beam and intracavitary therapy, followed by hysterectomy where possible (patients with late stage II disease). Five-year survival rates of 65 to 85 per cent are obtained for stage I, 50 per cent for stage II and 25 per cent for stage III disease.

For patients who are obese and unfit for surgery or external beam therapy, Heyman's technique of intracavitary irradiation may be used alone with 50 per cent survival at 5 years.

Regional anatomy

The uterus is supported by the levator ani muscles and is commonly anteverted and inclined forwards at an angle of 90° to the axis of the vagina (Fig. 32.1). The myometrial wall of the body of the uterus is lined by endometrium and covered externally by a reflection of the peritoneum. The base of the bladder is closely applied to the antero-inferior part of the uterus, and posteriorly the pouch of Douglas lies between the posterior fornix and the rectum. Loops of small bowel may lie in the pouch of Douglas, limiting the dose of irradiation which can be given.

Tumour may infiltrate locally through the myometrium and parametrium to involve other pelvic organs, or it may extend inferiorly to the endocervix and vagina. Lymphatic drainage from the corpus passes through the broad ligament to the obturator, presacral and external iliac lymph nodes, and via the round ligament to the superficial inguinal lymph nodes (Fig. 32.2). Spread may also occur in the ovarian vessels to the para-aortic nodes, and by retrograde lymphatic spread to the lower third of the vagina, particularly posterior to the urethra. If the endocervix is involved, lymphatic spread occurs through paracervical and parametrial pathways to pelvic lymph nodes.

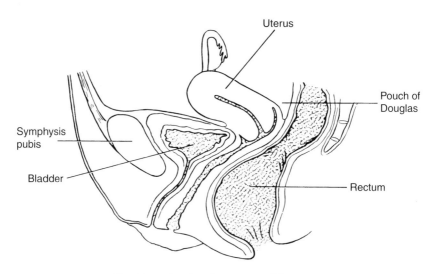

Fig. 32.1 Regional anatomy of the uterus.

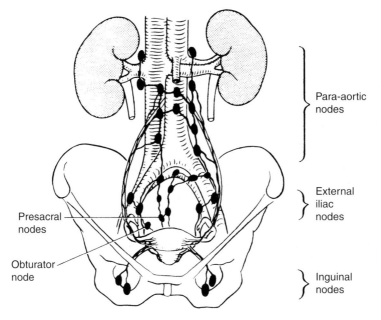

Fig. 32.2 Lymphatic drainage of the uterus.

Planning technique

ASSESSMENT OF DISEASE

Initial assessment involves examination under general anaesthesia for staging, and fractional curettage of the uterus and cervix to obtain histology. Intravenous urography is performed to detect ureteric obstruction from paracervical spread. CT scanning with intravenous contrast may delineate the thickness of the uterine wall and lymph-node involvement, and MRI may in addition predict the degree of myometrial tumour invasion. Assessment of patients to be treated post-operatively should take into account all surgical and histological information.

External beam irradiation

Where surgery reveals high-risk factors, pelvic irradiation is given with an anterior, posterior and two lateral fields to a volume encompassing the pelvic nodes to the level of the fifth lumbar vertebra, (or mid sacro-iliac joints for stage I), using the technique described in Chapter 30.

Intracavitary irradiation

A vaginal applicator (Fig. 32.3) may be used with sources afterloaded to treat the whole vaginal mucosa or the vaginal vault alone according to risk factors. For patients at low risk of pelvic recurrence, this may be given as the sole method of treatment; for those with high-risk factors, this treatment may be given subsequent to whole pelvic irradiation. With the patient anaesthetized, an EUA is performed and a urinary catheter inserted. A vaginal applicator is placed in the vagina and secured with sutures. The sources are then loaded into the applicator on the ward with an afterloading system, taking appropriate radiation-protective measures. Remote afterloading HDR brachytherapy can also be used. This can be delivered in a fractionated course on an out-patient basis.

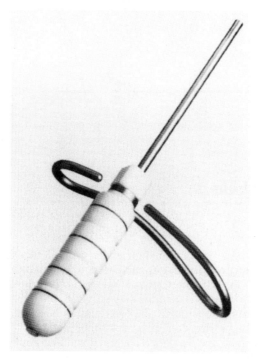

Fig. 32.3   Vaginal applicator for use with afterloading system.
(Courtesy of Nucletron.)

Heyman's packing technique

For obese unfit patients who may be unsuitable for either surgery or external beam radiation, Heyman devised a technique for packing the uterine cavity with beads containing radium. Originally a dose of 4000 mg-hours was prescribed. The technique has been superseded by remote afterloading techniques with more sophisticated dosimetry.

Under general anaesthesia the patient is examined and the cervical os widely dilated. The uterine cavity is then packed with small perspex capsules attached to afterloading catheters which protrude through the cervical os (Fig. 32.4).

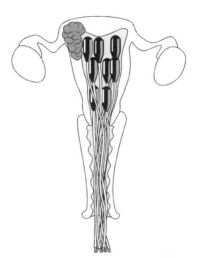

(a)

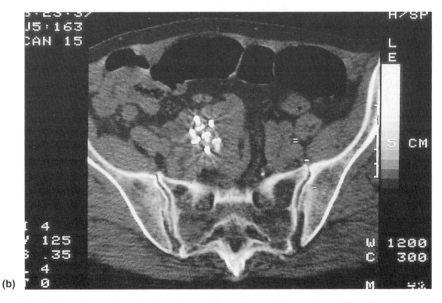

(b)

Fig. 32.4   Heyman's technique for packing the uterine cavity with radioactive sources. (a) Line diagram. (b) CT scan.

From 5 to 12 capsules are usually inserted, and AP and lateral radiographs and a CT scan are obtained which identify the sources and the relationship between them and the outer serosa of the uterus.

With HDR brachytherapy, 30 Gy are delivered to the serosa in 6 fractions which can be delivered twice daily. After 2 to 3 weeks the application is repeated and a further 30 Gy are delivered in 6 fractions.

Where there is evidence of tumour involving the cervix, the endometrial packing is combined with a vaginal ovoid.

If there is a need to irradiate the pelvic nodes in these patients, 40 Gy are given in 20 fractions over 4 weeks followed by brachytherapy treatment delivering 30 Gy in 6 fractions, in a single application.

Interstitial implantation

Suburethral recurrent deposits in the anterior vaginal wall may be suitable for iridium implantation using a template technique with a semicircular source configuration similar to that described for anal canal tumours (see Chapter 25).

Dose prescription

EXTERNAL BEAM IRRADIATION

40–50 Gy in 20–25 fractions given in 4.5 to 5 weeks.

INTRACAVITARY IRRADIATION

Vaginal applicator (e.g. Dobbie)

Low dose rate (1.2–1.5 Gy/hour):

30 Gy at 0.5 cm from the surface of the applicator.

High dose rate:

3 fractions of 4–5 Gy at 0.5 cm from the surface of the applicator.

Heyman's packing technique

See previous section.

Patient care

Diarrhoea may occur during external beam therapy and is usually controlled by dietary modification and loperamide hydrochloride. If it is severe, treatment is interrupted to allow recovery. Perineal skin reactions are treated with exposure to air and application of 1 per cent hydrocortisone cream.

Further reading

Bond, M.G., Workman, G., Martland, J. *et al.* 1997: Dosimetric considerations in the treatment of inoperable endometrial carcinoma by a high dose rate afterloading packing technique. *Clinical Oncology* **9**, 41–7.

Eifel, P.J., Ross, J., Hendrickson, M., Cox, R.S., Kempson, R. and Martinez, A. 1983: Adenocarcinoma of the endometrium: analysis of 256 cases with disease limited to the uterine corpus. Treatment comparisons. *Cancer* **52**, 1206–31.

CHAPTER 33

Ovary

Role of radiotherapy

The diagnosis of ovarian carcinoma is usually made at laparotomy when a total hysterectomy with bilateral salpingo-oophorectomy and omentectomy is performed with removal of any other macroscopic tumour. The disease is staged using the FIGO classification according to clinical examination and surgical findings. Approximately 70 per cent of patients have tumour spread beyond the ovary at the time of diagnosis, and the treatment of choice for the vast majority of patients is cytotoxic chemotherapy. Radiation can sometimes be useful for palliation after failure of primary chemotherapy.

Several treatment options are available for stage I disease. For well- and moderately differentiated stage IA tumours, no additional treatment is given after complete excision, and 5-year survival rates of up to 90 per cent are obtained. For other stage I tumours, chemotherapy is the usual first-line treatment. Intraperitoneal isotope therapy can be given unless adhesions are likely because of previous abdominal surgery or infection. Alternatively, external beam irradiation may be given to the whole abdomen with additional treatment to the pelvis, and this approach has been shown to reduce intra-abdominal relapse. However, its use is very controversial, but the technique is included here for the sake of completeness. The moving-strip technique of whole abdominal irradiation has been superseded by chemotherapeutic approaches. Patients with more advanced tumours are treated using chemotherapy, with radiotherapy given to residual pelvic disease. Five-year survival rates of only 10 to 20 per cent are achieved at present for stage III and IV disease.

Irradiation of the ovaries can be performed to induce an artificial menopause in the treatment of patients with breast cancer.

Regional anatomy

The ovaries lie on the posterior surface of the broad ligament attached to the uterus by the ovarian ligaments.

Ovarian tumours tend to present late when they have grown to a considerable size. Initial spread is within the pelvis to the uterus and Fallopian tubes, and not infrequently both ovaries are found to be involved by tumour. Transperitoneal spread is common and results in multiple seedlings of tumour on the pelvic organs, omentum, small bowel and the undersurfaces of the diaphragms.

Lymphatic spread occurs to the upper group of para-aortic nodes and renal hilar nodes as shown in Fig. 33.1. Where there is local pelvic involvement, spread to the external iliac nodes may occur.

Planning technique

ASSESSMENT OF PRIMARY DISEASE

The most important assessment of ovarian disease is that obtained at the initial laparotomy. An attempt at complete excision of tumour, total hysterectomy and bilateral salpingo-oophorectomy and omentectomy is undertaken. Ascites or peritoneal washings are sent for cytological examination and suspicious or enlarged abdominal lymph nodes are biopsied. Postoperatively, a general clinical and pelvic examination is performed and residual or metastatic disease may be defined by ultrasound examination of the abdomen, pelvis and liver. CT scanning is performed in order to assess residual macroscopic disease, pelvic and para-aortic lymph nodes and the renal tract.

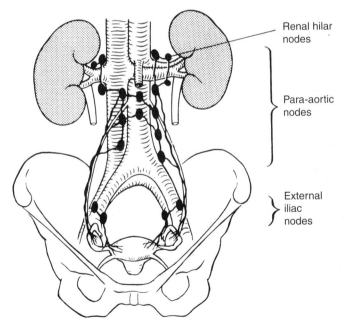

Fig. 33.1 Lymphatic drainage of the ovary.

DEFINITION OF TARGET VOLUME

Whole abdominal irradiation

The whole peritoneal cavity should be irradiated because of the high risk of transcoelomic spread. Radiation doses are limited by the tolerance of the kidneys, liver and small bowel. The kidneys must be protected after 15 Gy even though tumour may also be shielded. The entire liver is included within the target volume, since the peritoneal space between the dome of the right diaphragm and the superior surface of the liver is a common site for occult metastases. This limits the total dose which can be given to 25–30 Gy or less if the patient has received cytotoxic chemotherapy. The superior border of the target volume includes both diaphragms as screened during expiration. The inferior border extends to the lower margin of the obturator foramen to include the pelvic floor, and the lateral borders include the whole peritoneum with a margin of subcutaneous tissue.

LOCALIZATION

Most palliative treatments use simple parallel opposed fields. Ovarian cancer is not very sensitive to radiation, and doses of 30–40 Gy are necessary to achieve useful palliation of bulky disease. Where the whole pelvis must be irradiated, a four-field technique as described in Chapter 30 can be considered, provided that the target volume is adequately covered.

Whole abdominal irradiation

Simulator films are taken with the patient in the supine position at an extended FSD to obtain the required field length. If it is not possible to oppose the anterior field at an extended FSD with the patient lying supine, a change to the prone position is necessary for treatment of the posterior field, and further simulator films should be taken. The upper, lower and lateral borders of the volume are defined using a simulator, and a central tattoo is placed on the abdominal wall anteriorly and posteriorly. Lateral tattoos are placed over both iliac crests. Intravenous contrast is given in order to obtain a nephrogram, and the position of the kidney shields is defined. Shielding is also added inferiorly to protect the femora and subcutaneous tissues and superiorly to protect the left lung base (Fig. 33.2). Field margins and shields are either marked directly on to the patient's skin, or templates are made from the simulator films.

Whole pelvic irradiation

The target volume and localization technique are described in Chapter 30. A four-field 'brick' arrangement is chosen unless previous whole abdominal irradiation has been given, when a three-field technique is used to minimize the rectal dose.

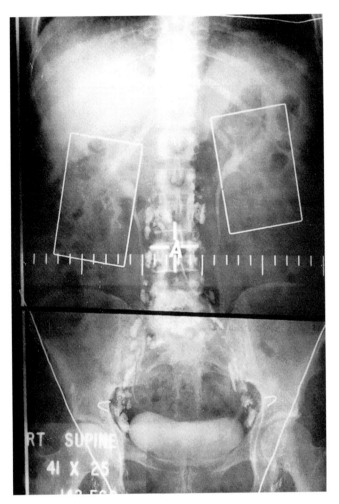

Fig. 33.2 Simulator film showing positioning of shielding when the whole abdomen is treated.

Radiation menopause

Irradiation is often given for ablation of ovarian function in the treatment of patients with breast cancer. The position of the ovaries can be very variable (Fig. 33.3), and to include most possibilities within the target volume the superior margin should be at the lower border of L5, the inferior margin at a line which traverses the middle of the femoral heads and the lateral border 1 cm lateral to the pelvic side-walls. Anterior and posterior opposing fields are used (about 12 $\times$ 12 cm^2) and localized with an AP simulator film.

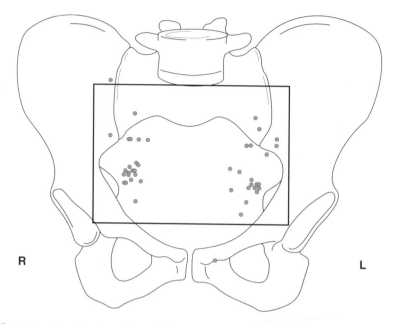

Fig. 33.3   Target volume for radiation menopause showing variable position of the ovaries. (Reproduced with permission from Counsell, R., Bain, G., Williams, M.V. and Dixon, A.K. 1996: Artificial radiation menopause: where are the ovaries? *Clinical Oncology* **8**, 250–3.)

Implementation of plan

Whole abdominal irradiation

The treatment is given with a linear accelerator at an extended FSD using lasers and skin tattoos to position the patient. Rotation is prevented by alignment of lateral tattoos. The treatment fields are aligned using skin marks or a template. An IPD measurement is taken at the centre of the volume in each position and used to calculate the mid-plane dose for the anterior and posterior fields. Shielding is placed on the tray fixed to the treatment head. Kidney shielding is introduced into both fields at a mid-plane dose of 15 Gy. Treatment of whole abdominal fields is sometimes prolonged because of bone-marrow suppression.

Dose prescription

Whole abdominal irradiation

25 Gy in 20 fractions of 1.25 Gy given in 4 weeks.

Pelvic boost

20 Gy in 10 fractions given in 2 weeks to give a total dose to the pelvis of 45 Gy in 30 fractions given in 6 weeks.

Whole pelvic irradiation alone

40–50 Gy in 20–25 fractions given in 4 to 5 weeks.

Radiation menopause

15 Gy in 5 fractions given in 7 days.

Patient care

Whole abdominal irradiation

Nausea, vomiting and diarrhoea are common. Adhesions between loops of small bowel following laparotomy may increase bowel reaction. Anti-emetics such as metoclopramide may relieve nausea, and codeine phosphate or loperamide hydrochloride are helpful for reducing diarrhoea. If the symptoms are severe, treatment may have to be suspended for several days until recovery takes place. Adequate fluid intake is important. Regular full blood counts are essential, since a large volume of bone marrow is included within the target volume. Weekly liver function tests are performed in order to monitor the liver response to irradiation, but transient abnormalities usually return to normal following treatment.

Further reading

Counsell, R., Bain, G., Williams, M.V. and Dixon, A.K. 1996: Artificial radiation menopause: where are the ovaries? *Clinical Oncology* **8**, 250–3.
Thomas, G.M. and Dembo, A.J. 1993: Integrating radiation therapy into the management of ovarian cancer. *Cancer* **7**, 1710–18.

CHAPTER 34

Vagina

Role of radiotherapy

Primary tumours of the vagina are rare, accounting for approximately 1 per cent of those arising in the female genital tract. Metastases in the vagina from tumours of the corpus uteri, bladder, ovary or rectum are more common. Radiotherapy is the treatment of choice for most patients because surgery would need to be extensive, resulting in considerable morbidity.

Carcinoma *in situ* may be treated with intracavitary or interstitial therapy alone, although lesions confined to the upper half of the vagina may be removed surgically. Small, superficial but invasive tumours less than 5 mm thick may be treated radically with intracavitary or interstitial therapy alone. All other stages of the disease require additional external beam therapy to the primary tumour and lymph nodes. Brachytherapy may be used to deliver an additional dose. If the size and thickness of residual disease after external beam radiation make treatment by a single intracavitary vaginal source possible, brachytherapy can be used as for radical treatment.

Where the thickness of residual disease is greater than 5 mm, interstitial treatment is needed to treat paravaginal tissues adequately. Palliative treatment of vaginal metastases and advanced primary tumours may be useful for controlling bleeding or pain.

Regional anatomy

Tumours of the vagina spread laterally into the paravaginal tissues and the pelvic side-walls, anteriorly to the bladder and posteriorly to the rectum. Lymphatic spread is common, from the upper part of the vagina to internal and external iliac lymph nodes, and from the lower part to the inguinal, femoral and iliac nodes. The anterior vaginal wall drains primarily to the lateral pelvic-wall nodes and the posterior vaginal wall drains primarily to the sacral and pararectal deep pelvic lymph nodes.

Planning technique

ASSESSMENT OF PRIMARY DISEASE

For patients with early-stage disease, the entire vaginal mucosa should be examined by colposcopy, and multiple biopsies of any suspicious areas performed. For patients with invasive carcinoma, staging and assessment must include cystoscopy, dilatation and curettage, cervical biopsy, bimanual examination and sigmoidoscopy where indicated. All areas of abnormality in the vaginal mucosa are biopsied. The inguino-femoral region is examined for lymphadenopathy, and needle aspiration of palpable nodes is performed in order to obtain cytology. CT scanning is used to detect ureteric compression and lymph-node involvement from primary vaginal tumours.

DEFINITION AND LOCALIZATION OF TARGET VOLUME

The initial target volume encompasses the primary tumour, the entire vagina and the pelvic nodes, including inguinal nodes for tumours of the lower third of the vagina. A barium swab is placed in the vagina, barium in the rectum and a marker at the introitus to define the target volume as shown in Fig. 34.1.

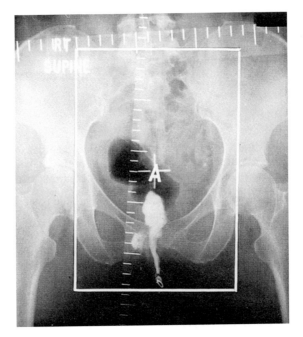

Fig. 34.1   Simulator film to show the target volume for external beam therapy of carcinoma of the vagina. Metal ring marks introitus.

A reduced target volume is used to treat the primary vaginal tumour and vaginal mucosa.

Field arrangements

INITIAL TARGET VOLUME

A four-field 'brick' technique is used as described in Chapter 30. If the inguinal nodes are to be treated, anterior and posterior opposing fields are used as described in Chapter 25 and shown in Fig. 25.6.

REDUCED VOLUME

For tumours arising in the upper third of the vagina, intracavitary treatment with an intravaginal applicator or uterine and vaginal sources may be used to deliver additional dose to the primary tumour. Lesions in the lower two-thirds of the vagina may be suitable for interstitial implantation using iridium wire.

For more advanced lesions where brachytherapy is not feasible, additional irradiation is given by external beam therapy.

INGUINAL NODES

In cases where there is lymph-node involvement, a further dose may be delivered by direct anterior electron fields as described in Chapter 25.

BRACHYTHERAPY TECHNIQUE

Intracavitary irradiation is given by means of a central vaginal source in a vaginal applicator using an afterloading Selectron. Lead or tungsten shielding can be used for part of the circumference to protect uninvolved mucosa.

Interstitial implantation is used where the lesion is more than 5 mm thick to treat the paravaginal tissues adequately. This can be done by implanting one or more iridium wire hairpins submucosally parallel to the axis of the vaginal wall, sometimes in combination with a single intravaginal source.

For thick tumours of the recto-vaginal septum or lateral vaginal walls, a boost can be given with a template implant similar to that described for anal canal tumours in Chapter 25.

Implementation of plan

Details of external beam irradiation are given in Chapter 30.

Dose prescription

Initial volume

40–45 Gy in 20–25 fractions given in 4 to 5 weeks.

Reduced volume

20–25 Gy at 0.5 cm from the surface of the applicator (intracavitary therapy)

or 20–25 Gy at 85 per cent reference isodose (interstitial therapy)

or 20–24 Gy in 10–12 fractions given in 2 to 2.5 weeks (external beam therapy).

Inguinal node irradiation

A further 15–20 Gy in 7–10 fractions given in 10–14 days (where inguinal nodes are involved).

Radical treatment by brachytherapy alone

65 Gy at 0.5 cm from the surface of the applicator.

Patient care

Patients may develop diarrhoea and tenesmus during treatment. These symptoms may be alleviated by drug therapy and dietary restrictions. If urinary symptoms develop, bacteriological examination of the urine is performed and a high fluid intake is encouraged, with antibiotics where appropriate.

Vaginal fibrosis is difficult to avoid when high tumour doses are given, but can be reduced by vaginal douching following irradiation, vaginal dilatation and oestrogen cream.

Further reading

Perez, C.A., Camel, H.M. and Galakatos, A.E. 1988: Definitive radiation in carcinoma of the vagina: long-term evaluation of results. *International Journal of Radiation Oncology, Biology and Physics* **15**, 1283–90.

CHAPTER 35

Bone and soft-tissue sarcomas

Role of radiotherapy

For osteosarcoma, Ewing's tumour and most soft-tissue sarcomas, surgery is the treatment of choice for control of local disease.

OSTEOSARCOMA

Initial treatment should be given with chemotherapy according to a standard or trial protocol. This is given to control micro-metastatic or overt disseminated disease, and to assess the chemosensitivity of the primary tumour.

Small lesions or lesions in limb bones may be suitable for conservative surgery with prosthetic replacement of bone. If a prosthesis is not appropriate, amputation may be necessary. Where resection is impossible (e.g. some primary tumours in pelvic or frontal bones, vertebral bodies or the base of the skull), radical radiotherapy may have to be used after chemotherapy. In patients who present with metastatic disease and for whom appropriate local treatment would be amputation, radiotherapy may be used to control the primary lesion until it is clear that metastases have been eradicated.

Whole-lung irradiation (see Fig. 36.3) is not indicated if there is overt lung disease, and has been shown to be of no benefit when given prophylactically, although it has been suggested that it might be given in conjunction with chemotherapy to reduce the overall duration of treatment. It may be considered in special individual cases if, for example, surgical excision of one or two metastases is impossible, or after chemotherapy and total resection of lung metastases where the excised lesions have shown evidence of persisting active disease, but these indications are very rare.

EWING'S SARCOMA

There is some evidence that surgical resection followed by radiotherapy produces optimal local control for Ewing's sarcoma. Where surgery is not possible for lesions in inaccessible sites, or where amputation would be necessary for local control, radiotherapy is the treatment of choice. It may also be used alone for local control in patients with metastatic disease at presentation for whom the prognosis remains poor.

PRIMARY LYMPHOMA OF BONE

Although radiotherapy has been given following chemotherapy for control of systemic disease, it does not appear to be necessary for good local control, and it may predispose to an increased risk of later fracture. For stage I low-grade disease, radiotherapy alone (or after surgery) may be given if it is desirable to avoid the toxicity of chemotherapy.

BENIGN TUMOURS OF BONE

Wherever possible radiotherapy is avoided in the treatment of benign tumours, in part because of the risk of induction of malignant change. Occasionally, giant-cell tumours in surgically inaccessible sites or where surgery would produce severe functional deficit may be effectively treated with radiation alone. Localized bone lesions of Langerhans' cell histiocytosis respond very well to low doses of irradiation, but since it is now uncertain whether these lesions represent a malignant process, other treatments such as intra-lesional steroids are preferred.

SOFT-TISSUE SARCOMAS

The prognosis of soft-tissue sarcomas is related to completeness of surgical excision, size and histological grade. Surgical removal may be by radical local resection, compartmental resection or amputation. Radiotherapy is indicated:

- pre-operatively if complete excision is unlikely to be possible. Such an approach is not commonly used unless these patients are assessed by a multidisciplinary team before any treatment is given;
- postoperatively if examination of the resection margin shows that excision has been incomplete or marginal. In these cases, repeat surgical excision should be considered before radiotherapy is started;
- following removal of recurrent local tumour, whether or not excision has been complete;
- some groups consider that postoperative irradiation is indicated for any patients with tumours of high-grade histology;
- when metastases are present and surgical excision of the primary tumour would result in unacceptable functional or cosmetic deficit.

Some groups also recommend postoperative radiotherapy for large low-grade tumours.

Radiotherapy may also be considered for the treatment of desmoid tumours and fibromatosis where surgical excision is impossible. There is some evidence that this reduces the rate of recurrence or progression of the disease.

Regional anatomy

OSTEOSARCOMA

These tumours usually occur in the metaphyses of long bones, especially the femur, tibia and humerus. The pelvis, jaw and fibula are less common sites, although any bone may be affected. A variable amount of local soft-tissue involvement is seen. Spread is predominantly haematogenous to the lungs. Bone metastases may also occur.

EWING'S SARCOMA

Approximately 40 per cent of lesions arise in the axial skeleton, 40 per cent in the distal extremities and 20 per cent in the proximal extremities. Bony change is usually accompanied by a significant soft-tissue mass. Metastases are most frequent in the lungs and other bones, and also occur in bone marrow, lymph nodes and other soft tissues.

SOFT-TISSUE SARCOMAS

These tumours may arise at any site. They spread by local infiltration through lymphatics to regional lymph nodes, and haematogenously to the lungs.

Assessment of primary disease

Plain X-ray of bone lesions is required to localize the tumour and to assess the stability of the bone. CT scanning and MRI are used to assess the extent of the primary lesion and to delineate associated soft-tissue masses. MRI is particularly useful for assessment of the local extent of soft-tissue sarcomas (Fig. 35.1). The extent of involvement of the medullary cavity of long bones is demonstrated by CT scanning.

Isotope bone-scanning is also useful for defining local involvement and excluding lesions in other bones. Arteriography may be necessary to plan surgical approaches. Metastatic lung disease is detected by chest X-ray and CT scanning.

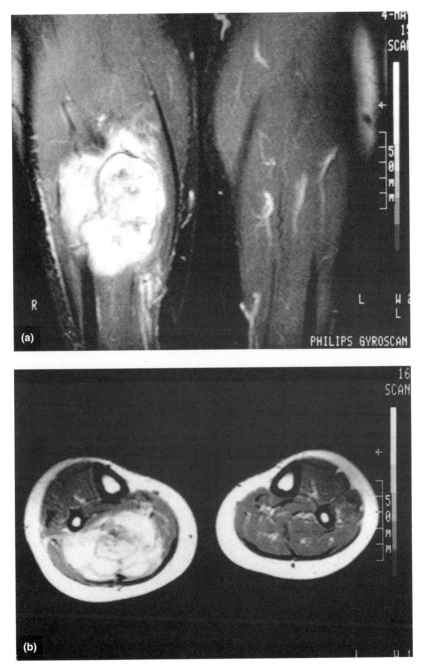

Fig. 35.1   MRI scans of malignant fibrous histiocytoma in the right calf at presentation. (a) Coronal. (b) Axial.

Definition of target volume

OSTEOSARCOMA (INOPERABLE OR METASTATIC)

The gross tumour volume is determined from plain X-rays, bone scans, CT and MRI investigations. A margin of 2–3 cm is then allowed around that volume.

EWING'S SARCOMA

Traditionally the whole tumour-bearing bone has been treated. It is not yet clear whether the more accurate localization of tumour with current scanning techniques and the primary use of effective chemotherapy make it safe to use reduced target volumes. At the very least, a generous margin (3–5 cm) should be left around the original tumour volume, taking full account of the extent of intramedullary spread. The epiphysis most distant to the tumour may usually be excluded. For primary lesions in the pelvis, the whole ipsilateral pelvic bone is included. For vertebral lesions, one vertebra above and one below the tumour are included.

LYMPHOMA, GIANT-CELL TUMOUR AND HISTIOCYTOSIS

The target volume includes only the known tumour with a small margin (approximately 1 cm).

SOFT-TISSUE SARCOMAS

For inoperable or incompletely excised tumours, the target volume encompasses the gross tumour volume defined by MRI scanning pre-operatively with a margin of 2–3 cm. Where the muscle compartment containing the lesion has not been breached, compartmental irradiation may be considered.

If the patient is assessed in a multidisciplinary clinic before treatment is started, the biopsy site will be removed by the definitive surgical procedure, and the position of the skin scar in relation to the tumour will be clearly known. In situations where the patient is seen postoperatively, the biopsy site may be at some distance from the operation scar, and irradiation of this site should be considered. Sometimes the length of the surgical scar precludes radical treatment to a sufficiently high dose, unless parts of the scar deemed to be at less risk of tumour implantation are excluded. Shrinking fields may be used to deliver a high dose to gross disease.

Localization

Immobilization should be ensured by using a perspex cast, vacuum bag, alpha cradle, foot rest or arm pole as appropriate. The optimal position for treatment should be assessed by the clinician before planning begins, e.g. to exclude the contralateral lower limb. This should ensure where possible that the scar is placed at right angles to the incident beam of radiation and that maximum sparing of normal tissues is obtained. Unless simple opposing fields are appropriate, localization is performed using CT scanning.

Field arrangements

These are chosen to cover the tumour and to minimize the dose to adjacent critical organs.

For limb lesions, opposing fields are normally used. A strip of normal tissue should be left on either side of the fields wherever possible to prevent late lymphatic obstruction and oedema. The fields should not cross joints unless it is essential to do so in order to cover tumour. Field edges should preferably be at a well-defined bony margin for tumours in other bones, e.g. intervertebral space rather than midvertebral, sacro-iliac joint or symphysis pubis.

In the pelvis, care should be taken to exclude as much bladder and bowel as possible. Spinal cord doses should be minimized when vertebral lesions are treated by using electron fields, shallow wedged fields or rotational techniques as appropriate. Field arrangements for soft-tissue lesions must be individualized according to the principles outlined above.

BRACHYTHERAPY

For patients with high-grade lesions, a local control advantage may be obtained by using postoperative brachytherapy. After complete surgical resection, afterloading catheters are implanted in the surgical bed according to the standard Paris rules. A drain is left *in situ* and the wound is closed. Iridium wires are loaded on the sixth postoperative day and removed after a dose of 45 Gy has been delivered in 4 to 6 days. Brachytherapy in combination with external beam therapy may also be used to deliver a boost if there is residual tumour following surgery.

Implementation of plan

Patients are treated in the appropriate position with immobilization. A linear accelerator delivering high-energy photons or electrons is used. In some cases a cobalt unit with lower exit doses and less skin-sparing effect may be advantageous. Photon treatments are given isocentrically treating all fields daily. For lesions in the upper part of the adductor compartment of the thigh, or in the sacral region, consideration should be given to shielding the testes and natal cleft if possible.

Dose prescription

Tumour control rates improve with increasing doses for all bone and soft-tissue sarcomas (except Ewing's sarcoma). The maximum dose possible should therefore be given. This dose will depend on the site of disease and adjacent normal tissues, and a shrinking-field technique may be needed. Severe fibrosis may occur with doses in excess of 55–60 Gy.

RADICAL TREATMENT

Osteosarcomas, soft-tissue sarcomas and fibromatosis

54–66 Gy in 27–33 fractions given in 5.5 to 6.5 weeks.

Ewing's sarcoma

55 Gy in 27 fractions given in 5.5 weeks.

Giant-cell tumour (and lymphoma)

45 Gy in 23 fractions given in 4.5 weeks.

Langerhans' cell histiocytosis

8–10 Gy in 4–5 fractions given in 1 week.

Palliative treatment (uncontrolled metastatic disease)

40–45 Gy in 15 fractions given in 3 weeks.

Patient care

Skin erythema may be troublesome during the last fractions of treatment, and can be minimized by cutting out the perspex shell if used, keeping the skin dry and using 1 per cent hydrocortisone cream. Diarrhoea may occur if large volumes of bowel are included in the field, and may be controlled with loperamide or codeine phosphate and a low-residue diet. Vigorous physiotherapy during treatment and for some months afterwards may help to maintain the mobility of joints and prevent muscle fibrosis.

Further reading

Bamberg, M. and Hoffman, W. 1994: Soft tissue sarcomas in adults – current treatment strategies. *International Journal of Cancer* **57**, 143–5.

Verweij, J., Pinedo, H. and Suit, H. (eds) 1997: *Soft tissue sarcomas: present achievements and future prospects*. Boston, MA: Kluwer Academic Publishers.

See also Further reading for Chapter 36.

Paediatric tumours

General considerations

Children who are cured of cancer have a long life expectancy, and treatment-related complications may have greater significance than those which occur in adults. Recognition of the late effects of radiotherapy has led to a reduction in its use, but approximately 50 per cent of children with malignant disease will still require radiotherapy for cure or palliation. Complications are related to the dose and volume of irradiation, and are inversely proportional to the age of the child at the time of treatment. Immature organs with high growth potential are more susceptible to radiation damage than their adult counterparts. Chemotherapy is usually given before or during radiotherapy, and therefore normal tissue tolerance may be altered. The dose given per fraction should be reduced in young children to 1.2–1.8 Gy/day in order to obtain the best cosmetic and functional results. Specific organ tolerances are listed in Table 36.1. The immature liver and kidneys are particularly sensitive to radiation damage, and care must be taken to minimize doses to these organs. Baseline measures of organ function should be taken before chemotherapy starts, and again before any radiotherapy is given. These baseline measures should include estimation of cardiac, renal, hepatic and hormonal function, and should also test vision and hearing if appropriate. Psychological assessment is indicated if brain irradiation is needed.

Patients and their parents should be cared for by a team with appropriate expertise in a children's unit.

Radiotherapy treatment should be planned before chemotherapy is started so that there is an accurate record of the initial extent of disease. The size of the target volume for radiotherapy will vary according to tumour site and histology, and response to chemotherapy. As a general principle, the smallest volume that encompasses residual disease alone is treated in order to minimize normal tissue damage. Treatment is planned using a CT scanner, taking into account all other imaging information, including that from MRI scanning. Treatment is delivered with a linear accelerator with good beam definition, or with electrons. Treatment fields are designed to maintain symmetry of growth of the musculo-skeletal system in order to avoid scoliosis or torticollis. Epiphyses are avoided where possible, and vertebrae are treated across their whole width, including transverse processes. Treatment to the neck should usually therefore be bilateral.

Dose reductions may be made for very young children, although there is no firm evidence for variation in the radiosensitivity of tumours with age. The dose

Table 36.1 Tolerance doses of specific organs to irradiation

Organ	Tolerance dose*	Note
Brain		
> 2 years	55 Gy	Endpoint is necrosis, functional deficit may be noted after doses of 15 Gy
< 2 years	45 Gy	Maximum weekly dose for infants is 7–8 Gy
Definitive hair loss	55 Gy	
Lens	6–8 Gy	
Lung	18–20 Gy	Daily fractions of 1.8 Gy
Kidney	12 Gy	Both kidneys
	15–20 Gy	One kidney only
Liver	20 Gy	Whole abdominal irradiation
	15–20 Gy	After chemotherapy or partial hepatectomy
	30 Gy	To one area only
Epiphyses	10 Gy	Partial growth impairment
Hypothalamus	30 Gy	
Ovary	6–15 Gy	
Testis	4–12 Gy	Endpoint spermatogenesis
	20 Gy	Endpoint hormone production

* The tolerance doses quoted for each organ are total doses given in daily fractions of 1.5–2 Gy/day which represent the best estimate of tolerance doses when radiation is used alone. However, this is rarely the case in paediatric radiotherapy, and the specific organ effects of different chemotherapy agents must also be taken into account.

given should be the minimum effective dose taking into account normal tissue tolerance.

Immobilization is essential for accurate treatment. Extra visits and time for play may be necessary to persuade young children to co-operate. For children under 2 years of age, treatment with ketamine (5–15 mg/kg) produces adequate, short-lasting, safe anaesthesia. An anaesthetist must be present throughout treatment, and careful monitoring carried out using remote systems such as pulse oximetry. Sedation with a cocktail of drugs, including those such as trimeprazine, droperidol and methadone, has proved less satisfactory, as the onset of sedation cannot be so accurately co-ordinated with treatment time and may leave the child in a sleepy state for longer periods. This may lead to problems with feeding. Acute toxicity such as nausea and vomiting may also produce dehydration or weight loss in young children, and intravenous or nasogastric feeding may be necessary. Treatment should therefore be carefully timed to avoid regular mealtimes, and if anaesthesia is required, treatment should be scheduled for early in the morning.

The trunk and limbs may be immobilized using perspex shells or moulded vacuum bags. Treatment in a prone cast (as for medulloblastoma treatment) requires particular care, and planning for complex set-ups may be best done under general anaesthesia, although for subsequent treatments the child may learn to co-operate well.

Invasive procedures such as lumbar punctures (for patients with leukaemia) may be performed under the same anaesthetic as that used for treatment, and daily induction of anaesthesia is facilitated by an indwelling Hickman or Porta-cath device.

Children are treated according to the protocols of the United Kingdom Children's Cancer Study Group (UKCCSG), the Children's Solid Tumour Group (CSTG) or the International Society of Paediatric Oncology (SIOP), and these protocols should be consulted.

Rhabdomyosarcoma

ROLE OF RADIOTHERAPY

Systemic therapy is required for all patients in order to prevent the development of metastatic disease, and it produces survival rates of 70 per cent. Chemotherapy is given as the first treatment unless complete excision of the primary tumour is possible at presentation without any mutilation. Studies from the American Intergroup Rhabdomyosarcoma Group and SIOP have reached different conclusions about the role of radiotherapy, the American group favouring more aggressive local treatment at an earlier stage and to large volumes. SIOP studies have shown that radiotherapy can be successfully omitted from the treatment of a proportion of children in whom complete remission is obtained by chemotherapy. Although local relapse rates are higher than when radiotherapy is given systematically, some children treated with this approach will be spared the late sequelae of radiation. Further data are needed to determine whether salvage of patients who suffer local relapse can be satisfactorily obtained without increased toxicity from treatment (as, for example, from intensification of chemotherapy). If complete remission is not obtained with chemotherapy, local therapy with either surgery or radiotherapy is chosen according to which of these agents will cause the least functional and cosmetic deficit. The timing of radiotherapy remains controversial, as patients with relatively chemoresistant disease may benefit from early radiotherapy, but where a good response is obtained there is no proof that this is necessary. These tumours appear to have a tendency to shrink down towards their point of origin after successful chemotherapy, and therefore treatment of residual tumours with a margin of 2–3 cm is adequate for local control. Brachytherapy with iridium wires should be considered as an alternative to external beam radiotherapy if feasible.

REGIONAL ANATOMY

Rhabdomyosarcomas may occur at any site, but are commonest in the genitourinary tract (the bladder, prostate, vagina, uterus, urethra and paratesticular region). Lesions occur in the limbs and in the head and neck region, where they are classified as parameningeal (nasopharynx, nasal cavity, paranasal sinuses, middle ear and mastoid, pterygopalatine or infratemporal fossa) or non-parameningeal (orbit, parotid, cheek, etc.). Prognosis is related to site and probably size and histology. Spread is local, to regional lymph nodes and by the bloodstream to bones, lung and bone marrow.

PLANNING TECHNIQUE

Assessment of primary disease

The extent of the primary lesion is documented by clinical examination, and regional nodal areas are palpated carefully. CT scanning is used to define more precisely the extent of the primary lesion, any impalpable nodes and small-volume lung metastases. Bone scanning is used to exclude bone metastases with appropriate local X-rays if a positive result is obtained. For head and neck primary tumours a CT brain scan is performed, and if there is evidence of intracranial extension, cerebrospinal fluid must be examined in order to exclude involvement.

Definition of target volume

Provided that the response to chemotherapy has been adequate, residual tumour is treated with a margin of 2–3 cm. For parameningeal sites with intracranial extension, irradiation is given to the initial volume of disease, and if the cerebrospinal fluid is positive for malignant cells, whole neuraxis irradiation may be given.

FIELD ARRANGEMENTS

The simplest field arrangement which encompasses the tumour and contains least normal tissue should be used. Opposing fields are often suitable. For extremity lesions, irradiation of the whole compartment may not be feasible. When the limb is treated, some of the circumference of normal tissue on either side of the limb should be spared in order to prevent late fibrosis and oedema. For rhabdomyosarcoma arising in the eyelids or the muscles of the orbit, the whole orbit should be treated (see Fig. 15.3). The eye should be kept open during treatment to prevent build-up of dose on the cornea.

DOSE PRESCRIPTION

45–50 Gy in 25–28 fractions (1.8 Gy/fraction) given in 5 to 6 weeks.

(Doses may be reduced to 40 Gy for good-prognosis disease.)

Neuroblastoma

ROLE OF RADIOTHERAPY

Patients with early-stage disease (stage 1,2) do not benefit from the addition of radiotherapy after surgery, although chemotherapy may confer a survival advantage after incomplete excision in patients with unfavourable biological features (n-myc amplification, chromosome 1_p deletion, etc).

Many patients present with metastatic disease (stage 4) and are initially treated with chemotherapy. Residual abdominal disease after chemotherapy (which is common) should be removed surgically where feasible. Postoperative radiotherapy may be given when excision is incomplete. Meta-iodobenzylguanidine I-131 (MIBG) may be used in targeted therapy.

Some centres give whole body irradiation as part of high-dose consolidation therapy in patients with poor-prognosis stage 4 disease, although the benefit of this approach has not yet been fully demonstrated in randomized trials. Radiotherapy also appears to be effective in local control and in improving survival in stage 3 disease after chemotherapy.

Palliation of metastases that recur after chemotherapy may be achieved with fractionated radiotherapy or by single-fraction treatments in cases where the prognosis is very poor.

In patients with stage 4s disease, emergency radiotherapy to shrink the liver is occasionally necessary, but is usually avoided by chemotherapy treatment.

PLANNING TECHNIQUE

Assessment of disease

Staging is carried out by clinical examination of the primary site, estimation of urinary catecholamines, CT scan of the abdomen and chest, bone scan, bone-marrow aspirate and trephine and MIBG scanning where available.

Definition of target volume

This is determined by surgical documentation of disease extent and CT scanning of the residual mass. For patients with stage 4s disease, only part of the liver need be treated in order to produce regression.

FIELD ARRANGEMENTS

Anterior and posterior opposing fields often produce a satisfactory dose distribution, although care must be taken to limit the dose to the spinal cord and contralateral kidney. The whole width of the vertebrae should be included.

For emergency irradiation of the liver, two lateral fields are used, the posterior borders of which lie in front of both kidneys.

CT scanning with three-dimensional planning using beam's-eye view and an inverse planning approach provides the best hope of achieving good tumour dose distributions with acceptable doses to critical normal tissues such as the liver, kidneys and spinal cord.

DOSE PRESCRIPTION

Control may be age related, with lower doses being needed for younger children.

Primary residual disease

25 Gy in 1.8-Gy daily fractions (age < 2 years).

35–40 Gy in 1.8-Gy daily fractions (age > 2 years).

Metastatic disease

8-Gy single fraction.

20 Gy in 5 fractions given in 7 days.

30 Gy in 10 fractions given in 2 weeks.

Hepatic disease (4s)

4.5 Gy in 3 daily fractions

or 10 Gy in 5 daily fractions.

MIBG

Targeted radiotherapy with the catecholamine precursor MIBG labelled with iodine-131 can be used in the treatment of those tumours which are shown to take up the agent during diagnostic scanning. Various approaches have been tried. This technique may be used as the first treatment in patients with stage 4 disease (as recommended by the Amsterdam Group) and followed with chemotherapy. Other groups recommend its use in combination with external beam therapy to reduce normal tissue toxicity, as part of a combined strategy of intensive therapy that includes TBI with bone-marrow or stem-cell rescue and external beam therapy for poor-risk stage 4 disease, or for palliation after chemotherapy. Although it is undoubtedly an effective agent, optimal scheduling and incorporation into treatment protocols have not yet been determined. Activities of 7–10 megabecquerels are usually given, but this can result in widely differing doses to tumour and normal tissue depending on the specific uptake in an individual patient. Uptake cannot yet be accurately predicted from pre-treatment diagnostic scans.

Wilms' tumour

ROLE OF RADIOTHERAPY

Wilms' tumour is a malignant embryonal tumour of the kidney which is very sensitive to chemotherapy and radiotherapy. The interrelationship of these two modalities has been explored by a series of studies from the American National Wilms' Tumour Study Group. Radiotherapy does not improve survival or local control rates when added to chemotherapy in stage I disease, and intensification of chemotherapy appears to have removed the need for radiotherapy in stage II disease, where regional tumour extension is completely excised at surgery. In patients with stage III disease, where there is residual tumour postoperatively or the peritoneum has been grossly contaminated, localized or whole abdominal radiotherapy improves control rates. These studies have also shown that tumours with favourable histology can be controlled with reduced doses of radiotherapy.

In children with metastatic lung disease at presentation, whole-lung irradiation (after complete remission has been obtained with chemotherapy) improves survival by about 20 per cent.

Irradiation of other sites of metastatic disease may also be needed. Development of metastatic disease (in the lung or brain) may be successfully treated, but control of bone or liver disease is less likely. Palliation of symptomatic metastatic disease can usually be obtained with low-dose radiotherapy.

REGIONAL ANATOMY

The kidneys lie lateral to the twelfth thoracic and first and second lumbar vertebrae. The renal hilum usually lies along the line of the lateral vertebral pedicles, but rotation of the kidney may produce marked variations in position. Tumour invasion of the renal vein, sometimes extending into the inferior vena cava, is a common route of spread, as is lymph-node involvement of the para-aortic nodes at the level of T10–L2. Involvement of the peritoneum may lead to transcoelomic spread.

PLANNING TECHNIQUE

Assessment of disease

Abdominal disease is assessed with ultrasound, which will show a solid mass involving the kidney and determine whether there is tumour extension into the renal vein or the inferior vena cava. CT scanning is used to assess extrarenal spread, retroperitoneal node involvement, the contralateral kidney and the liver. Pulmonary metastases are excluded by a thoracic CT scan. Bone scanning is indicated when histology shows a clear cell sarcoma or rhabdoid tumour. A CT brain scan may be performed for rhabdoid tumours which are associated with primary central nervous system tumours. Planning for treatment should be based on the initial staging investigations, taken in conjunction with surgical findings.

Definition of target volume

Tumour bed

The entire initial tumour extent is covered, including the renal vein to its entry to the inferior vena cava and the regional lymph nodes (Fig. 36.1). On the left, the upper border is at the diaphragm. On the right, the initial tumour extent is encompassed with due regard to the amount of liver included in the target volume. The lower and lateral borders are determined by the initial CT scan. Medially, the volume is extended to cover the whole width of the vertebral bodies and pedicles in order to minimize scoliosis and to include bilateral para-aortic nodes. The position of the kidneys is defined from CT scans, and is checked using intravenous contrast. The contralateral kidney should be excluded from the target volume.

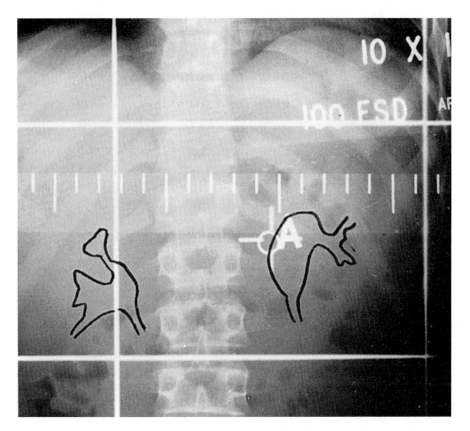

Fig. 36.1 Planning film taken before surgery to define field margins for irradiation of the left renal bed and para-aortic lymph nodes with the entire width of the vertebrae included.

Whole abdominal irradiation

The target volume extends from the domes of the diaphragms to the lower border of the pubis and laterally to include the abdominal wall. Some sparing of pelvic bones may be achieved by suitable shielding (Fig. 36.2). The kidneys should be shielded from both fields after doses of 12–15 Gy, and a single kidney may be shielded posteriorly throughout treatment. After chemotherapy, hepatic doses should be limited to 15 Gy by appropriate shielding.

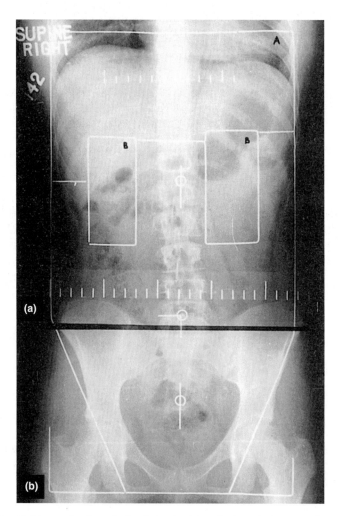

Fig. 36.2 Field margins for whole abdominal irradiation. A shows inclusion of left lung base on inspiration. B indicates kidney shields (inspiratory film).

Whole-lung irradiation

The whole of both lungs are included in the target volume, from the apices to the pleural reflection inferolaterally (usually at T11–12), making allowance for movement of the diaphragm with respiration. Laterally, the chest wall is encompassed. The heads of the humeri and shoulder joints are shielded as shown in Fig. 36.3.

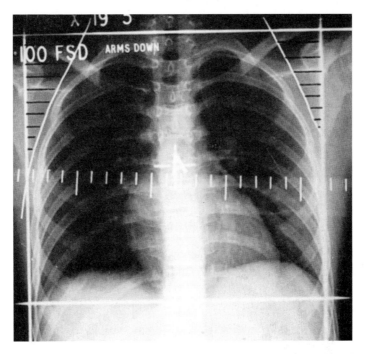

Fig. 36.3 Field margins for whole lung irradiation with shielding to shoulder joints (inspiratory film).

Localization

Simulator films are taken with the child lying in the supine position.

For irradiation of the tumour bed, the position of the kidneys or of the remaining kidney is determined from CT scanning and marked on the simulator film as shown in Fig. 36.1.

Although, in adults, whole-lung or abdominal fields may need an extended FSD, children are usually small enough for the machine to be used at its standard FSD. For whole abdominal irradiation, the kidney position is defined as described above. A template should be prepared, on to which shielding should be marked (Fig. 36.2). This should then be checked after giving intravenous contrast in order to verify the position of the kidneys during respiration, and a film is taken as a permanent record.

For both whole-lung and whole abdominal treatments, the position of the diaphragms during inspiration and expiration should be noted by screening, and the position of the liver defined. Shielding of the humeri is added to the lung template as shown in Fig. 36.3.

A lateral simulator film is taken to localize the lungs for inhomogeneity corrections, or CT scanning may be used to produce a direct density correction. Any residual metastases can be localized for additional 'boost' treatments.

Anterior and posterior opposing fields are used to minimize the integral dose, facilitate shielding and maintain symmetry.

DOSE PRESCRIPTION

Tumour bed

20 Gy in 10 fractions of 2 Gy given in 2 weeks (stage 3 favourable histology).

30 Gy in 20 fractions of 1.5 Gy given in 4 weeks (stage 3 unfavourable histology).

Whole abdominal irradiation

Stage 3 with peritoneal contamination or recurrent disease:

20 Gy with daily fractions of 1.5 Gy.

The kidneys are shielded at 12–15 Gy and the liver at 15 Gy.

Whole lung

12 Gy in 8 fractions of 1.5 Gy given in 2 to 3 weeks.

Boost to residual metastases

10 Gy in 5–6 fractions given daily.

Hodgkin's and Non-Hodgkin's lymphoma

ROLE OF RADIOTHERAPY

Hodgkin's disease

Approaches to the treatment of Hodgkin's disease vary widely, but overall survival rates are very similar. In most centres in the UK, staging laparotomy has not been used for many years and studies have been directed towards the aim of maintaining cure rate and reducing toxicity. For clinical stage I disease, radiation to the whole neck may be given, with chemotherapy reserved for patients who will relapse. The side-effects of a thin neck and hypothyroidism from this approach must be balanced against the side-effects of chemotherapy, which will produce equally good control rates. In stage II–IV disease, involved-field radiotherapy given to sites of residual disease after chemotherapy improves local control rates.

Non-Hodgkin's lymphoma

In childhood, most disease is of the diffuse type and is appropriately treated by systemic chemotherapy. Local radiotherapy to primary sites of disease does not confer any benefit, and CNS-directed therapy is increasingly being given by systemic and intrathecal chemotherapy. Cranial irradiation may be used where there is initial CNS involvement, or as part of the conditioning regimen before bone-marrow or stem-cell transplantation. If cranial irradiation and total body irradiation are both likely to be given, care should be taken to leave an adequate time interval (6–12 months) between treatments, or to give both at the same time (see Chapter 37).

Primary lymphoma of bone is adequately controlled with chemotherapy alone. Radiotherapy may be given for disease that is recurrent at the primary or a single site after chemotherapy, or for palliation of uncontrolled advanced disease.

PLANNING TECHNIQUE

Definition of target volume

If radiotherapy is used for stage I Hodgkin's disease, the target volume includes the site of primary disease and the adjacent cervical nodes on both sides of the neck. This is important for maintaining symmetry of muscle and bone growth. The upper border of the volume is at the tip of the mastoid processes, and the lower border extends to below the clavicles and encompasses supraclavicular nodes. Shielding is added to clavicles and lung as shown in Fig. 36.4. If there is involvement of the antrum or nasopharynx, the whole of Waldeyer's ring is included. Infradiaphragmatic presentations (which are very rare) may be treated by inguinal node irradiation alone.

Localization

A supine cast is made with the head slightly extended to facilitate treatment of the upper cervical nodes with some sparing of the buccal mucosa.

FIELD ARRANGEMENTS

Anterior and posterior opposing fields are used to treat the neck. The cervical spine may be shielded posteriorly at a dose of 15–20 Gy unless there is involvement of the posterior or occipital nodes.

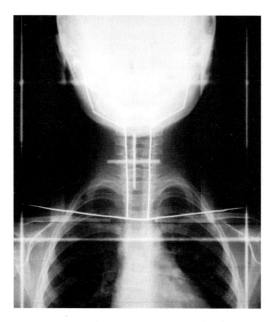

Fig. 36.4 Bilateral neck irradiation for Hodgkin's disease in the left side of the neck.

Additional shielding covers the buccal mucosa, the alveoli and teeth, and the clavicles and lung.

For other sites, templates may be made for 'mantle' or 'inverted Y' treatments which are given as described in Chapter 22. For mediastinal irradiation where opposing fields are used, two lateral tattoos are made in the mid-axillary line and used for alignment to prevent lateral rotation.

IMPLEMENTATION OF PLAN

The patient lies supine in a cast on the treatment couch, and shielding is aligned according to the template or tattoos. For extended fields where there may be variations in tissue thickness throughout the target volume, doses to nodes in different areas must be determined separately and the prescription made taking these variations into account.

DOSE PRESCRIPTION

No previous chemotherapy

30–35 Gy MPD or to a specified depth of nodes in 15–18 fractions given in 3 to 4 weeks.

After chemotherapy

20–30 Gy MPD or to a specified depth of nodes in 10–15 fractions given in 2 to 3 weeks.

Treatment is given daily at 2 Gy per day, but the fraction size may be reduced to 1.8 Gy in children under 10 years old, or where there are special risk factors.

PATIENT CARE

Patients should see a dentist before treatment for advice about dental care. Side-effects are usually minimal during treatment and are limited to mild mucosal reactions or gastrointestinal upset. Skin reactions may occur after some chemotherapy combinations (e.g. adriamycin, bleomycin, etoposide, methotrexate), and may be exacerbated by loss of skin sparing from the shell and high exit doses. There may be marked temporary posterior hair loss in the upper part of the fields.

Other tumours

The treatment of retinoblastoma is discussed in Chapter 15, and treatment of intracranial tumours is discussed in Chapter 21. Hepatic tumours are treated by chemotherapy and surgery. Radiotherapy is rarely used for palliation alone.

Further reading

Halperin, E.C., Kun, L.E., Constine, L.S. and Tarbell, N.J. 1989: *Paediatric radiation oncology*. New York: Raven Press.

Voute, P.A., Rodary, C. and Barrett, A. (eds) 1998: *Cancer in children*, 4th edn. Oxford: Oxford University Press.

CHAPTER 37

Systemic irradiation

Role of systemic irradiation

Total body irradiation (TBI) is used as part of the preparative regimen for bone-marrow transplantation (BMT) or stem-cell transplantation in patients with leukaemia, lymphoma and some solid tumours. It may be used in conjunction with a variety of chemotherapy schedules such as high-dose alkylating agents (cyclophosphamide or melphalan) or combinations, including etoposide, cyto-sine arabinoside, carboplatin, etc.

The aim of treatment is to reduce the number of any residual malignant cells and to permit engraftment of donor marrow. For tumour control, the total dose of radiation should be as high as possible within the limits of normal tissue tolerance. Ease of engraftment is related to the type of marrow infused. Less immune suppression is needed when autologous marrow is reinfused than when compatible allogeneic marrow is used, and high doses of TBI appear to facilitate engraftment of marrow which is not fully compatible (mismatched or matched unrelated transplants).

The role of BMT for many malignant diseases is still unclear, although indi-vidual patients may benefit strikingly. Patients with acute myeloid leukaemia in first remission are often considered for transplantation and, in selected groups, 5-year disease-free survival rates may be improved from an expected 20 per cent with chemotherapy alone to 65 per cent. In patients with acute lymphatic leukaemia, relapse remains a problem, but intensive treatment with BMT may be beneficial in some patients with high-risk disease. Many groups are currently investigating this approach in patients with relapse of lymphoma, particularly where the disease remains chemosensitive.

Remission should be obtained before total body irradiation and BMT, as the treatment is ineffective when there is overt disease.

For patients with lymphatic leukaemia, 'boosts' may be given in conjunction with TBI to 'sanctuary sites', either prophylactically or when there has been pre-vious relapse in these areas. Patients with lymphoma who achieve a good response after chemotherapy may have residual disease at sites of initial bulky involvement, and boosts may be considered. Boosts to the mediastinum increase the risk of pneumonitis and, if considered essential, only a low dose is recom-mended. Similarly, TBI given after previous mediastinal (or cranial) irradiation will be associated with a higher risk of complications. In other situations, boosts can be given safely and most conveniently in a few treatments before TBI. Total doses are determined according to the age of the patient, the time interval since previous irradiation, and the type and amount of previous chemotherapy given. Young age, short time interval (less than 6 months) and high doses of chemotherapy are generally associated with increasing toxicity.

High-dose single-fraction half-body irradiation is given as palliative treatment for widespread painful bony metastases from carcinoma, usually of the breast, bronchus or prostate, or occasionally for widespread drug-resistant lymphoma. Symptomatic relief is excellent and often long-lasting, although survival is not affected.

Fractionated systemic irradiation may be given for some non-Hodgkin's lymphomas, either electively with radical intent after remission has been induced with chemotherapy, or palliatively for widespread disease. Sequential half-body irradiation is better tolerated than TBI and is therefore preferred. Bone-marrow involvement with lymphoma is a relative contraindication to palliative treatment, and severe thrombocytopenia may develop.

High-dose total body irradiation (TBI)

A number of TBI regimens have been shown to be safe and effective, using the endpoints of rate of engraftment, tumour control and incidence of pneumonitis (the most common dose-limiting toxicity). From radiobiological first principles, a TBI regimen should use the highest tolerable dose to control tumour, and a low dose rate or fraction size to minimize normal tissue damage. Variability in parameters of the tumour, growth characteristics, radiosensitivity and differences in the number of occult residual tumour cells at the time of TBI will make it difficult to determine the 'best' schedule for any individual patient. However, data from the Seattle and UK Medical Research Council Studies suggest that doses of 13.2–14.4 Gy given in 1.8-Gy fractions treating twice daily may be recommended from experience and on theoretical grounds.

Homogeneity of dose distribution, which is of major importance in most radiotherapy treatments, is not necessary for TBI. The aim should rather be to deliver as high a dose as possible to all areas without causing damage. Compensation to areas of high dose (such as the neck and ankles) is not essential as doses do not exceed tolerance. Lung shielding can be safely omitted if maximum doses to the lung do not exceed those quoted above. Shielding may be undesirable as it may protect tumour cells in the ribs and lung. Techniques that combine lung shielding and electron boost to the ribs may result in lung doses as high as those received when no shielding is applied. Reproducibility and maintenance of positioning of lung shields are difficult to ensure, and only about two-thirds of the lung volume can be shielded effectively.

For fractionated treatments, the critical factor is probably the dose per fraction to the lung. The dose should be prescribed for the lung according to measurements made there. If measurements made at the abdomen are used for prescription, each fraction will then deliver a higher dose to the lung because of increased transmission of radiation.

The whole body is treated using anterior and posterior fields with the patient lying on his or her side (Fig. 37.1). No shielding is used. An attempt is made to position the arms across the chest to provide some compensation for increased radiation transmission through the lungs. A cobalt unit or linear accelerator is used at an extended SSD to give a field size sufficient to cover the whole body. When single treatments are given with cobalt, a suitable filter is inserted in the beam to give a dose rate of 0.02–0.04 Gy/min. A 1-cm thickness of perspex is needed to deliver a 100 per cent dose to the skin. The field margins within which the patient must be confined are checked from the light projection of the beam on to the wall beyond the patient.

Before treatment is given, or during the first treatment for fractionated TBI, the distribution of dose in the body is measured using lithium fluoride thermoluminescent dosimetry or silicon diodes. Lithium fluoride capsules are placed on the skin and a known dose of radiation is delivered (Fig. 37.2).

Any necessary changes in treatment times are made after checking the doses received during this test period.

CRANIAL BOOST

Opposing lateral fields are set up using Reid's baseline. No perspex shell or eye shielding is necessary (since the eye cannot be spared the subsequent TBI dose).

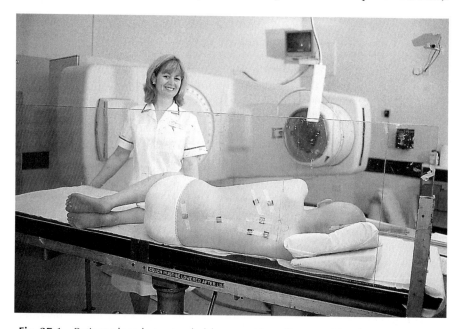

Fig. 37.1 Patient placed at extended focus – skin – distance (FSD) for TBI treatment with dosemeters positioned on her back to measure upper and lower lung, mediastinal, abdominal and pelvic doses.

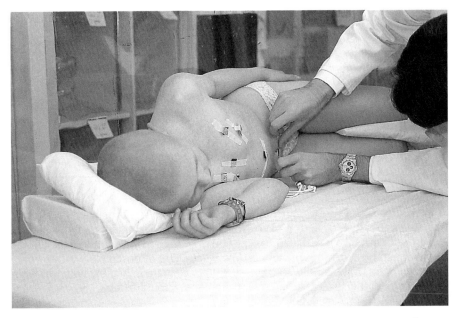

Fig. 37.2   Patient dosemeters placed on front of patient in positions corresponding to those in Fig. 37.1.

TESTICULAR BOOST

A single direct field of orthovoltage radiation or electrons is used with the penis taped as far out of the field as possible.

POSITIONING OF LITHIUM FLUORIDE DOSEMETERS

Dosemeters should be placed as far as possible at right angles to the incident beam. In the lateral position, anterior dosemeters are placed as described below and posterior dosemeters are placed opposite them. In all patients readings should be obtained from the following:

- skull – middle of the forehead;
- upper lung – just below the mid-point of the clavicle;
- mediastinum – 4 cm below the suprasternal notch in the mid-line;
- lower lung – in the mid-clavicular line at the level of the xiphisternum;
- abdomen – in the mid-line half-way between the xiphisternum and the superior iliac crest;
- pelvis – over the anterior superior iliac spine;
- thigh – at the mid-point between the groin and the knee;
- ankle – on the anterior surface at the level of the malleoli.

Additional measurements may be taken to correlate with specific organ function at the following sites:

- neck – overlying the thyroid;
- bladder – in the mid-line just above the pubic symphysis;
- ovary – at the mid-point between the pelvis and bladder dosemeters;
- parotid – over the parotid gland at the level of the tragus;
- eye – on the closed eyelid.

Dose prescription

From the lithium fluoride measurements a dose distribution is obtained. The dose is prescribed to the maximum lung dose which is normalized to 10.5 Gy for single treatments and 14.4 Gy for fractionated treatments. If dosemeters have been correctly positioned, there should be a good correlation between the anterior and posterior dosemeters and between pairs of dosemeters in the upper and lower part of the lung. Variations of ± 5 per cent are inevitable with this technique, but readings suggesting larger differences should be checked.

Patient care

For fractionated treatments, a maximum dose of a serotonin antagonist such as ondansetron should be given orally 30 min before each fraction of treatment. Vomiting may occur between treatments, starting after the second or third fraction. If necessary, hydrocortisone ($80\,mg/m^2$) or phenobarbitone ($80\,mg/m^2$) can be added. With single-fraction treatments, nausea and vomiting may be minimized by overnight fasting and intravenous hydration in addition to the above drug regimen.

Parotid swelling may occur within 24 hours of starting irradiation, and subsides spontaneously. Mild diarrhoea occurs from 4 to 5 days after the start of treatment. Reversible hair loss, if not already present, starts after 10 to 14 days. Recovery of engrafted marrow begins from day 7 to 21. A somnolence syndrome of anorexia, lassitude, nausea or headache may occur from 6 to 8 weeks after irradiation and is self-limiting. Sterility and cataract may be expected as late effects. Hormone replacement therapy will be necessary for many patients.

Radiation pneumonitis with cough and breathlessness occurs in less than 5 per cent of patients treated with this schedule. However, chest symptoms are common. Their aetiology is multifactorial and effective treatment depends on accurate diagnosis.

Half-body irradiation (HBI)

Fields extend from the head or feet to cover the upper or lower half of the body. The other border of the field is determined by the site of the disease, but is usually at the level of the iliac crests. Lateral tattoos are placed over the iliac crests with the patient in the supine position, and these tattoos are used to match fields if necessary. Treatment is given with a linear accelerator working at an extended FSD to give an adequate field size. The patient lies supine on the couch with their legs bent if necessary, and treatment is given with opposing lateral fields. If the patient is short, an adequate field size may be obtained with them lying prone and supine on the floor, using anterior and posterior fields. With this technique, the upper half of the body is treated with a field at a gantry angle of $0°$, and the bottom half is treated with the gantry angled $24°$ away from the junction in order to minimize field overlap and give a slightly larger field size. For fractionated half-body treatment, a similar set-up to that for TBI may be used with the patient lying supine on the couch, which is placed at extended FSD against the wall of the treatment room. Tattoos are marked laterally at the level of the iliac crest, and sequential treatment fields are matched at the skin mark. Test doses may be given as for TBI with an extra measurement at the field edge. From knowledge of the approximate machine output at the FSD corresponding to the mid-plane dose, an estimated dose of 0.3 Gy is given. The following day, measured doses are checked and any necessary adjustments made. The patient is then treated by right and left lateral fields daily.

Patient care

Preparation and sedation are given as for whole-body treatments. Nausea and vomiting may occur from the end of treatment for 4 to 6 hours. Diarrhoea is rare. Dry mouth and taste disturbance are frequent. Treatments of the upper half of the body may cause hair loss which begins at 10 to 14 days.

Blood count nadirs are reached at 10 to 14 days, but pancytopenia may persist for 6 to 8 weeks. The blood count must be checked carefully before starting the other HBI. Interstitial pneumonitis presenting with cough, breathlessness and hypoxia may occur at about 6 weeks after treatment (range 1–6 months). Lethargy and weakness are sometimes marked.

Dose prescription

SINGLE-FRACTION TOTAL BODY IRRADIATION

10.5 Gy MPD (measured at the lungs from lithium fluoride dosemeters) at a dose rate of 0.05 Gy/min.

FRACTIONATED TOTAL BODY IRRADIATION

14.4 Gy in 8 fractions over 4 days (1.8 Gy/fraction) twice daily, dose specified to the maximum lung dose.

Testicular boost (if used before TBI)

5.4–6 Gy in 3 fractions.

Cranial boost (individualized)

Usually 5.4–6 Gy in 3 fractions.

Mediastinal boost (bulk disease with residuum after chemotherapy – no previous radiation)

10–10.8 Gy in 5–6 fractions.

HALF-BODY IRRADIATION

Upper half body

6 Gy MPD (with lung correction) in a single fraction.

Lower half body

8 Gy MPD in a single fraction specified at the mid-point of the pelvis.

FRACTIONATED HALF-BODY IRRADIATION

3 Gy in 10 fractions given in 2 weeks (0.3 Gy/fraction).

If treatment to the other half of the body is to be given subsequently, an interval of 6 to 8 weeks should elapse to allow time for bone-marrow recovery.

Further reading

Appelbaum, F.R. 1993: The influence of total dose, fractionation, dose rate and distribution of TBI on bone marrow transplantation. *Seminars in Oncology* **20** (Suppl. 4), 3–10.

Gale, R.P., Butturini, A. and Bortin, M.M. 1991: What does TBI do in bone marrow transplants for leukaemia? *International Journal of Radiation Oncology, Biology and Physics* **20**, 631–4.

CHAPTER 38

Emergency irradiation

Urgent palliative radiotherapy may be needed to treat various symptoms from either primary disease or metastases when cure is not possible. Elective palliative treatments are described in the appropriate chapters. However, certain medical conditions may require emergency radiotherapy to relieve life-threatening symptoms or to prevent the development of irreversible damage.

Superior vena caval obstruction (SVCO)

Patients with SVCO often present with acute dyspnoea and tachypnoea, which are exacerbated by lying flat, facial or upper limb oedema and distension of veins in the neck with evidence of a collateral circulation.

In the majority of cases, this obstruction is due to a primary bronchogenic carcinoma, although 10 per cent may be due to lymphoma. Other rare tumours such as thymoma, T-cell acute lymphatic leukaemia or mediastinal germ-cell tumours may also present in this way. Confirmation of the histological nature of the tumour is important, and can usually be obtained by biopsy of the primary tumour at bronchoscopy or mediastinoscopy, or by removal of a cervical lymph node, if necessary using local anaesthesia. Bone-marrow examination and estimation of serum alpha-fetoprotein or human chorionic gonadotrophin may sometimes be helpful. The choice of treatment will depend on the tumour type.

Chemotherapy will produce a rapid response with small-cell carcinoma, lymphoma, leukaemia and germ-cell tumours.

Radiotherapy is preferred for other bronchogenic carcinomas. After a diagnosis has been established, dexamethasone is given to relieve oedema, and the dose is gradually decreased as a response to radiotherapy occurs.

Treatment may have to be given with the patient sitting upright using a direct anterior field from a cobalt-60 unit. The field margins are determined from clinical examination and chest X-ray appearances (to include the mediastinal mass and the superior vena cava), and are transferred to the patient's skin by reference to fixed landmarks such as the suprasternal notch. Field sizes of approximately 12 × 12 cm are usually adequate. The IPD of the patient is measured at the centre of the field. For this field size and an IPD of 20 cm (assuming that the tumour lies in the mid-plane) the percentage depth dose for a cobalt-60 unit at 10 cm is approximately 60 per cent. An applied dose of up to 4 Gy is usually given daily until the patient can be treated in the supine position with opposing fields. For palliation, total doses of 20 Gy in 5 fractions (or 30 Gy in 10 fractions) are usually adequate, and may be preferred to single-fraction high-dose treatment because of the risk of increasing oedema.

Obstruction of the upper and lower airways may also present with acute dyspnoea, often associated with cough, wheezing or stridor. The site of the obstruction must be determined and histology obtained. Upper airways obstruction may be caused by lymphomatous involvement of Waldeyer's ring, tumours of the thyroid, and cervical or paratracheal lymphadenopathy. Lower airways obstruction is usually due to bronchial occlusion by a primary lung carcinoma. Dexamethasone is given and palliative radiotherapy used to treat the smallest volume that will encompass the tumour. The total dose and fractionation schedules depend on the histology of the lesion. Alternatively, the obstruction may be relieved with laser treatment, followed by endobronchial brachytherapy (see Chapter 18).

Spinal cord compression

Spinal cord compression may occur in about 5 per cent of patients with cancer, and is most commonly associated with primary tumours of the lung, prostate, breast and kidney.

The onset of spinal cord compression may be insidious, with asymmetric limb weakness, patchy sensory changes, and disturbances of gait, bowel or bladder function. Back pain or radicular nerve root pain commonly accompany and may precede these symptoms. A high index of suspicion is needed to detect early cases while the functional status is still good. If left untreated, the condition will progress to the syndrome of symmetrical spastic paraparesis, sensory loss below a well-defined spinal cord level, and loss of bowel and bladder function. Where the disease occurs below L2, a different syndrome may result with lower motor neurone motor signs and, frequently, with asymmetrical sensory loss. However, paraplegia may develop rapidly with few or no preceding symptoms. This constitutes one of the few true emergencies in radiotherapy practice, where a delay even of only a few hours may drastically influence the functional outcome. Complete sudden paraplegia is usually associated with vascular damage, and is irreversible. Radiotherapy is therefore not indicated unless the patient also has severe pain.

Thorough neurological history and examination are needed to determine the rate of onset and the spinal level involved. X-rays of the spine may show involvement with malignant disease and the presence of crush fracture of the vertebral column. MRI is the investigation of choice, since it is the most informative and non-invasive technique. The whole length of cord should be imaged because there is frequently involvement at multiple levels. CT is the best technique for showing local soft-tissue extension and bone destruction, and it may be of help before surgical intervention.

A diagnosis of malignant disease may already have been made, or this may become obvious from a general examination. Simple investigations such as chest X-ray and sputum cytology may reveal the primary source. If a diagnosis of malignancy has not been established, an attempt should be made to obtain histology, either by needle biopsy of the spinal lesion, or at open operation for decompression.

Dexamethasone at a high dose (16 mg daily) should be given to all patients at presentation. Its usefulness lasts only 3 to 4 days, whereafter it should be reduced rapidly.

It is not clear whether routine surgical decompression, with or without postoperative radiation, gives better results than radiotherapy alone. Most patients with an established histological diagnosis should therefore be treated initially with radiotherapy. If a diagnosis of lymphoma or other chemosensitive disease is made, primary chemotherapy may be appropriate. Surgery is indicated for patients who present with a rapidly deteriorating neurological condition or with mechanical vertebral collapse, for those who deteriorate during radiotherapy, and for those who have already received radiotherapy to the site of compression. Some patients with vertebral body collapse may be made worse by posterior decompression, and frequently are not helped by radiotherapy either. The optimal treatment for selected patients in this group is anterior decompression and stabilization. Although surgical decompression may produce rapid relief of symptoms, it is not usually an adequate antitumour treatment, and postoperative radiotherapy is indicated.

Because of the depth of the cord and vertebral body, megavoltage radiotherapy should be used (Table 38.1) to give adequate doses at depth. Treatment should be planned on a simulator, using the imaging information obtained previously. If the upper and lower limits of the tumour are known, a field can be used which extends 5 cm above and below these. If this information is not available, fields should be generous enough to cover the estimated tumour, and lengths of at least 15 cm are often needed. A field width of 6–8 cm is used or width is determined by CT scan where available. If treatment is planned on the basis of clinical findings alone, it must be remembered that the sensory level detected in a skin dermatome arises from compression of the corresponding cord segment, which lies at a higher level than the vertebral body of the same number; e.g. a sensory level at T10 on the skin arises from compression of its cord segment at the level of the T8 vertebra.

Table 38.1 Treatment depth for spinal cord or vertebral metastases and percentage depth doses from megavoltage treatment

Site	Depth (cm)	Percentage depth dose	
		Cobalt-60	6 MV
Cervical and thoracic canal	4.5–6.0	82–74	88–82
Lumbar canal	5.5–7.0	76–69	84–78
Lumbar vertebral body	9–10	61–57	70–66

Ideally the patient is treated prone, using a direct posterior field marked with a central tattoo. Otherwise, the supine patient is treated with an undercouch beam with the reference tattoo placed on the anterior skin surface. Doses of 20 Gy in 5 fractions (or 30 Gy in 10 daily fractions) are usually satisfactory, and may be preferred to single-fraction treatment because of the risk of increasing oedema and neurological deficit.

Occasionally, spinal cord compression is due to a primary tumour (e.g. plasmacytoma). It is important to establish this diagnosis early, with complete staging, since high-dose local radiotherapy, appropriately planned and fractionated, may produce permanent local control or even cure. In these conditions doses of 35–45 Gy in 1.8-Gy fractions are recommended, using a planned homogeneous dose distribution with wedged posterior oblique fields or electron therapy (Fig. 38.1).

The most important prognostic variable in spinal cord compression is the neurological status at the time of treatment. Urgent diagnosis and treatment of the deteriorating patient are essential. Early physiotherapy is also important to prevent, as far as possible, the muscle-wasting and contracture that accompany compression of the spinal cord, so giving the patient the best chance of becoming or remaining ambulant.

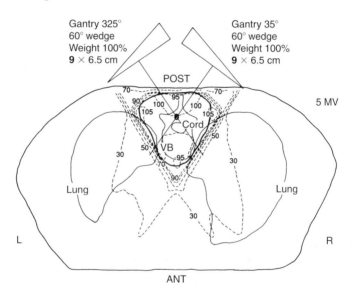

Fig. 38.1 Posterior wedged oblique fields used to treat tumour of vertebral body (VB).

Haemorrhage

Bleeding from advanced tumours of the breast, bladder or bronchus may be treated with radiotherapy. Simple field arrangements such as opposing anterior and posterior fields for treatment of the bronchus or bladder or small tangential fields for breast lesions are desirable.

Single treatments of 8 Gy may be adequate to control some very superficial haemorrhagic lesions, or weekly fractions of 6 Gy may be used for patient convenience (breast and bladder) to a dose of 30 Gy, or less if control is achieved sooner. For carcinoma of the bronchus, a split-course treatment of 20 Gy in 5 daily fractions may be repeated after 1 month if necessary (with shielding of the spinal cord).

Bone pain

Pain from bone metastases may be transient and adequately treated by analgesia. More persistent pain can be successfully relieved by radiotherapy in up to 80 per cent of patients. Because it is desirable to relieve pain as quickly as possible, this topic is discussed here.

When a patient first presents with pain, a full evaluation of sites of metastases by isotope bone-scanning is important in order to determine whether local or systemic therapy is appropriate. If local treatment is indicated, the site of origin of the pain must be confirmed by local tenderness, X-ray or bone-scan abnormalities. For example, pain in the knee may arise from disease in the spine, the hip or the femur, and rib pain is frequently referred from a vertebral body.

If the cortex of the bone is eroded in relation to an osteolytic metastasis in a limb, surgical stabilization should be considered to prevent fracture. Postoperative radiotherapy should then be given.

Lesions of the upper cervical vertebrae are best treated with the patient lying supine using opposing lateral fields with margins chosen to avoid as much of the oral cavity and pharynx as possible. Lower cervical, thoracic and lumbar vertebrae are treated with a direct posterior field with the patient prone if possible, using a 4 to 6-MV linear accelerator. If a cobalt-60 beam is used, opposing fields may be needed to ensure an adequate dose to the anterior border of the vertebra, which may be in the mid-line in the lumbar region. The upper and lower borders of the field should lie in an intervertebral space. It is usual to include one or two vertebrae above and below the site of involvement.

Anterior and posterior opposing fields are used to treat pelvic metastases. The field should be chosen to avoid small bowel, but consideration must be given to the possible need for treatment of adjacent sites in the future. Limb metastases are also usually treated with opposing fields.

Treatment margins are marked on the patient's skin with a reference tattoo for a permanent record. Photographs, machine check films or simulator films should also be taken, as these will be needed if further treatment has to be given to avoid overlap of fields.

Most treatments are given with a cobalt-60 machine or a linear accelerator, although the latter may give a better dose distribution for pelvic or spinal treatments in large patients. Ribs, clavicles or limb lesions in thin patients may be treated with electron or orthovoltage therapy. Single fractions of 8–10 Gy are adequate for most situations. For large fields, where survival is likely to be prolonged, or where a long segment of spinal cord is included in the field, fractionated treatment may be preferred using 20 Gy in 5 daily fractions or 30 Gy in 10 fractions.

Further reading

Faul, C.M. and Flickinger, J.C. 1995: The use of radiation in the management of spinal metastases. *Journal of Neuro-oncology*, **23**, 149–61.

Abbreviations

AAPM	American Association of Physicists in Medicine
AFP	α-fetoprotein
AP	Antero-posterior
β-HCG	β-subunit of human chorionic gonadotrophin
BED	Biological effective dose
BMT	Bone-marrow transplantation
BSF	Back-scatter factor
BSI	British Standards Institute
CHART	Continuous hyperfractionated accelerated radiotherapy
CNS	Central nervous system
CSF	Cerebrospinal fluid
CSTG	Children's Solid Tumour Group
CT	Computed tomographic scanning
CTV	Clinical target volume
DCIS	Ductal carcinoma *in situ*
DICOM	Digital imaging communication in medicine
D_{max}	Dose at the depth of maximum build-up
DMLC	Dynamic multileaf collimation
DNA	Deoxyribonucleic acid
DRR	Digitally reconstructed radiographs
DVH	Dose–volume histogram
ENT	Ear, nose and throat
EORTC	European Organization for Research and Treatment of Cancer
ESQUAN	European Society Quality Assurance Network
ESR	Erythrocyte sedimentation rate
ESTRO	European Society for Therapeutic Radiology and Oncology
EUA	Examination under anaesthetic
FAD	Focus axis distance
FIGO	Federation Internationale de Gynecologie et d'Obstetrique
FNA	Fine-needle aspirate
FSD	Focus skin distance
GA	General anaesthetic
GTV	Gross tumour volume
Gy	Gray
HBI	Half-body irradiation
HDR	High dose rate
HIV	Human immunodeficiency virus

HVL	Half value layer
ICRU	International Commission on Radiation Units and Measurements
IM	Internal margin
IMRT	Intensity-modulated radiation therapy
IPD	Interplanar distance
ITV	Internal target volume
LD	Limited disease
LDR	Low dose rate
LQ	Linear quadratic
MeV	Mega-electronvolts
MDR	Medium dose rate
MIBG	Meta-iodobenzylguanidine
MLC	Multileaf collimator
MPD	Mid-plane dose
MRI	Magnetic resonance imaging
MV	Megavolts
NSD	Nominal standard dose
NSCLC	Non-small-cell lung cancer
NTCP	Normal tissue complication probability
PA	Postero-anterior
PACS	Picture archiving and communication system
PCI	Prophylactic cranial irradiation
%DD	Percentage depth dose
PEG	Percutaneous endoscopic gastrotomy
PET	Positron emission tomography
PRV	Planning organ at risk volume
PSA	Prostate-specific antigen
PTV	Planning target volume
PUVA	Psoralens plus ultraviolet A
QA	Quality assurance
QC	Quality control
SCLC	Small-cell lung cancer
SDR	Surface dose rate
SF	Surviving fraction
SIOP	International Society of Paediatric Oncology
SM	Set-up margin
SOF	Stand-off
SPECT	Single positron emission computed tomography
SSD	Source skin distance
SVCO	Superior vena caval obstruction
SXRT	Superficial X-ray therapy
TBI	Total body irradiation
TCP	Tumour control probability
TIN	Testicular intra-epithelial neoplasia
TL	Tolerance level
TLD	Thermoluminescent dosemeter

TNM	Tumour, nodes, metastases
TRAK	Total reference air kerma
TRUS	Transrectal ultrasound
TURP	Transurethral resection of prostate
UICC	Union International Contre le Cancer
UKCCSG	United Kingdom Children's Cancer Study Group
WHO	World Health Organization

Index